Color Atlas of Veterinary Pathology

Huaitao Chen

Color Atlas of Veterinary Pathology

Volume 1

Springer

Huaitao Chen
Department of Veterinary Pathology
Gansu Agricultural University
Lanzhou, China

Jointly published with China Agriculture Press

ISBN 978-981-96-7616-3 ISBN 978-981-96-7617-0 (eBook)
https://doi.org/10.1007/978-981-96-7617-0

This Springer imprint is published by the registered company Springer Nature Singapore Pte Ltd.
The registered company address is: 152 Beach Road, #21-01/04 Gateway East, Singapore 189721, Singapore

Preface

On the occasion of the publication of the first volume of "Color Atlas of Veterinary Pathology," we would like to express our deep gratitude to the National Scientific and Technical Academic Works Publishing Foundation Committee and China Agriculture Press for their great support and assistance.

Veterinary pathology is a bridge between basic veterinary medicine, clinical and preventive veterinary medicine, and plays a connecting role in the field of veterinary medicine. To study veterinary pathology, we should not only deeply understand its important theory but also master the basic pathological changes in the diseased animals and the characteristic pathological changes of various diseases. It is necessary to understand these changes for the in-depth study and accurate diagnosis of animal diseases. As a true portrayal of pathological changes, pictures can play an important role in the teaching of veterinary pathology, which is difficult to be replaced by other teaching methods. In view of the lack of comprehensive and systematic works in this field in China, and the needs of the majority of veterinary students, we compiled the *Color Atlas of Veterinary Pathology*.

The *Color Atlas of Veterinary Pathology* includes the first volume and the second volume. The first volume is related to basic pathology, such as cell and tissue lesion, localized disturbances of blood circulation, inflammation, tumor and pathology of various systems and organs. The second volume is pathology of diseases, including diseases of various animals. Basic pathology is an introduction to the study of veterinary pathology, and is especially useful for young veterinary scientists who have not yet mastered this knowledge. They can compare the results of their experimental studies with these typical lesion pictures to improve their understanding level and discernment, to enrich and deepen their research content.

A total of 1995 pictures were selected for this atlas, including 565 pictures showing basic pathological changes. All these pictures were provided by Chinese veterinarians. In order to respect the achievements of the original producers and suppliers of the pictures and protect their intellectual rights, each picture in the book has been signed after the annotation.

The compilation of the first and second volume of the *Color Atlas of Veterinary Pathology* was carried out under the guidance and help of the older generation of veterinary pathology experts such as Zhu Xuanren and Zhu Kunxi. Professor Chen Huanchun, academician of the Chinese Academy of Engineering, is very concerned about the discipline construction of veterinary pathology, and strongly supports and contributes to the completion of this important work. Ninety-one experts and professors participated in the preparation and review of the manuscript, and hundreds of veterinary scientists provided pictures and other materials. The Board of Veterinary Pathology Branch of the Chinese Society of Animal Husbandry and Veterinary Medicine also gave active support and enthusiastic encouragement for the preparation and publication of this book. Therefore, the successful publication of this monograph is the result of the joint efforts of the majority of veterinary pathologists and related veterinary science and technology workers, and is the crystallization of their knowledge, wisdom, and labor. Here, I would like to express my gratitude to the above experts, professors and colleagues, as well as to all the staff who have supported and cared about the preparation and publication of this atlas.

This atlas is an important teaching material and reference book of veterinary pathology, and I hope that the majority of veterinary pathologists and students will enjoy it.

Although we have put a lot of effort into the compilation of this Atlas, due to our limited academic level and practical experience, we sincerely hope that readers can criticize and correct the errors and shortcomings in this book.

Lanzhou, China Huaitao Chen

Editorial Board

Contents

About the Author

Huaitao Chen is a Professor of veterinary pathology and a supervisor of Ph.D. students from Gansu Agricultural University. Professor Chen was born in August 1938 in Huayin, Shaanxi province. From 1979 to 1981, he was a visiting scholar in N. Bălcescu College of Agriculture and other institutions in Romania to study veterinary pathology. He has been the deputy director of the College of Veterinary Medicine of Gansu Agricultural University, the director of the Department of Veterinary Pathology, and the director of the Department of Basic Veterinary Medicine. He has presided over and participated in many national and Gansu Provincial Natural Science Foundation projects, and has won more than 10 scientific and technological progress awards at provincial and national levels, such as researches in horse asthma, animal pneumoconiosis, animal tumor ecology, and the histology of Bactrian camels. He is the chief editor for more than 20 monographs and textbooks such as veterinary pathology, diagnostic pathology of animal diseases, veterinary pathological anatomy, and color atlas of animal tumors, and he has published more than 150 scientific papers.

Lesion of Cells and Tissues

1

1 Ultrastructural Pathology

1.1 Ultramicroscopic Lesions of the Nucleus

1.1.1 Changes in the Size and Shape of the Nucleus (Figs. 1.1, 1.2, and 1.3)

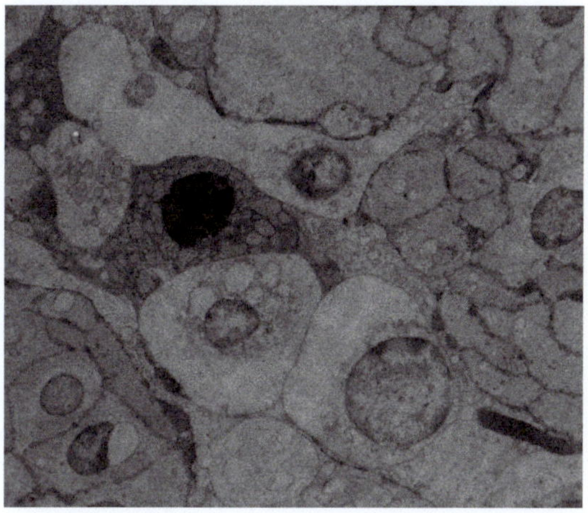

Fig. 1.1 Pyknosis. Plasma cells in the lamina propria of camel ileum: the nuclei of plasma cells are condensed and smaller, with a marked increase in electron density; the electron density of the cytoplasm is also increased. ×3000. (Wang Wenhui)

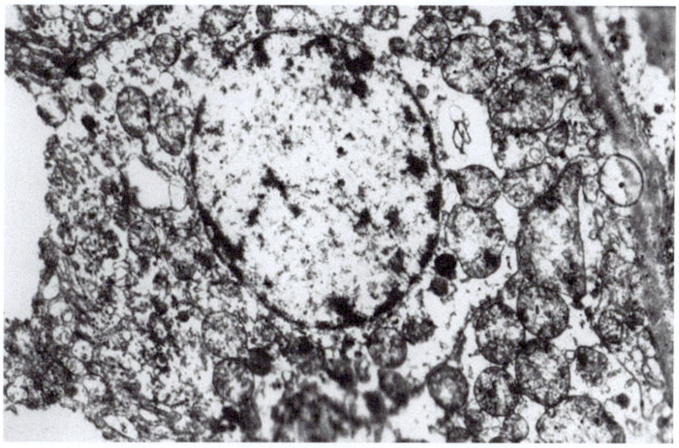

Fig. 1.2 Nuclear enlargement. Renal tubular epithelial cells are edematous, with enlarged nuclei, translucent nuclear fluid, and sparse chromatin. ×5000. (Chen Huaitao)

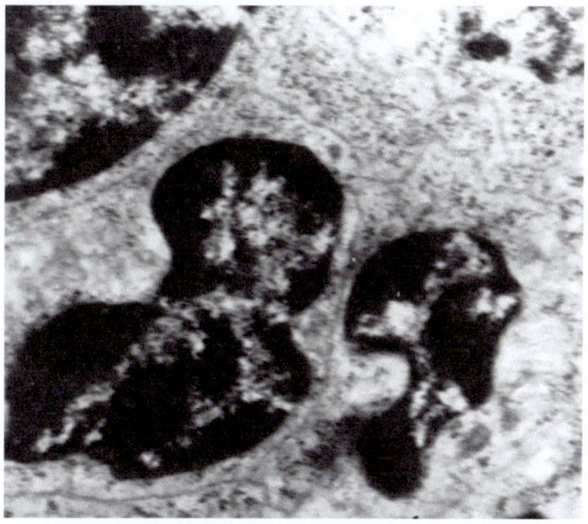

Fig. 1.3 Nuclear deformation. Spleen of copper-poisoned ducklings: the nuclei of lymphocytes are deformed and dumbbell-shaped. ×13,000. (Cui Hengmin)

H. Chen, *Color Atlas of Veterinary Pathology*, https://doi.org/10.1007/978-981-96-7617-0_1

1.1.2 Changes in the Nuclear Membrane (Fig. 1.4)

1.1.3 Changes in the Nucleolus (Figs. 1.5, 1.6, and 1.7)

1.1.4 Changes in Chromatin (Figs. 1.8, 1.9, 1.10, and 1.11)

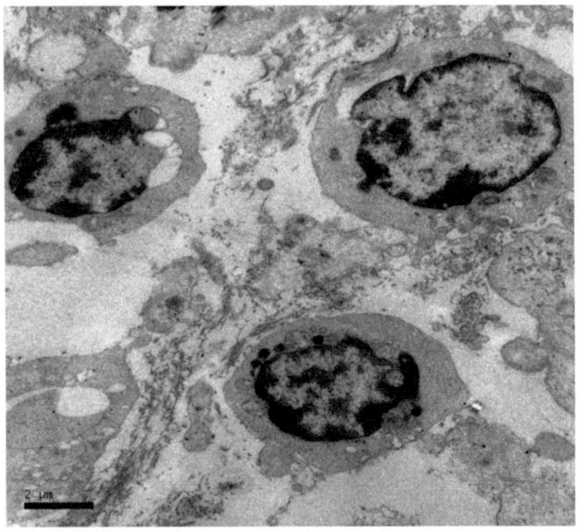

Fig. 1.4 Dilation of the perinuclear space. Lymphocytes in the lamina propria of the abomasum cardia gland area of Bactrian camel: mild local dilatation of the perinuclear gap. ×8000. (Wang Wenhui)

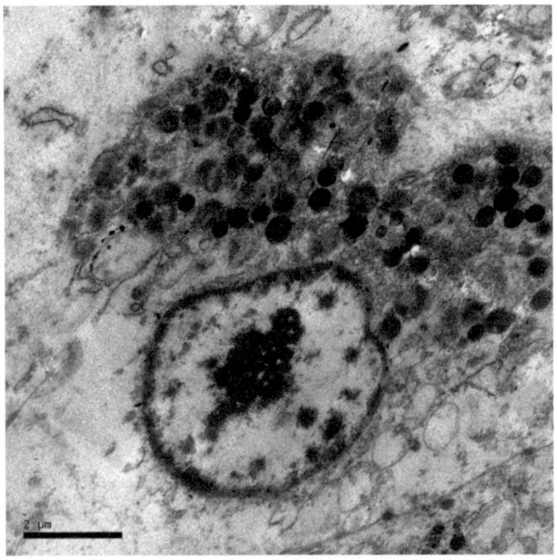

Fig. 1.5 Enlarged nucleolus. Glandular epithelial cells in the cardia gland of Bactrian camel: the nuclei are significantly enlarged in size. ×12,000. (Wang Wenhui)

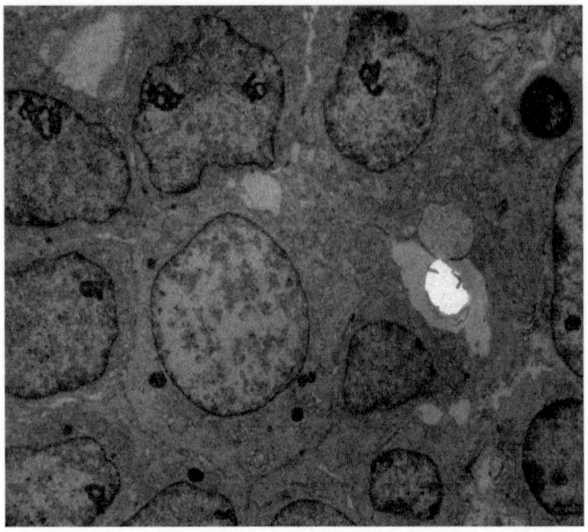

Fig. 1.6 Nucleolar margination. The nucleolar margination is present in nucleoli of several cells at the upper left of the figure. ×5000. (Wang Wenhui)

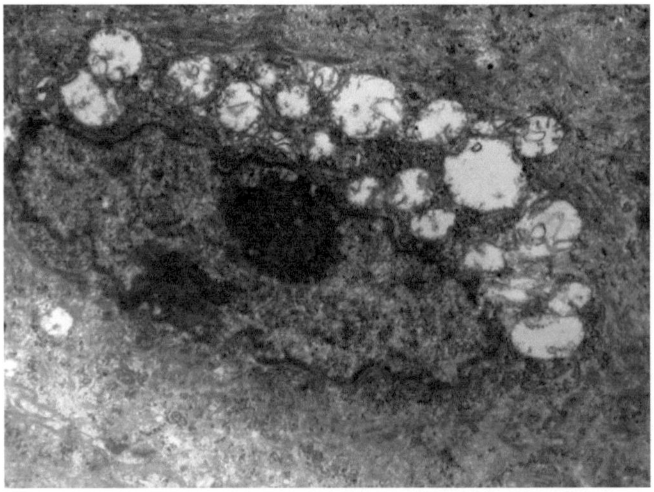

Fig. 1.7 Enlarged nucleoli and nucleolar margination. Bovine tongue mucosal epithelial spine cells: the nucleolus is enlarged with nucleolar margination, and mitochondria are heavily swollen. ×6600. (Wang Wenhui)

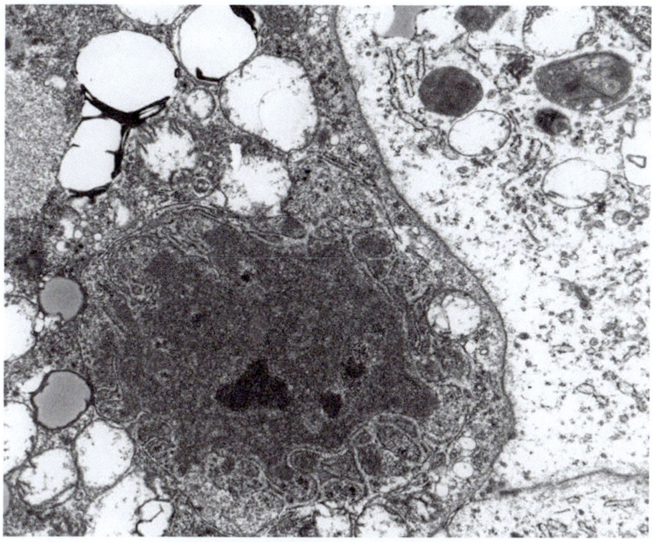

Fig. 1.8 Karyopyknosis. Type II alveolar epithelial cells infected with sheep adenovirus: chromatin gather and karyopyknosis are obvious. Mitochondria are swelling. (Deng Puhui)

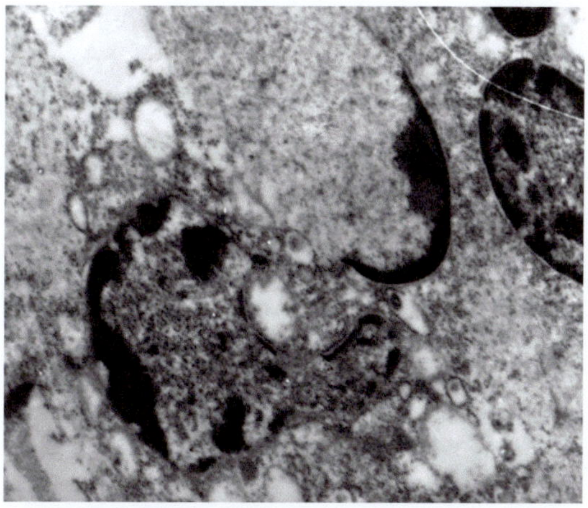

Fig. 1.9 Karyolysis. Thymus of copper-poisoned duckling: karyolysis of lymphocyte, localized chromatin lysis, and disappearance. ×15,000. (Cui Hengmin)

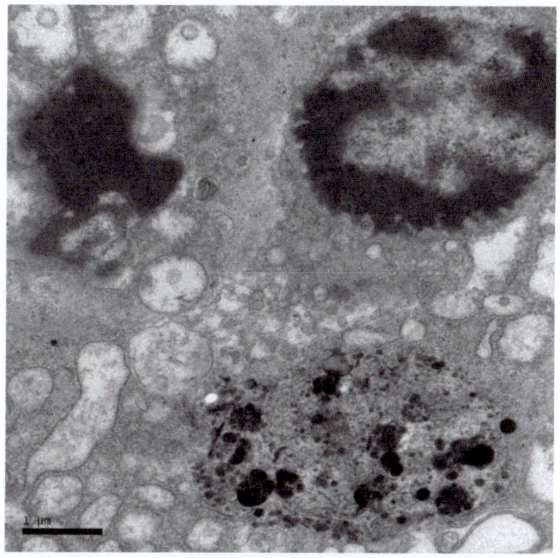

Fig. 1.10 Karyorrhexis. Glandular epithelial cells in the cardia gland of Bactrian camel: karyorrhexis. Nuclear chromatin of the glandular cells is cleaved into fragments of variable sizes; the nucleus of the upper left cell is condensed, deformed, and reduced in size. ×20,000. (Wang Wenhui)

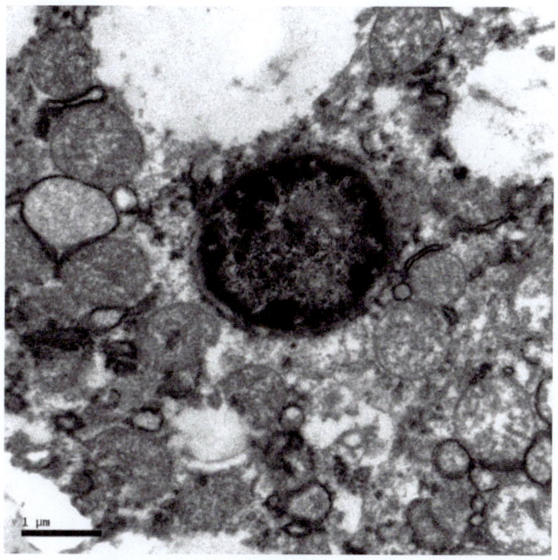

Fig. 1.11 Chromatin margination. Chicken liver: chromatin margination of hepatocyte; mitochondria are swelling with disappearance of cristae. ×20,000. (Wang Wenhui)

1.1.5 Nuclear Inclusion (Figs. 1.12, 1.13, and 1.14)

1.2 Ultramicroscopic Lesions of the Cytoplasm

1.2.1 Changes in Mitochondria (Figs. 1.15, 1.16, 1.17, 1.18, 1.19, 1.20, and 1.21)

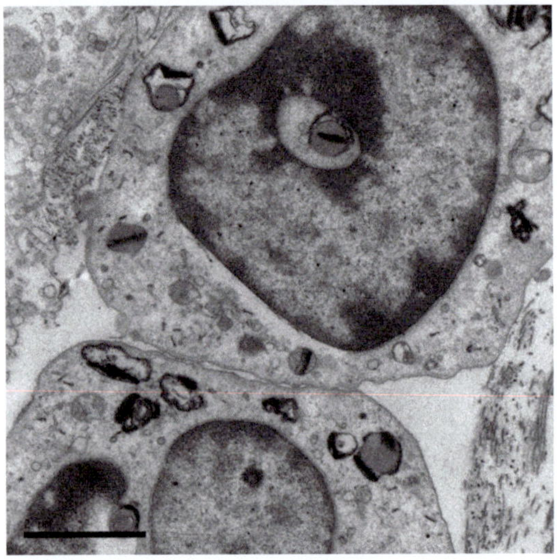

Fig. 1.12 Inclusion of nuclei. The cardia gland area of Bactrian camel. Nuclear inclusions are present in eosinophils in the lamina propria: the nucleus contains specific granules of eosinophils and some other cytoplasmic components, which are encapsuled by the nuclear membrane. ×15,000. (Wang Wenhui)

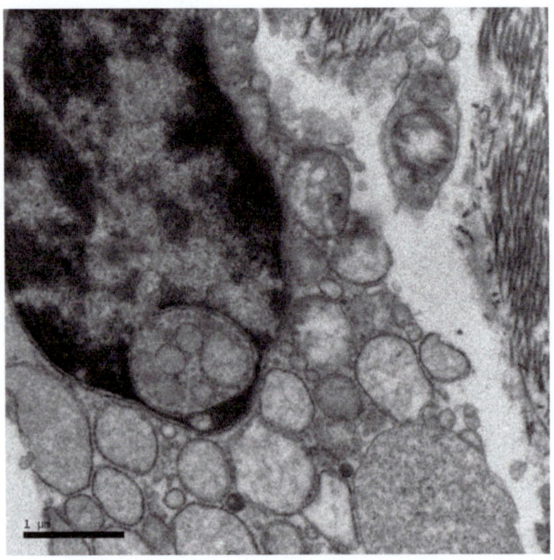

Fig. 1.13 Nuclear inclusion. Plasma cells in the lamina propria of the cardia gland area of Bactrian camel: a nucleus with an inclusion consisting of multiple organelles wrapped by a membrane and a small amount of cytoplasmic components. ×25,000. (Wang Wenhui)

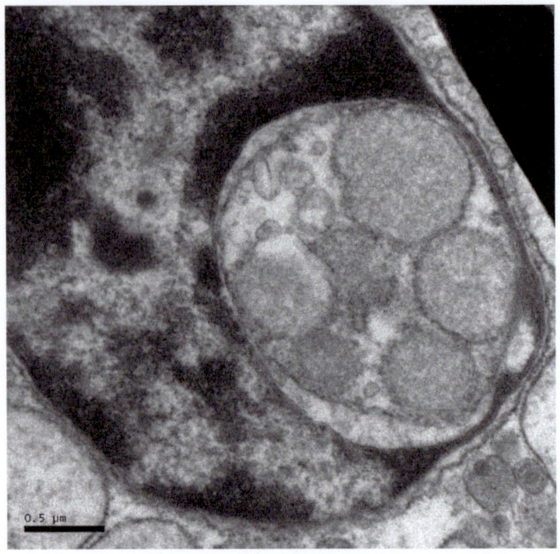

Fig. 1.14 Nuclear inclusion. Local magnification of the upper image: there is a clear boundary between inclusion and chromatin. ×40,000. (Wang Wenhui)

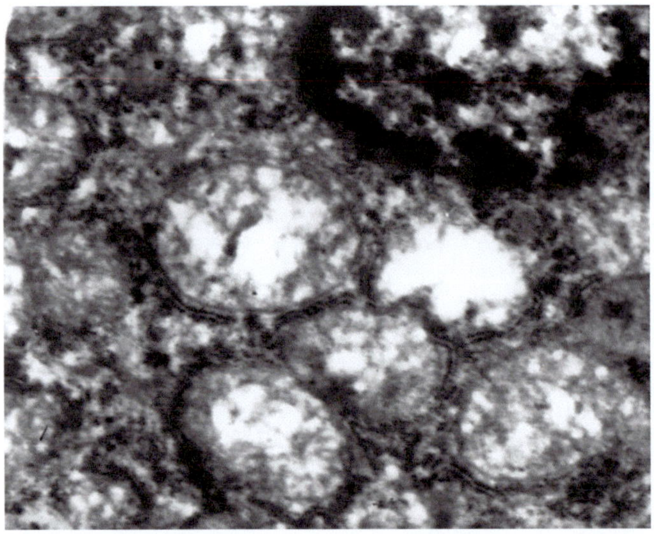

Fig. 1.15 Mitochondrial swelling. Liver of copper-poisoned ducklings. The mitochondria of the hepatocytes are swelling with cristae fragmented and dissolved. ×12,000. (Cui Hengmin)

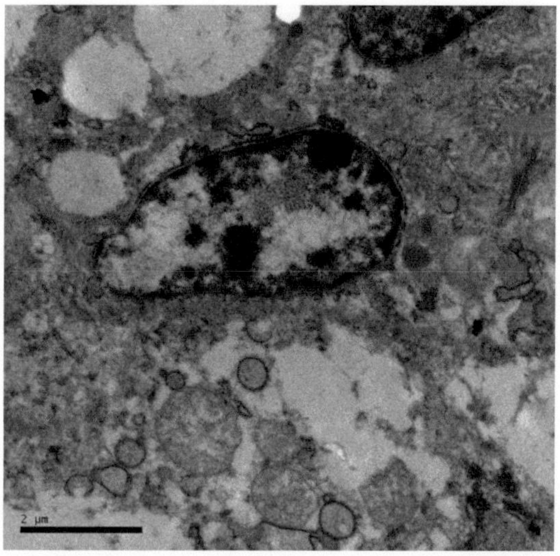

Fig. 1.16 Mitochondrial swelling. Chicken liver. Mitochondria of hepatocytes are heavily swollen, with cristae detached and dissolved, leaving mitochondria vacuolated with nucleolar margination. ×15,000. (Wang Wenhui)

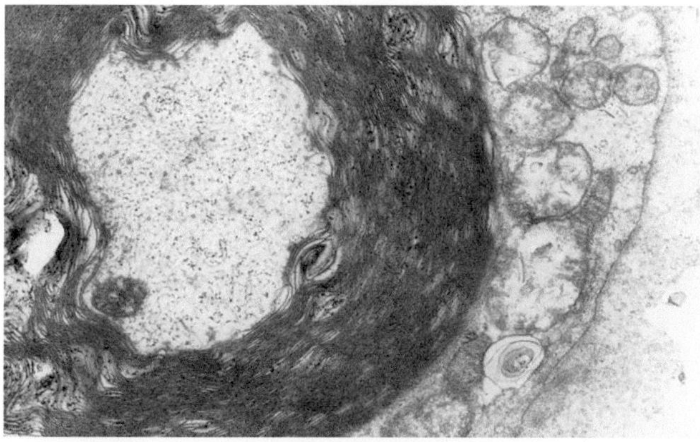

Fig. 1.17 Mitochondrial swelling. Chicken sciatic nerve (riboflavin deficiency). Mitochondria in Schwann's cells are swollen and deformed, and some cristae are detached and dissolved. ×20,000. (Wang Wenhui)

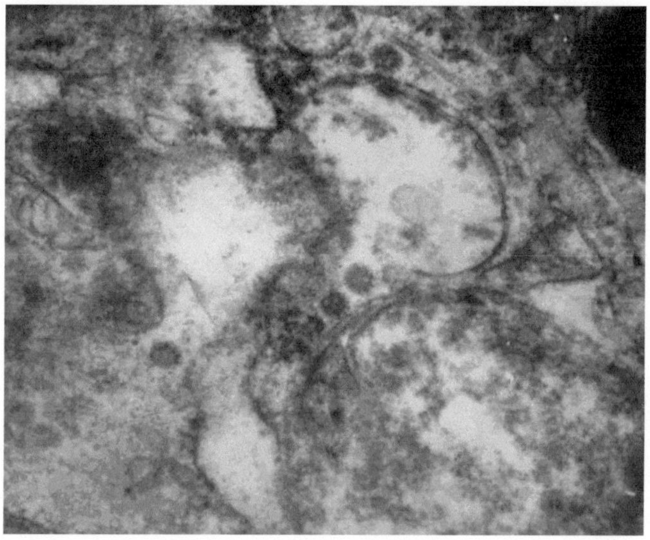

Fig. 1.18 Mitochondrial swelling. Epithelial spine cells of the mucosa of the tongue of cattle with foot-and-mouth disease: mitochondria are swollen with rupture, lysis, and indistinctness of local membrane; there are small amount of foot-and-mouth disease virus particles in cytoplasm. ×26,000. (Wang Wenhui)

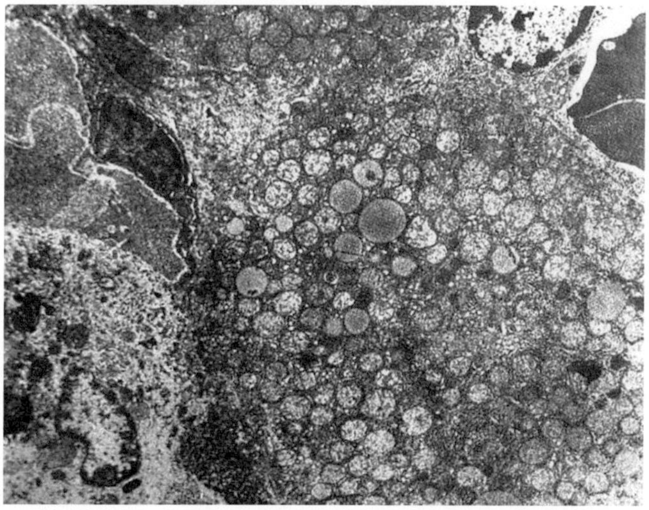

Fig. 1.19 Mitochondrial hyperplasia. Mitochondrial hyperplasia is present in hepatocytes with a significant increase in number. ×5600. (Xu Yimin)

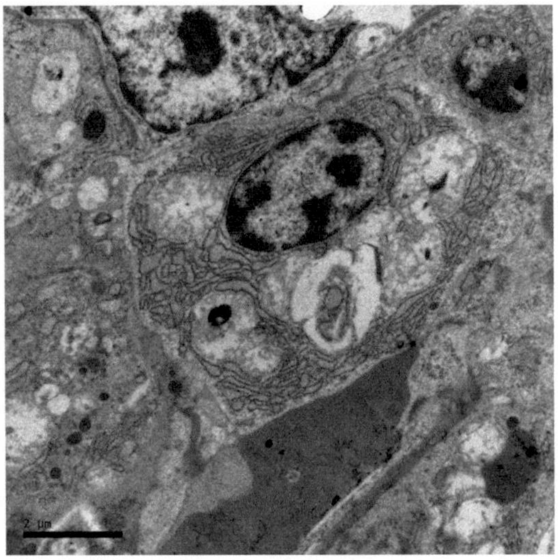

Fig. 1.20 Mitochondrial inclusion. Chicken plasma cells: mitochondria are swollen containing inclusion of high electron-density. ×12,000. (Wang Wenhui)

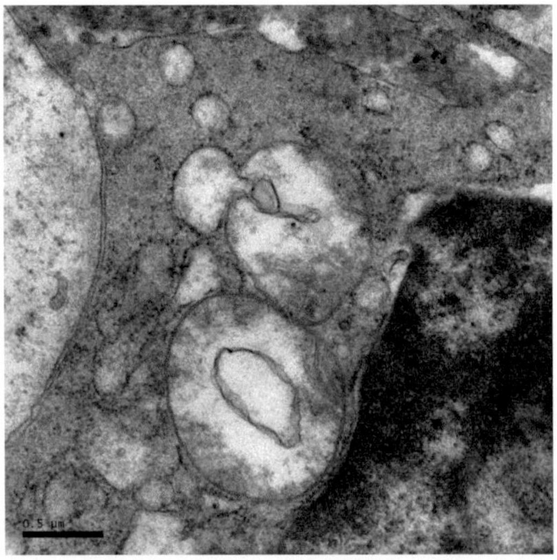

Fig. 1.21 Mitochondria and rough endoplasmic reticulum embedding (riveting). Plasma cells in the lamina propria of the cardia gland area of bactrian camel: One rough endoplasmic reticulum is locally embedded in a neighboring mitochondrion, and the other one contains membranous inclusion. ×40,000. (Wang Wenhui)

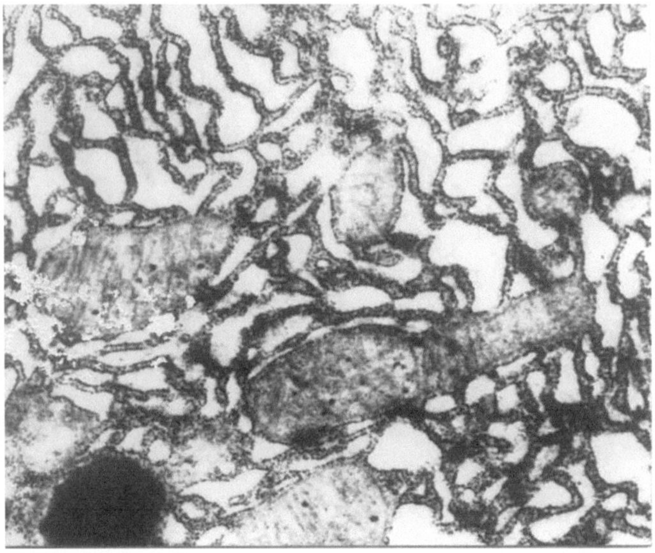

Fig. 1.22 Dilation of the endoplasmic reticulum. Selenium deficiency in chickens. Expansion of rough endoplasmic reticulum of pancreatic epithelial cells, which are like vesicles of variable sizes; mitochondria are swollen with cristae broken and structure indistinct. ×12,000. (Cui Hengmin)

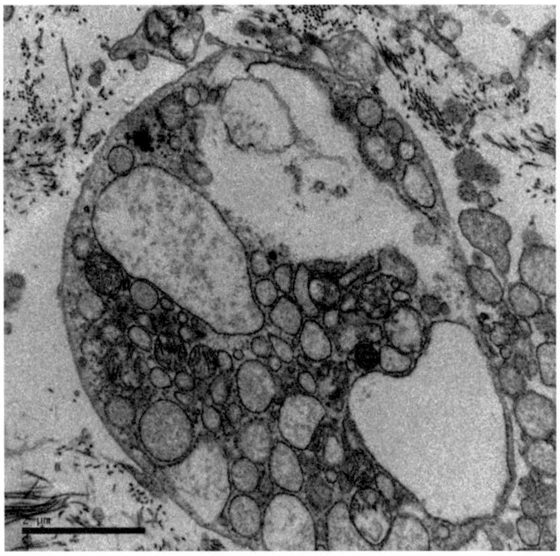

Fig. 1.23 Dilation of the endoplasmic reticulum. Plasma cells: some endoplasmic reticula are extremely dilated, being like a vesicular pool containing flocculent material. ×15,000. (Wang Wenhui)

1.2.2 Changes in the Endoplasmic Reticulum (Figs. 1.22, 1.23, 1.24, 1.25, 1.26, 1.27, 1.28, 1.29, and 1.30)

1.2.3 Changes in Lysosomes (Figs. 1.31 and 1.32)

1.2.4 Cytoplasmic Inclusion (Figs. 1.33, 1.34, 1.35, and 1.36)

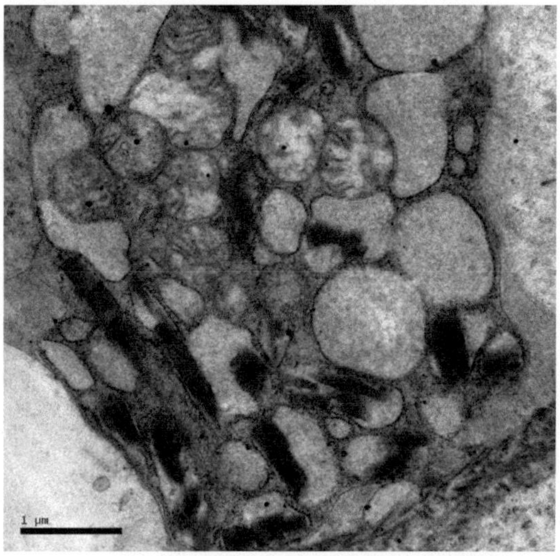

Fig. 1.24 Endoplasmic reticulum inclusion. Plasma cells: The high electron-density protein crystals are visible in rough endoplasmic reticula, as which is the Russel body; the rough endoplasmic reticula also contain a large amount of flocculent material. ×25,000. (Wang Wenhui)

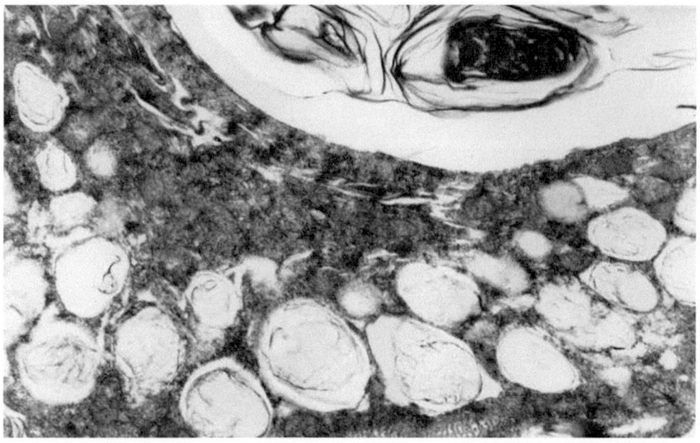

Fig. 1.25 Endoplasmic reticulum inclusion. Riboflavin deficiency in chickens. The number of endoplasmic reticulum containing membranous material is increased in sciatic nerve Schwann's cells. ×10,000. (Wang Wenhui)

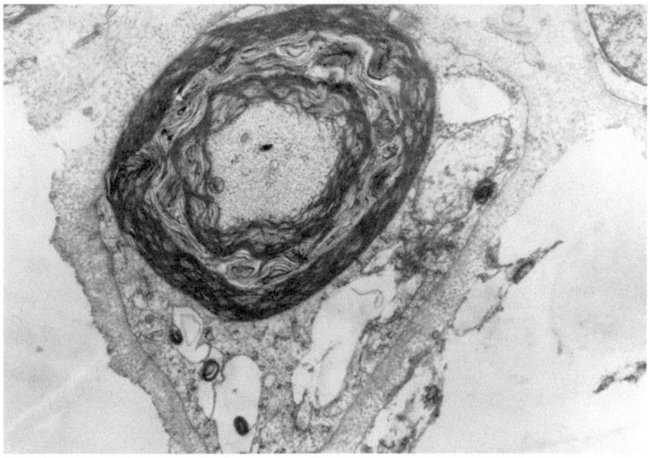

Fig. 1.26 Dilation of the endoplasmic reticulum. Chicken riboflavin deficiency. Significant expansion of the smooth endoplasmic reticula in sciatic nerve Schwann's cells containing myelin-like bodies with high electron density. ×8300. (Wang Wen-Hui)

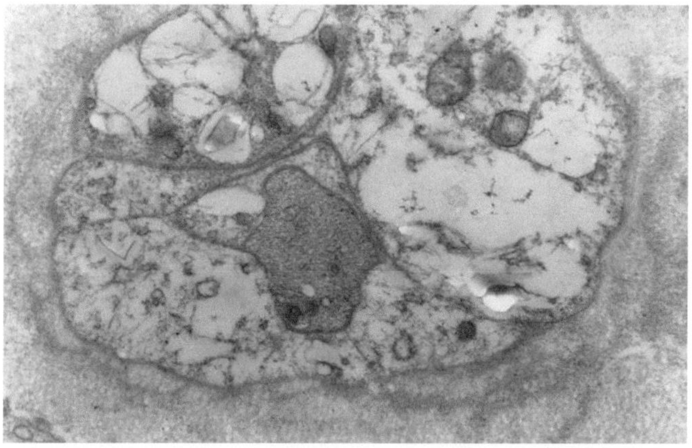

Fig. 1.27 Dilation of the endoplasmic reticulum. Chicken riboflavin deficiency. Extreme expansion or disintegration of the smooth endoplasmic reticula in sciatic nerve Schwann's cells caused a significant decrease in cytoplasmic electron density and resulted in a vacuolated appearance. ×13,000. (Wang Wen-Hui)

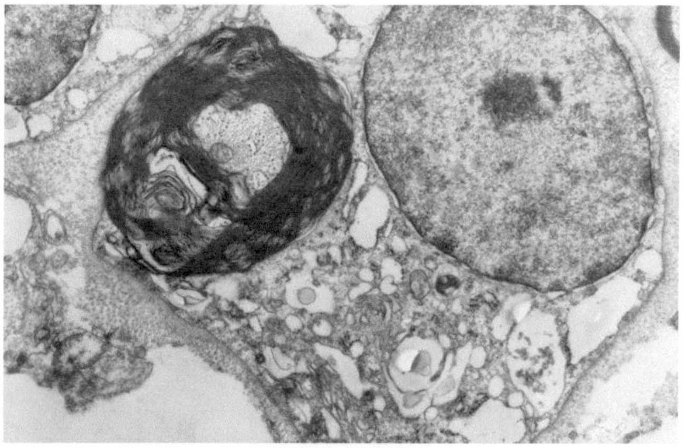

Fig. 1.28 Endoplasmic reticulum hyperplasia. Chicken riboflavin deficiency. The number of smooth endoplasmic reticulum in sciatic nerve Schwann's cells was significantly increased and the endoplasmic reticula were dilated. ×8300. (Wang Wen-Hui)

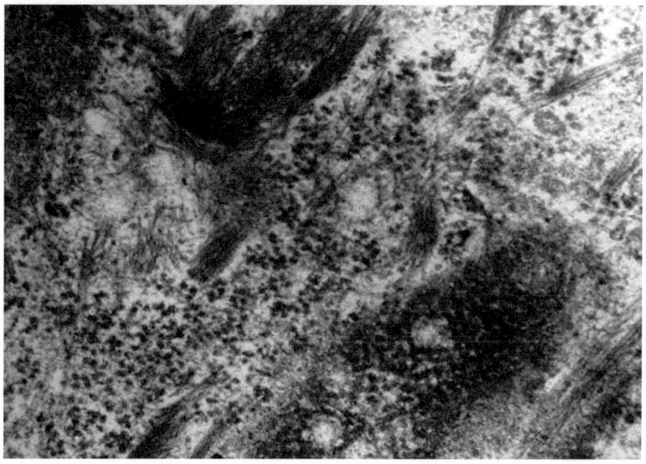

Fig. 1.29 Ribosome aggregation. Bovine soft palate epithelial spiny cells: ribosomes are abundant in the cytoplasm. ×33,000. (Wang Wen-Hui)

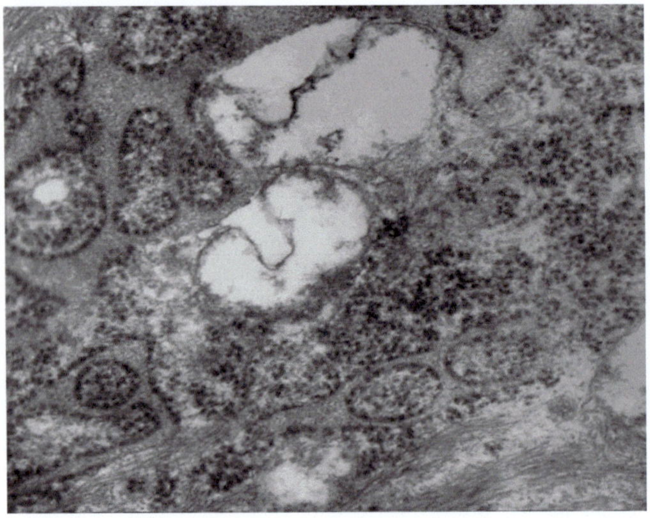

Fig. 1.30 Ribosome aggregation. Epithelial echinocytes (spiny cells) of the tongue: there is a large amount of rough endoplasmic reticula in the plasma with plenty of free ribosomes visible in its lumen and surrounding cytoplasm; some rough endoplasmic reticula contain rough endoplasmic reticula; mitochondria are heavily swollen with cristae detached and dissolved. ×26,000. (Wang Wen-Hui)

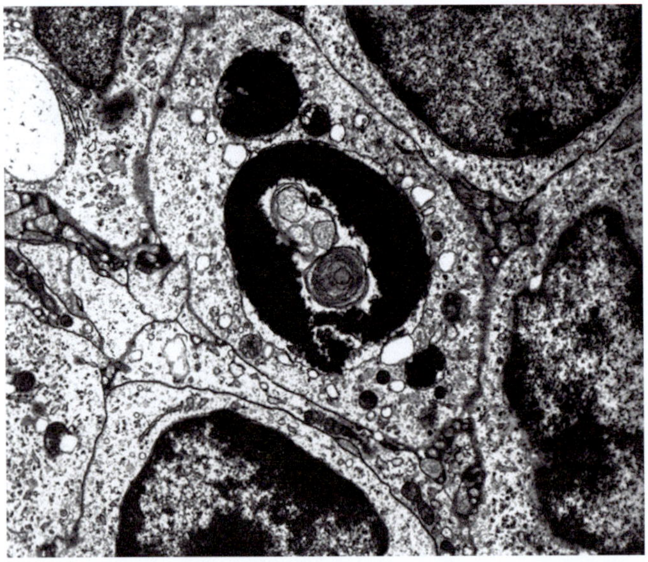

Fig. 1.31 Secondary lysosomes. Chronic progressive pneumonia in sheep. Secondary lysosomes in mastitis acinar cells contain endoplasmic reticula and cytoplasmic vacuoles. (Deng Puhui)

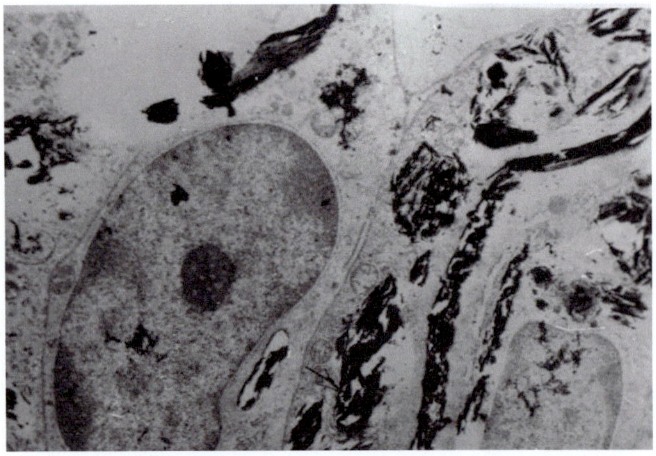

Fig. 1.32 Lysosomal overload. Equine pneumoconiosis. Macrophages in the alveolar septum (dust cells): secondary lysosomes containing aluminosilicate crystals are present in the cytoplasm. Some lysosomes are disrupted with dense electron crystallites located in the cytoplasm. × 12,000. (Chen Huaitao)

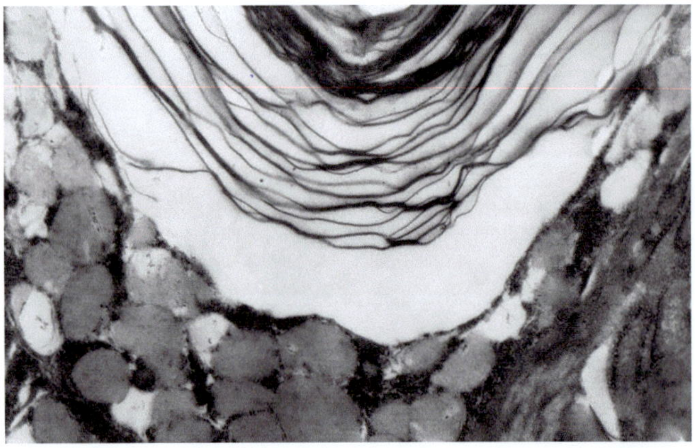

Fig. 1.33 Lipid Inclusion. Riboflavin deficiency in chickens. A large amount of lipid inclusions with varying electron density are present in the cytoplasm of sciatic nerve Schwann's cells. Myelin sheaths of myelinated nerve fibers are loose. ×16,000. (Wang Wenhui)

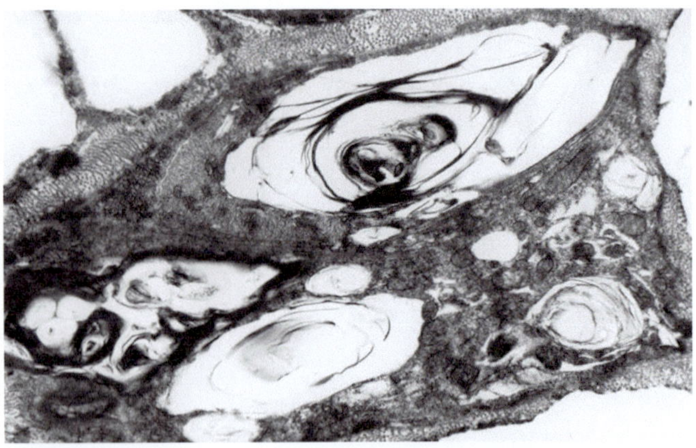

Fig. 1.34 Myelin-like body inclusion. Riboflavin deficiency in chickens. Morphologically diverse myelinoid bodies are present in the cytoplasm of sciatic nerve Schwann's cells. ×8300. (Wang Wenhui)

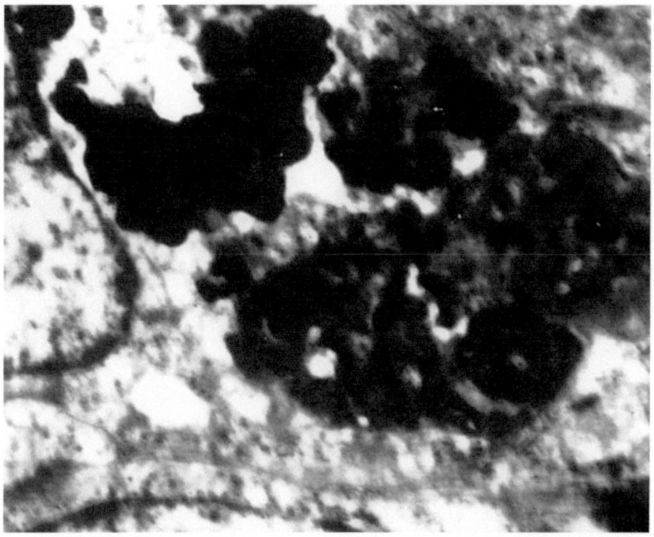

Fig. 1.35 Copper inclusion. Copper-poisoned ducklings. Copper deposits with very high electron density are present in the hepatocyte plasma. ×10,000. (Cui Hengmin)

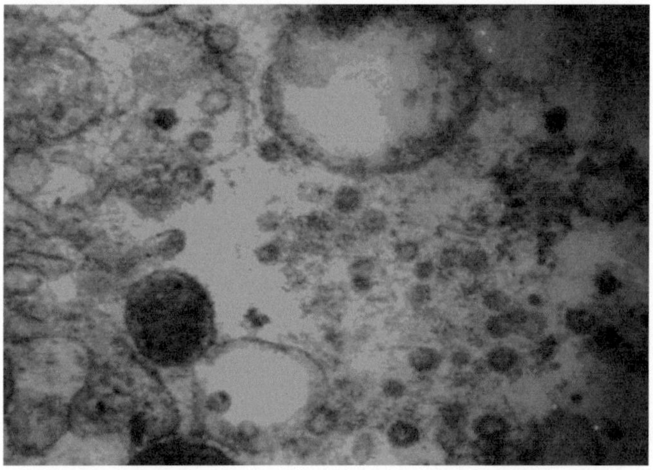

Fig. 1.36 Viral inclusion. Bovine foot-and-mouth disease. Foot and mouth disease virus (viral inclusions) are present in the cytoplasm of epithelial spinous cells of tongue mucosa, which are approximately consistent in morphology and size. ×33,000. (Wang Wenhui)

1.3 Ultramicroscopic Lesions of the Cell Membrane (Figs. 1.37, 1.38, and 1.39)

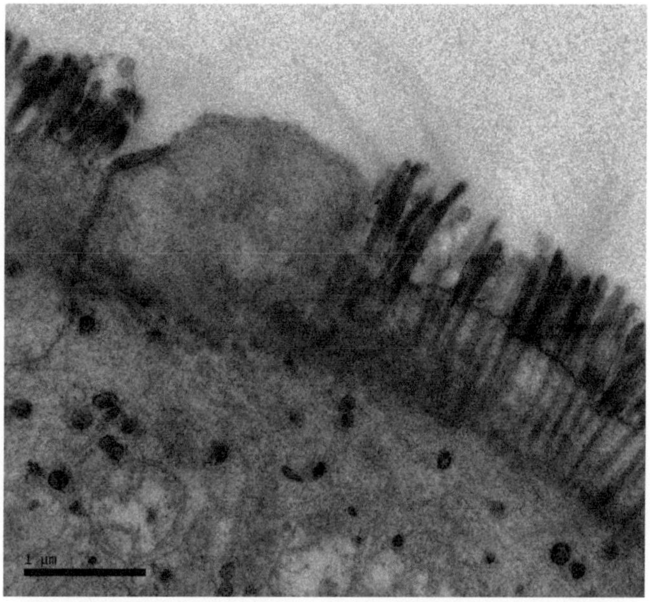

Fig. 1.37 Blistering of the cell membrane. Colonic mucosa epithelium of Bactrian camel: localized microvilli at the free end of the cell disappeared and formed a large blister of moderate electron density. ×25,000. (Wang Wenhui)

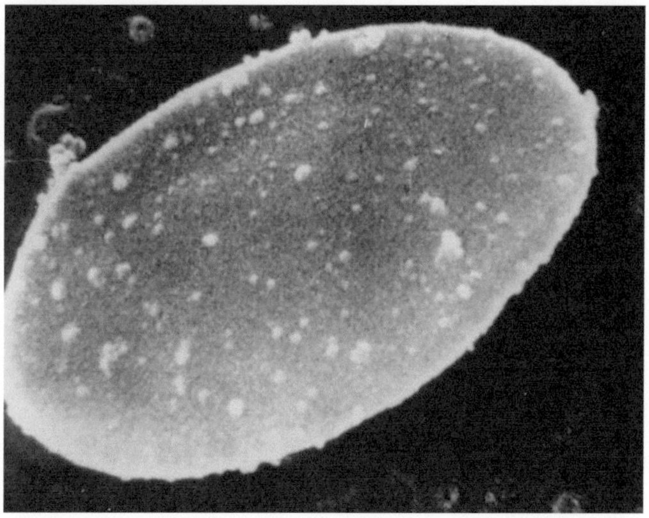

Fig. 1.38 Cell membrane protrusions. After a heavy drink of water or when erythrocytes are placed in hypotonic solutions, camels have markedly enlarged erythrocytes and many protrusions of varying sizes formed on the cell membranes. ×10,000. (Chen Huaitao)

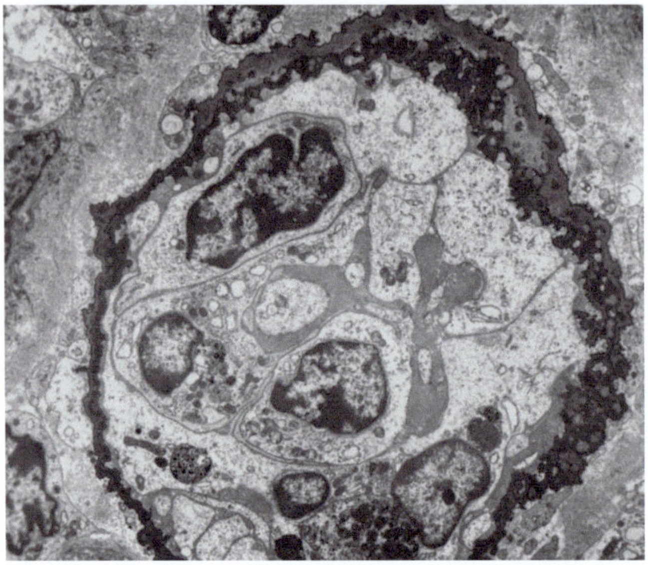

Fig. 1.39 Basement membrane thickening. Chronic progressive pneumonia in sheep. Mastitis: the acinar basement membrane is markedly and unevenly thickened. (Deng Puhui)

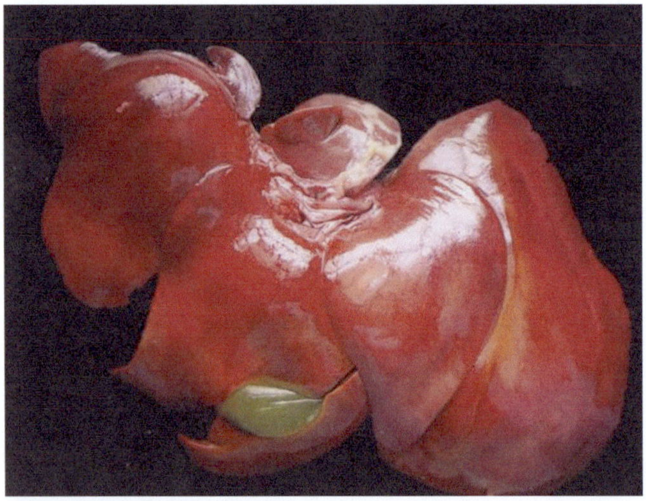

Fig. 1.40 Granular degeneration of liver. Canine parvovirus infection. The liver is enlarged, brittle, and soft with a reddish-yellow color. (Chen Huaitao)

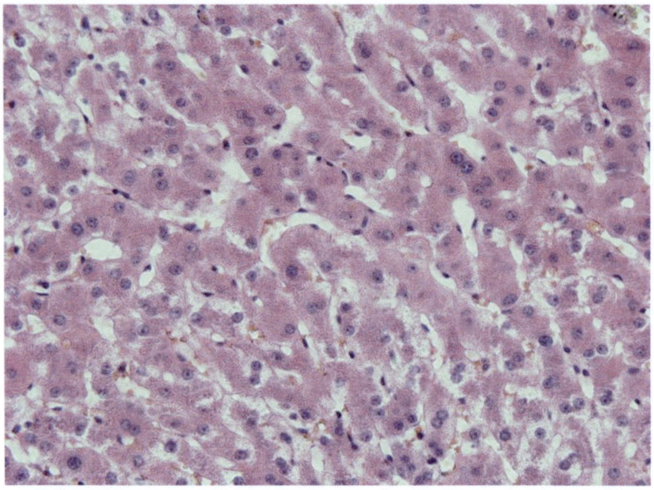

Fig. 1.41 Granular degeneration of liver. Hepatocytes are enlarged with many eosinophilic granules in the cytoplasm, and the hepatic sinusoids are narrowed. HE ×400. (Chen Huaitao)

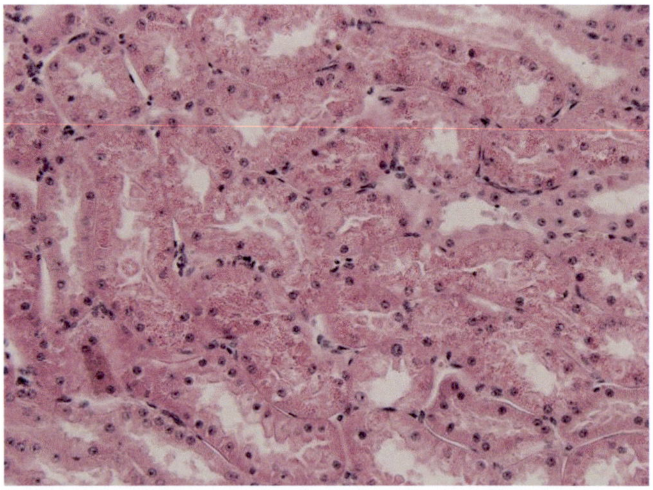

Fig. 1.42 Renal granular degeneration. A large amount of red proteinaceous granules are present in the cytoplasm of epithelial cells of the renal tubule, and the epithelial cells are swollen and protrude into the tubular lumen, resulting in reduced lumen volume to resemble a shape of fissure or star, and in some cases there is a small amount of proteinaceous material in the lumen. HE ×400. (Chen Huaitao)

2 Degeneration

2.1 Granular Degeneration (Figs. 1.40, 1.41, 1.42, and 1.43)

2.2 Vacuolar Degeneration (Figs. 1.44, 1.45, 1.46, 1.47, and 1.48)

Vacuolar degeneration is also known as hydropic degeneration.

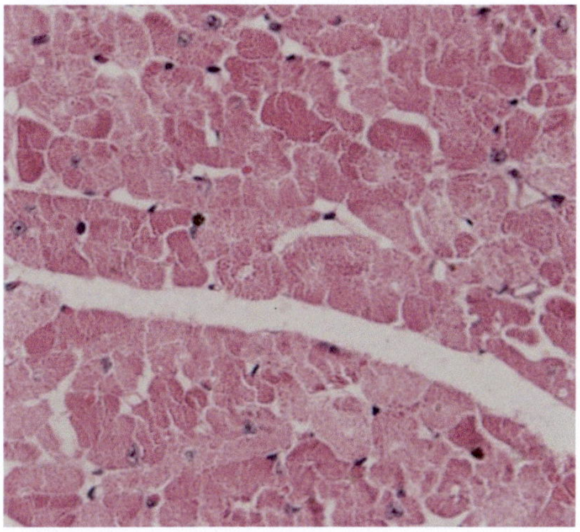

Fig. 1.43 Heart granular degeneration. Cardiac myocytes are enlarged and numerous red proteinaceous granules are present in the cytoplasm (cross-section of myocardial fibers), with some cells necrotized. HE ×400. (Chen Huaitao)

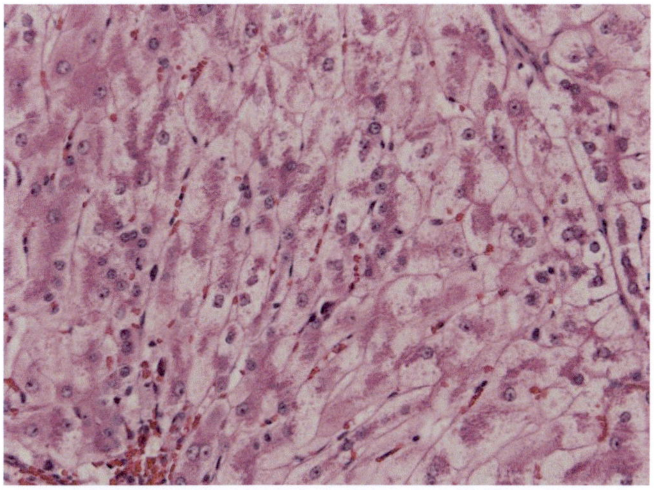

Fig. 1.44 Hepatic vacuolar degeneration. Hepatocytes are enlarged with uneven cytoplasmic staining, and the cells are mostly translucent and lightly stained, but the position of the nucleus is often unchanged. HE ×400. (Chen Huaitao)

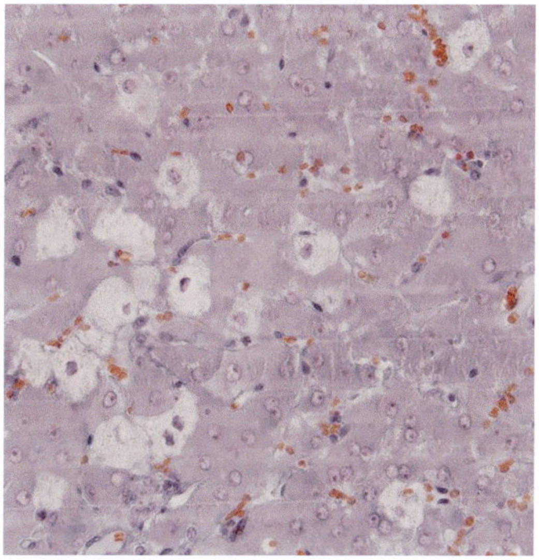

Fig. 1.45 Hepatic vacuolar degeneration. Some of the hepatocytes are enlarged, lightly stained, in the shape of large vesicles, resembling balloons, so it is called ballooning degeneration. HE ×400 (Chen Huaitao)

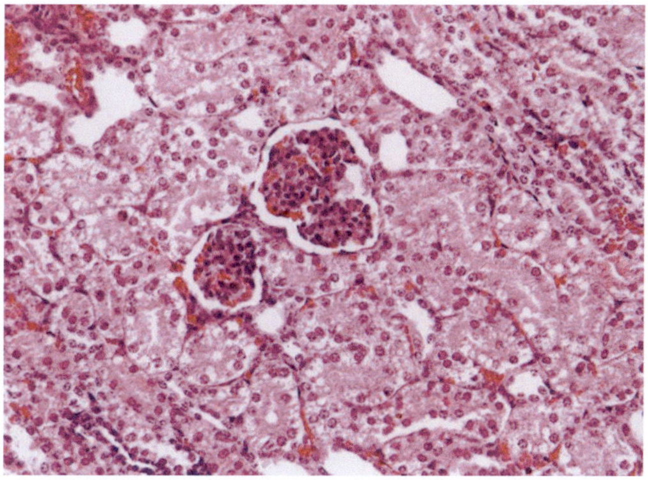

Fig. 1.46 Renal vacuolar degeneration. The tubular epithelial cells near the glomerulus are swollen with lightly stained cytoplasm. HE ×400. (Chen Huaitao)

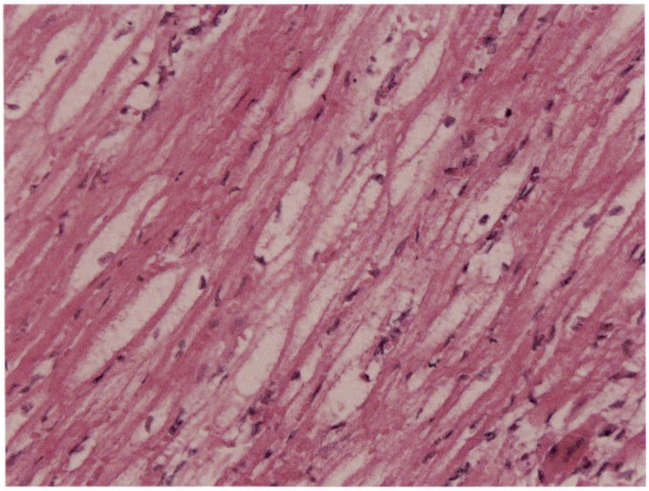

Fig. 1.47 Cardiac vacuolar degeneration. Cardiac myocytes are swollen and lightly stained with some cells vacuolated. HE ×400. (Chen Huaitao)

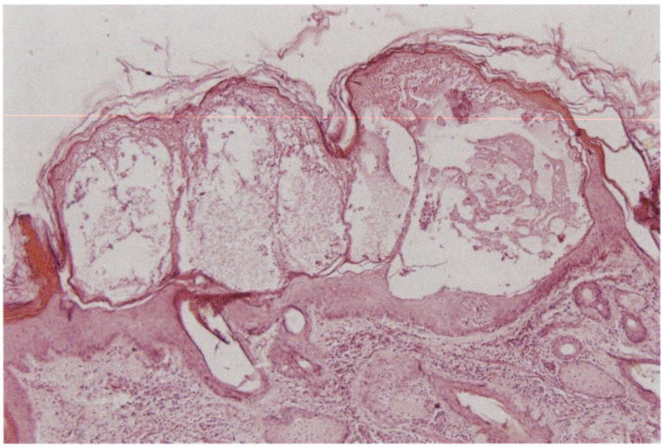

Fig. 1.48 Skin vacuolar degeneration. Vacuolar degeneration of epidermal cells, which results in the disintegration and fusion of cells to form large blisters filled with serum and necrotic material. HE ×100. (Chen Huaitao)

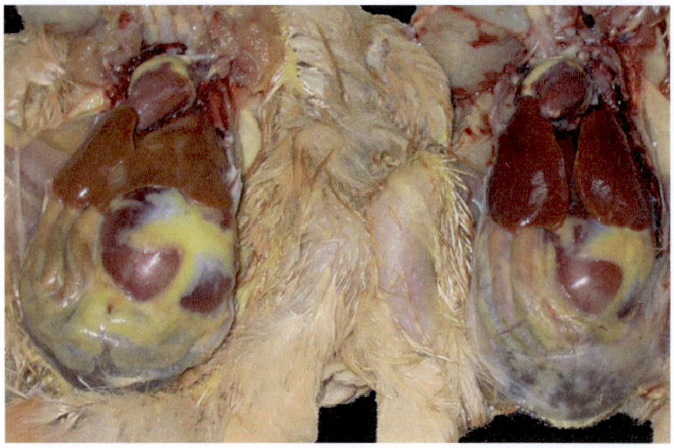

Fig. 1.49 Fatty degeneration in the liver. Fatty degeneration to the chicken liver is shown on the left side, which is in a yellowish brown color, while the liver on the right side is the normal control. (Wang Wenhui)

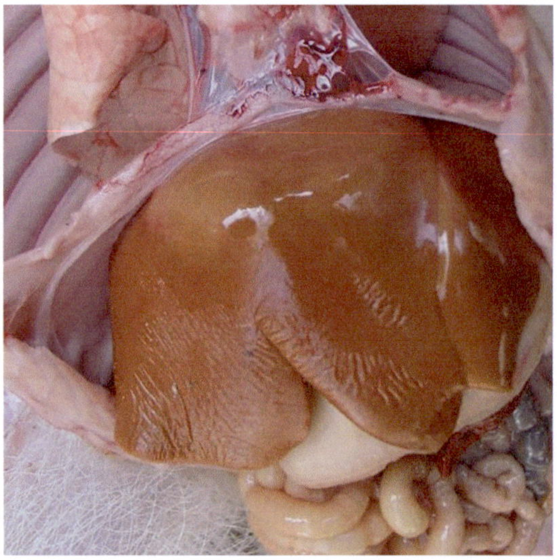

Fig. 1.50 Fatty degeneration in the liver. Pig liver. The liver is enlarged, with blunted edges and a marked yellowish color. (Wu Bin)

2.3 Fatty Degeneration (Figs. 1.49, 1.50, 1.51, 1.52, 1.53, 1.54, 1.55, 1.56, 1.57, and 1.58)

Fatty degeneration often occurs in the liver, kidney, and heart.

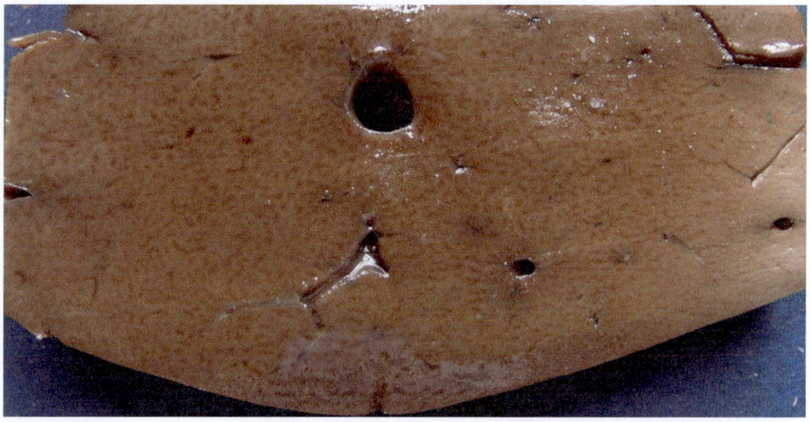

Fig. 1.51 Fatty degeneration in the liver. The liver with fatty degeneration is also congested, resulting in a red and yellow pattern on the liver surface, resembling a cut surface of betel nut, hence it is called betel nut liver or nutmeg liver. (Chen Huaitao)

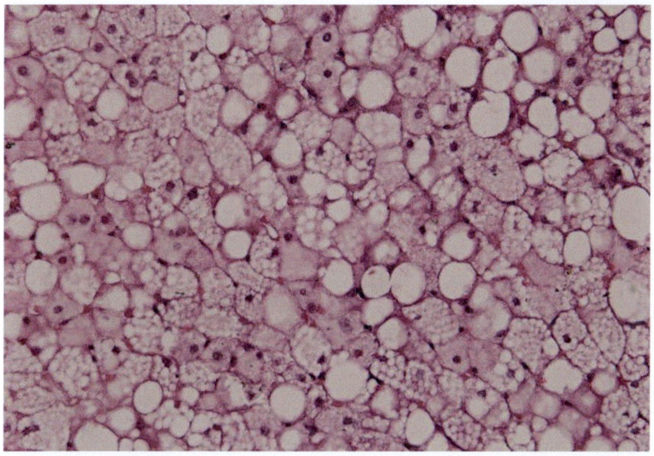

Fig. 1.52 Fatty degeneration in the liver. The hepatocytes are filled with a large number of small lipid droplets (the droplets were dissolved during the preparation of paraffin sections and left as vacuoles) or occupied by large lipid droplets, and the nuclei are squashed to one side; the hepatic sinusoids are narrowed. HE ×400. (Chen Huaitao)

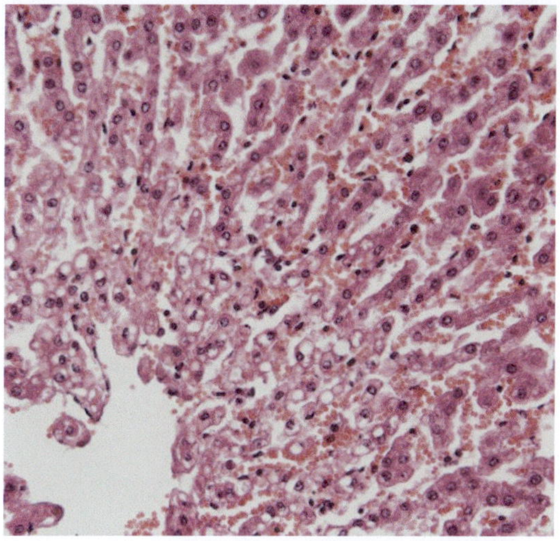

Fig. 1.54 Fatty degeneration in lobular center. Fatty degeneration occurred mainly in the hepatocytes around the central vein, and fat droplets of varying sizes are present within the cells; hepatocytes in the periphery of the lobules are mostly without significant changes. HE ×400. (Chen Huaitao)

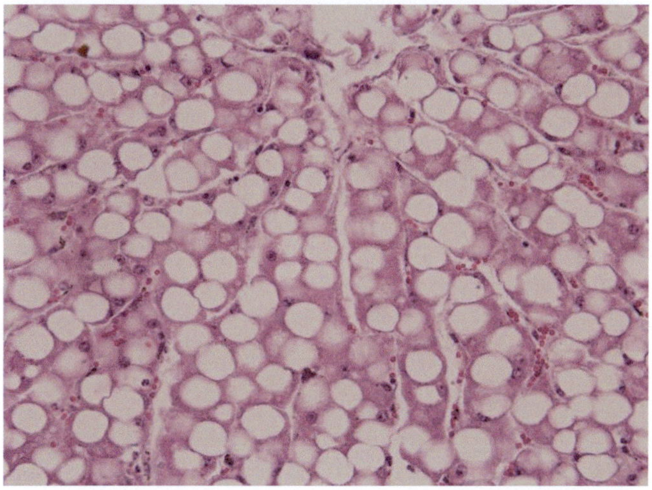

Fig. 1.53 Fatty degeneration in the liver. The hepatocyte cytoplasm is occupied by very large lipid droplets, the cytoplasm is scarce and squashed to the margin of the cells, and the nucleus is squashed to one side. HE ×400. (Chen Huaitao)

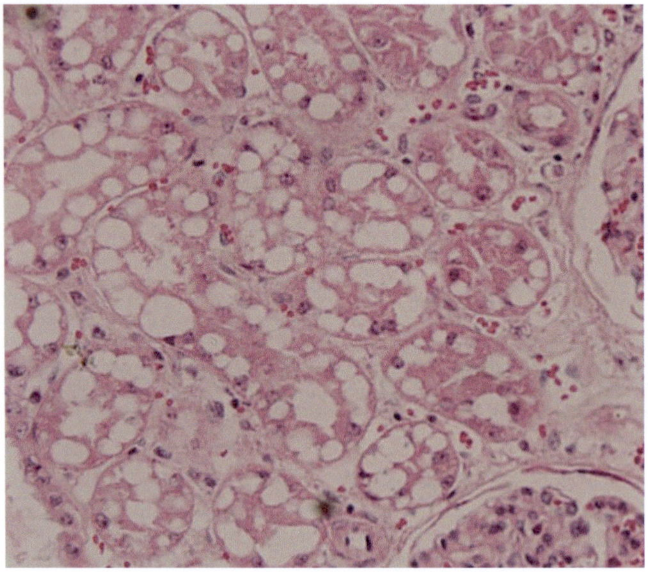

Fig. 1.55 Renal fatty degeneration. The epithelial cells of the renal tubules are filled with lipid droplets of different sizes, and the fat droplet vacuoles are clearly defined and the nuclei are often squeezed to one side. The tubular lumen of the renal tubules is reduced and in an irregular shape. HE ×400. (Chen Huaitao)

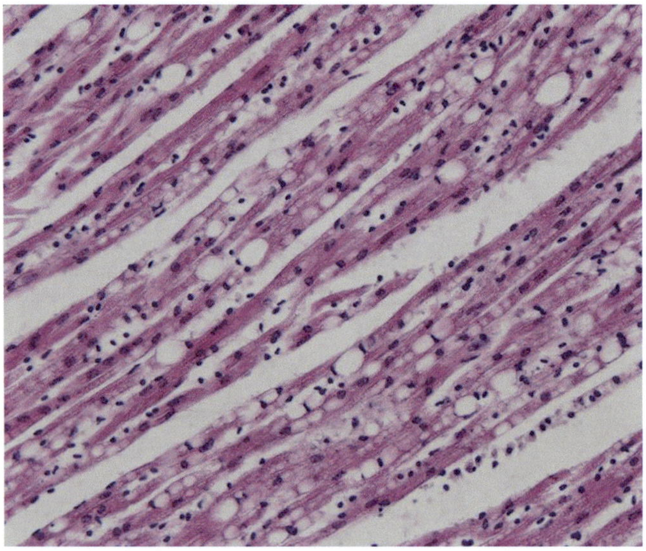

Fig. 1.56 Cardiac fatty degeneration. The lipid droplets of different sizes are beading arranged in the myocardial cell plasma, resulting in reduced cytoplasm

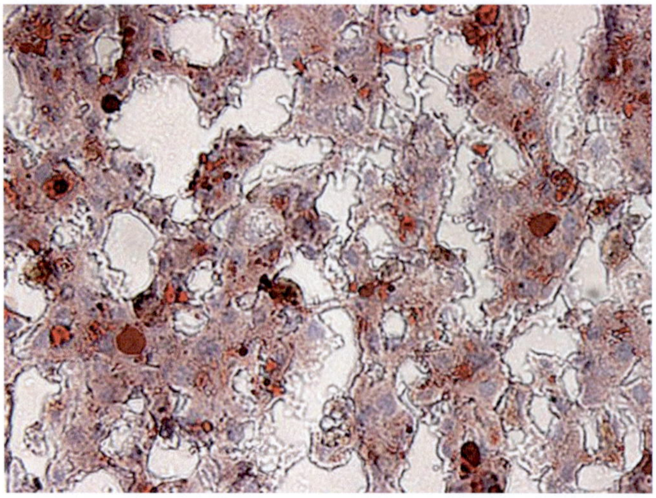

Fig. 1.57 Hepatic fatty degeneration. Frozen section of liver. Lipid droplets of varying sizes within the hepatocytes were stained orange. Sudan III staining ×400. (Cui Hengmin)

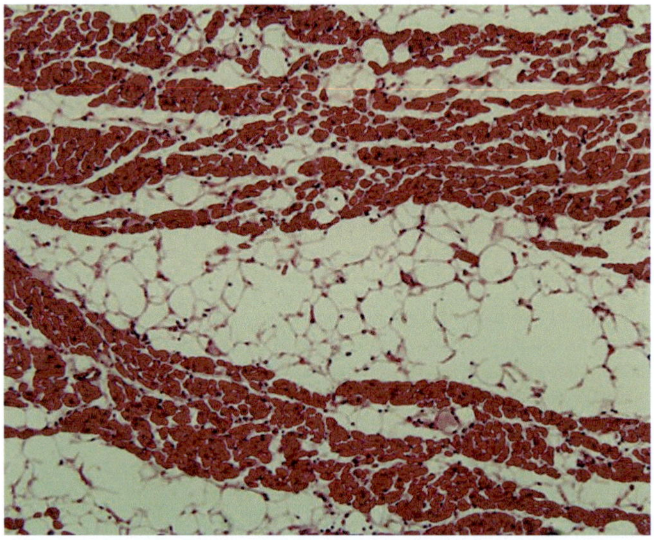

Fig. 1.58 Heart fat infiltration. There is severe infiltration of adipose tissue between the myocardial bundles, so the gaps between the bundles are widened. HE ×100. (Chen Huaitao)

2.4 Myelinic Degeneration (Figs. 1.59 and 1.60)

2.5 Hyaline Degeneration (Figs. 1.61, 1.62, 1.63, 1.64, and 1.65)

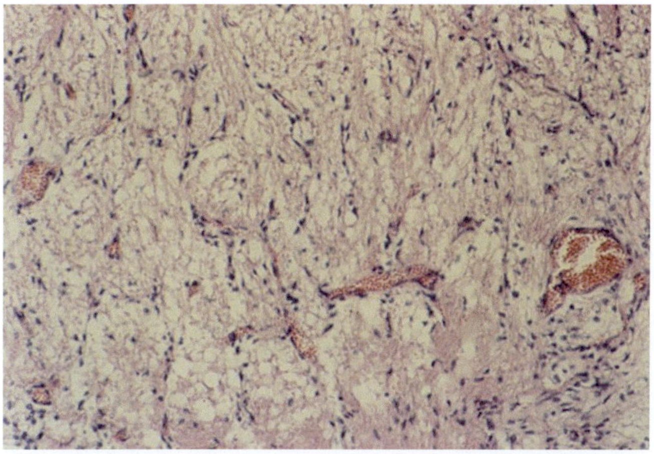

Fig. 1.59 Demyelination. Optic nerve: nerve fibers are demyelinated, so the nerve structure is loose and reticulate; the blood vessels are congested, and Schwann's cells are still present. HE ×200. (Chen Huaitao)

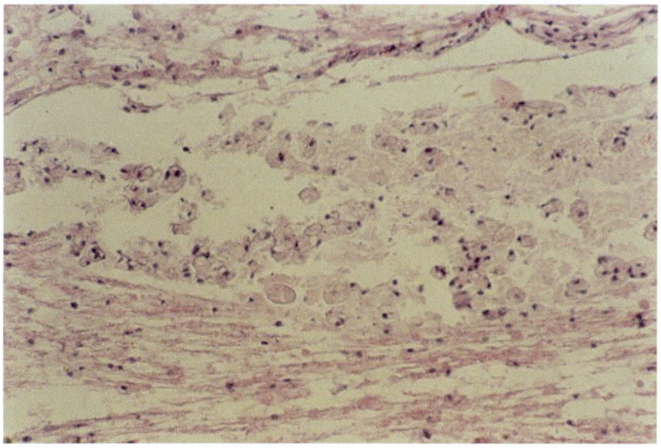

Fig. 1.60 Foam cells. Optic nerve: In the lower part of this figure, remnants of demyelinated nerve fiber axons are still visible, while most of the nerve fibers in the area have been completely necrotic and disintegrated, turning into structureless material containing myelin. Macrophages phagocytosed the phospholipids and turned into foam cells (gitter cells) of different sizes. HE ×400. (Chen Huaitao)

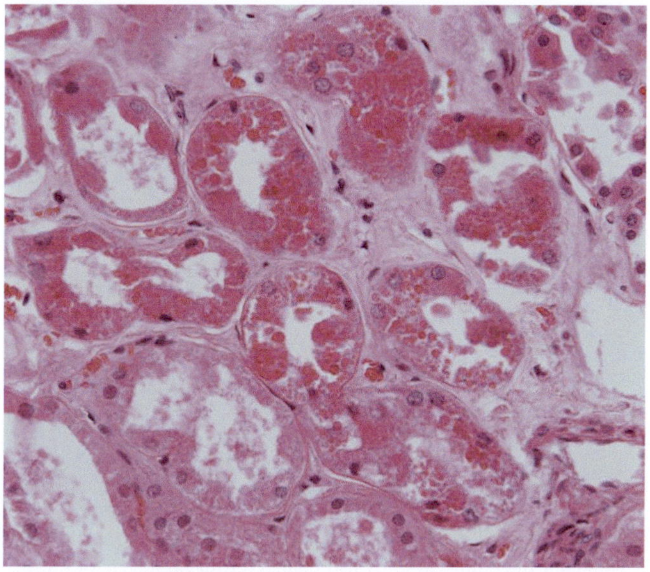

Fig. 1.61 Renal hyaline degeneration. Red, round, glassy droplets of varying sizes are present in the epithelial cells of the renal tubules, and droplets are also present in the renal tubules. HE ×400. (Chen Huaitao)

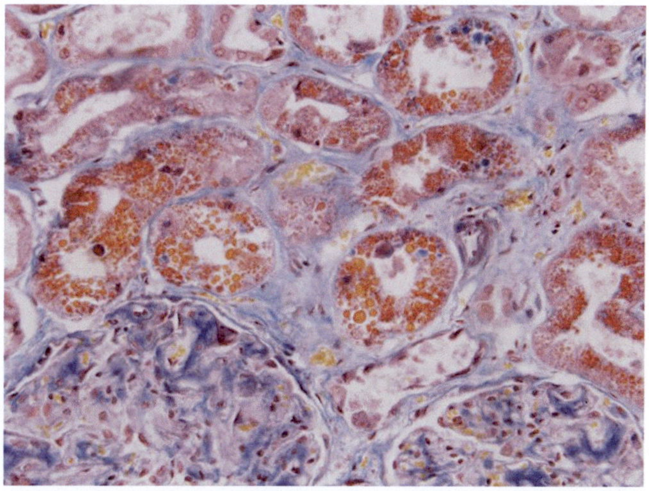

Fig. 1.62 Renal hyaline degeneration. Red, round, glassy droplets of variable size are present in the epithelium and lumen of the renal tubules. Mallory ×400. (Chen Huaitao)

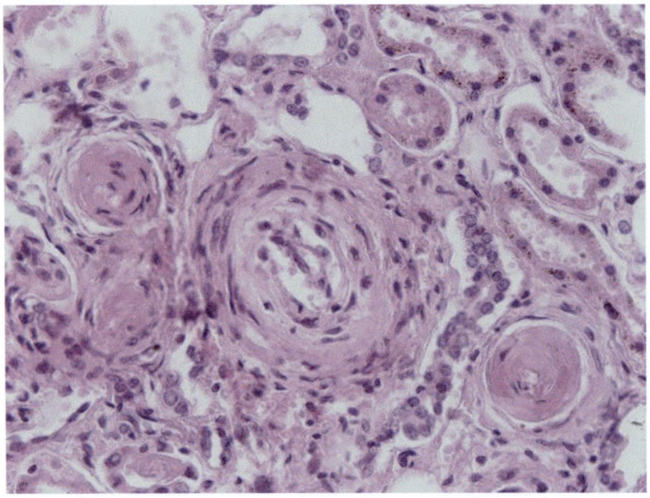

Fig. 1.63 Hyaline degeneration of small arterial wall. The walls of the small renal interstitial arteries had changed to a homogeneous structureless glassy material with little cellular component, and the lumen of the arteries had become small or even occluded. HE ×400. (Chen Huaitao)

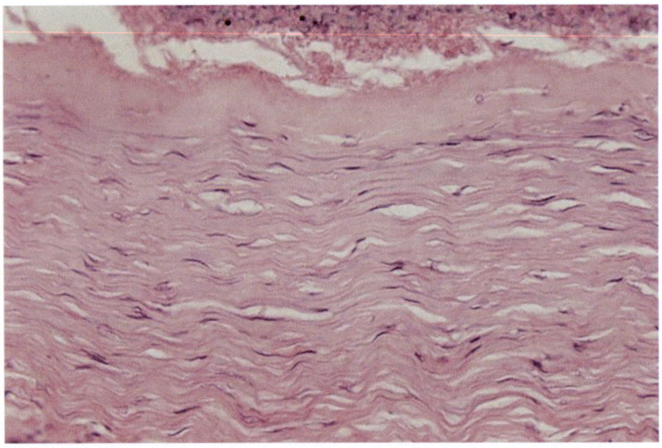

Fig. 1.64 Hyaline degeneration of connective tissue. The connective tissue of the abscess capsule undergoes hyaline degeneration and the collagen fibers fuse into a homogeneous reddish glassy material with few elongated fibroblast nuclei. HE ×400. (Chen Huaitao)

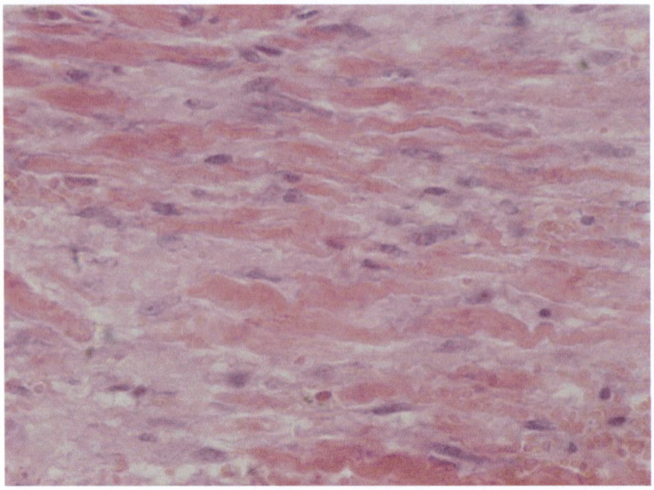

Fig. 1.65 Hyaline degeneration of connective tissue. Collagen fibers in connective tissue fuse and undergo hyaline degeneration; the collagen fibers are in strips of varying size, homogeneous, and deeply eosin stained. HE ×400. (Wang Wenhui)

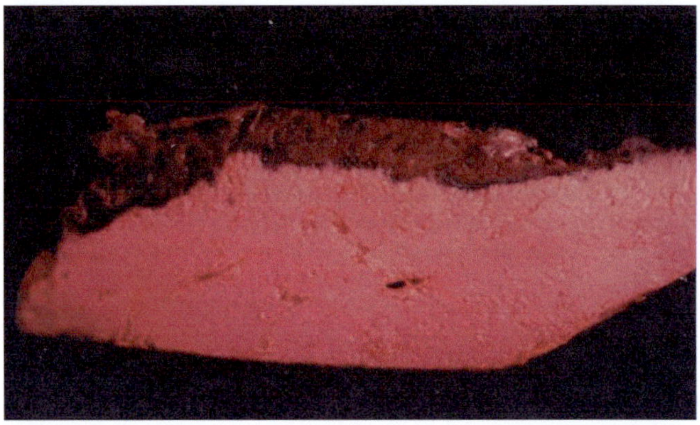

Fig. 1.66 Hepatic amyloid degeneration. Hepatic amyloid degeneration in horses for serum producing: the liver is pale, brittle, and hemorrhagic due to liver rupture; the dark red area in the upper part of the figure is the blood clot formed after bleeding. (Veterinary Pathological Unit, Gansu Agricultural University)

2.6 Amyloid Degeneration (Figs. 1.66, 1.67, 1.68, 1.69, 1.70, 1.71, 1.72, 1.73, and 1.74)

Amyloid degeneration is also known as amyloidosis.

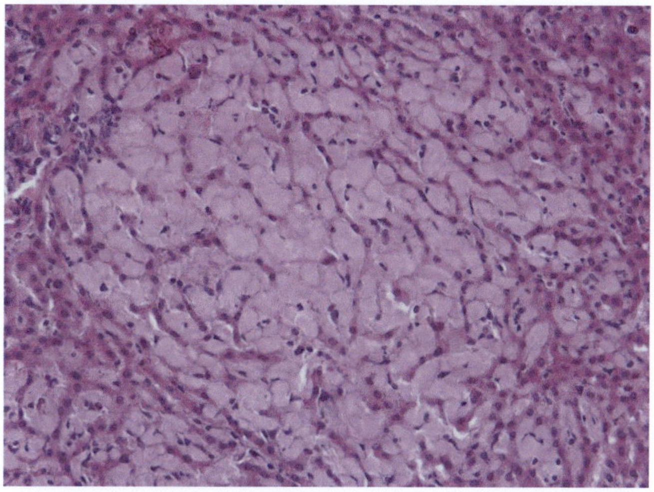

Fig. 1.67 Hepatic amyloid degeneration. A large amount of homogeneous reddish amyloid material accumulates between the hepatocyte cords and the hepatic sinusoids, and the hepatocyte cords are compressed and atrophied. HE ×400. (Chen Huaitao)

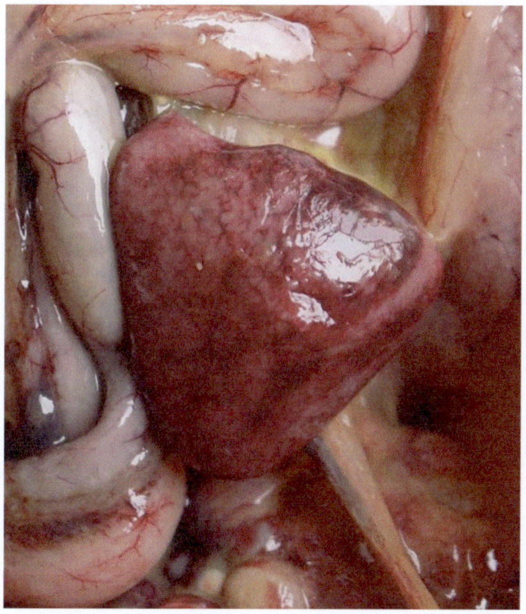

Fig. 1.68 Splenic amyloid degeneration. Duck spleen. The spleen is obviously enlarged and the areas with amyloid deposits are grayish in color. (Hu Xueying)

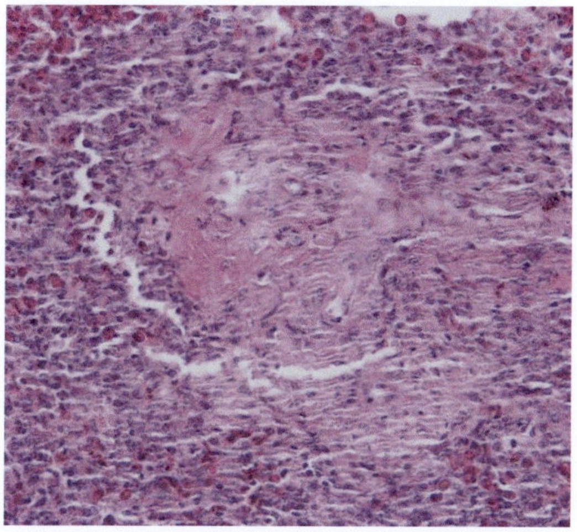

Fig. 1.69 Splenic amyloid degeneration (focal type). A large amount of amyloid deposit on the reticular fibers of the lymphoid follicles of the spleen with a reddish homogeneous appearance. HE ×400. (Chen Huaitao)

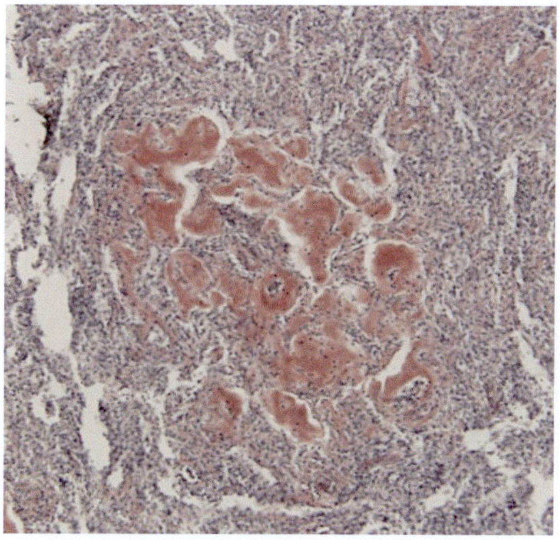

Fig. 1.70 Splenic amyloid degeneration (focal type). The amyloid material is mainly deposited in the lymphoid follicular area of the spleen with red color and homogeneity. Congo red stain ×400. (Chen Huaitao)

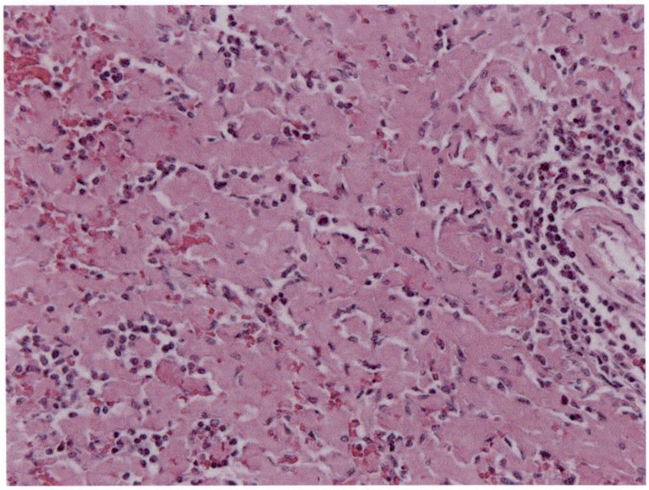

Fig. 1.71 Splenic amyloid degeneration (diffuse type). Pale red amyloid material is diffusely deposited between splenic medullary cells and on reticular fibers in irregular masses or cords, with lymphoid tissue reduced or even absent. HE ×400. (Chen Huaitao)

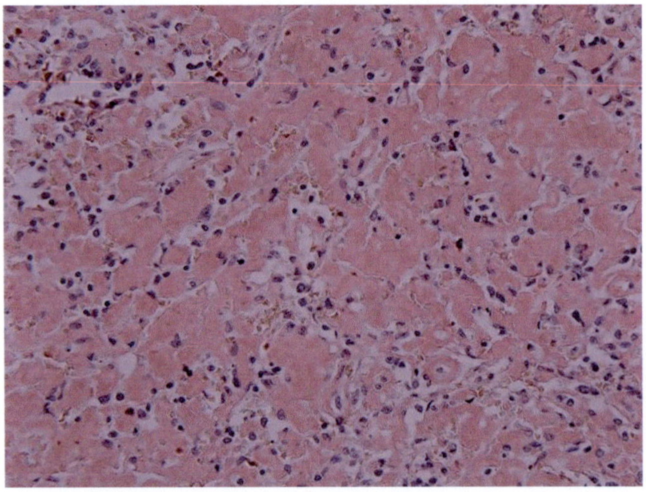

Fig. 1.72 Splenic amyloid degeneration (diffuse type). Diffusely deposited amyloid material in spleen tissue is stained red; massive deposition of amyloid material disrupts the spleen structure, with only a few lymphocytes scattered. Congo red staining ×400. (Chen Huaitao)

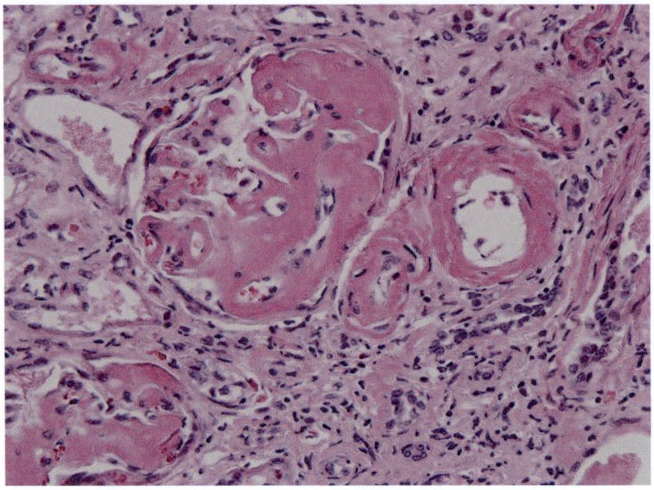

Fig. 1.73 Renal amyloid degeneration. There is a reddish homogeneous amyloid deposition on the glomerular capillary basement membrane and small arterial vessel walls, so the glomeruli and small arterial walls are indistinct. HE ×400. (Chen Huaitao)

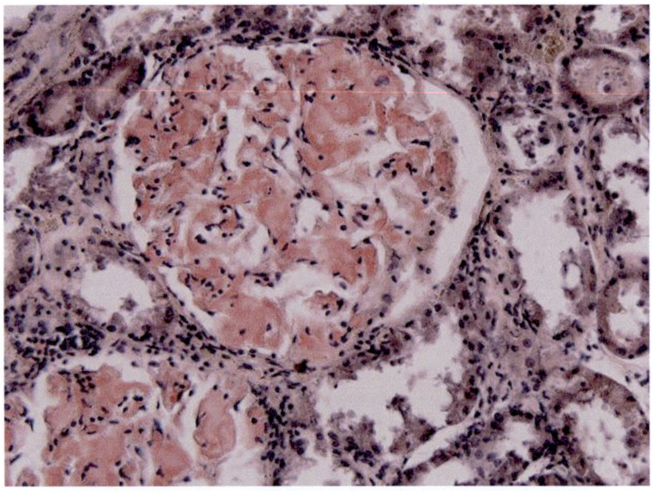

Fig. 1.74 Renal amyloid degeneration. The red-stained homogeneous amyloid material is deposited on the basement membrane of glomerular capillaries. Congo red staining ×400. (Chen Huaitao)

2.7 Mucoid Degeneration (Fig. 1.75)

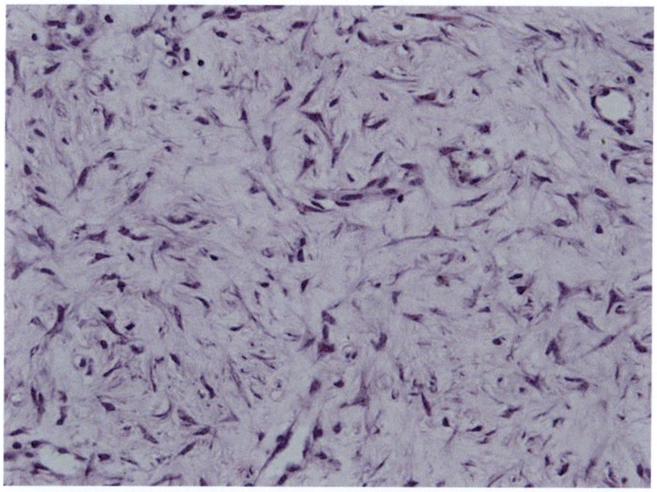

Fig. 1.75 Mucoid degeneration. A large amount of mucus-like material deposits between polygonal fibroblasts with a pale blue-red color. HE ×400. (Chen Huaitao)

2.8 Fibrinoid Degeneration (Figs. 1.76 and 1.77)

Fibrinoid degeneration is actually a necrotic change in connective tissue or the wall of small blood vessels, so it is also called fibrinoid necrosis.

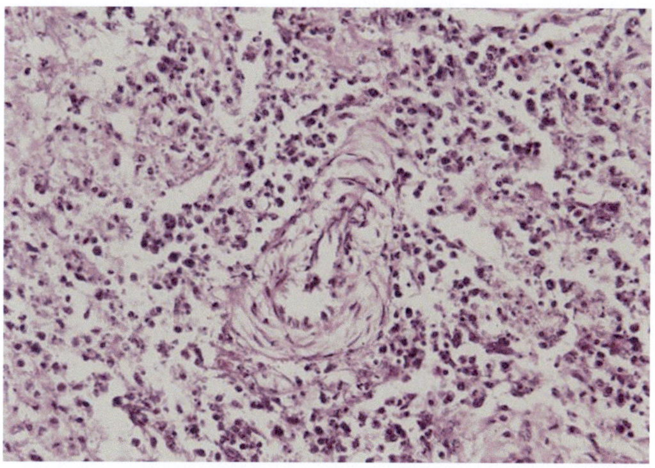

Fig. 1.76 Fibrinoid degeneration of the vessel wall. Necrosis of the vessel wall with a loose structure and a fuzzy fibrin-like substance. HE ×400. (Chen Huaitao)

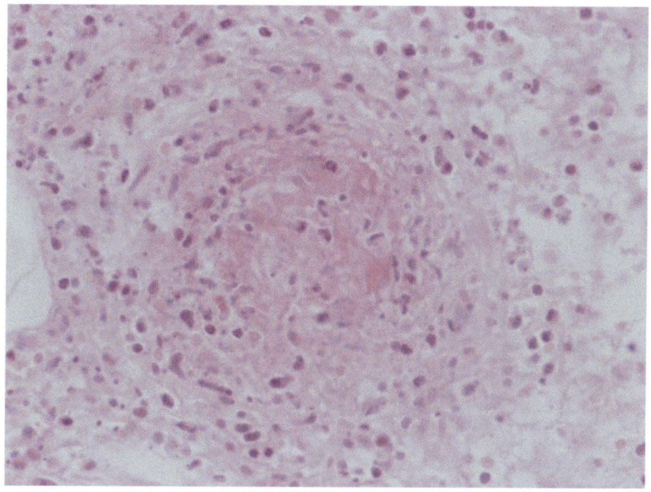

Fig. 1.77 Fibrinoid degeneration of the vessel wall. Porcine submandibular lymph node. The outline of the small arterial blood vessel wall is faintly visible, but the tissue structure is disrupted and disintegrated, and the necrotic material is mixed with a few inflammatory cells. HE ×400. (Wang Wenhui)

3 Necrosis

3.1 Changes in the Nucleus during Necrosis (Fig. 1.78)

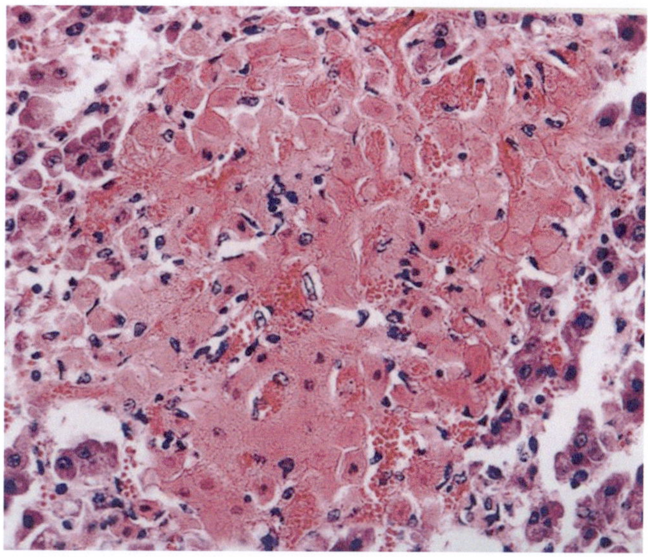

Fig. 1.78 Changes in the Nucleus. A foci of coagulative necrosis in bovine liver. The hepatocyte cytoplasm is coagulated and red-stained, and the histology is recognizable, but the necrotic hepatocyte nuclei show multiple changes: nuclear pyknosis, nuclear karyorrhexis, nuclear karyolysis, and nuclear disappearance. HE ×400. (Chen Huaitao)

3.2 Coagulative Necrosis

3.2.1 Renal Anemic Infarction (Figs. 1.79, 1.80, and 1.81)

3.2.2 Waxy Necrosis (Figs. 1.82 and 1.83)

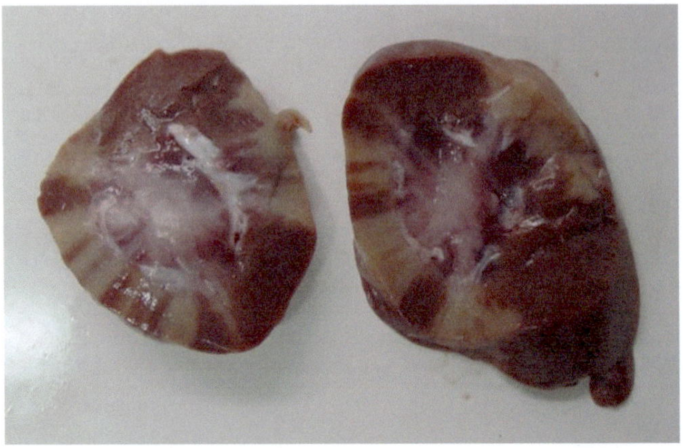

Fig. 1.79 Renal Anemic Infarction. In the renal section, the infarcted area is mostly wedge-shaped, earthy yellow in color, and clearly bounded from the surrounding area. (Xueying Hu)

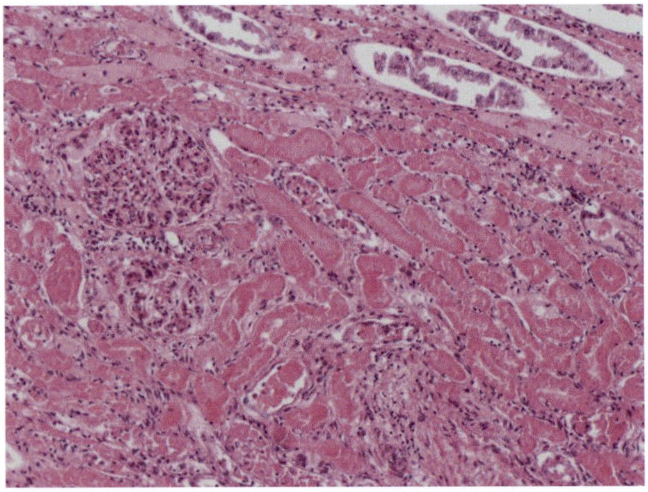

Fig. 1.80 Renal anemic infarction. The outline of the renal tubules in the infarcted area is still present, the cytoplasm is coagulated and deeply eosin-stained, but the nuclei are disappeared; the interstitial cells are mostly still alive. HE ×100. (Wang Wenhui)

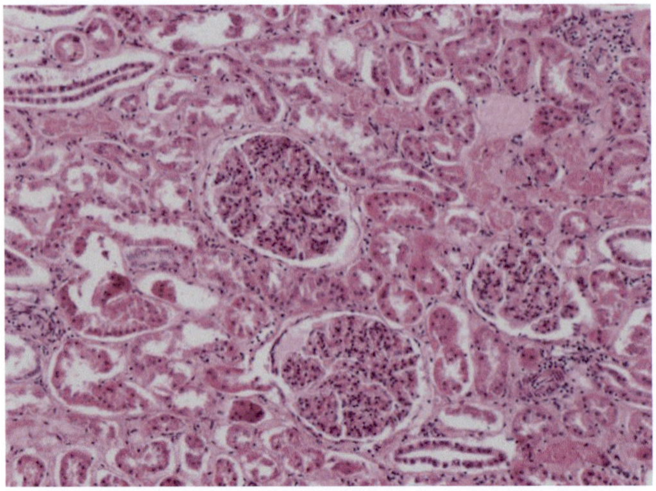

Fig. 1.81 Renal anemic infarction. In mild infarction, the nuclei of renal tubular epithelial cells are mostly present but concentrated and deeply stained. HE ×400. (Wang Wenhui)

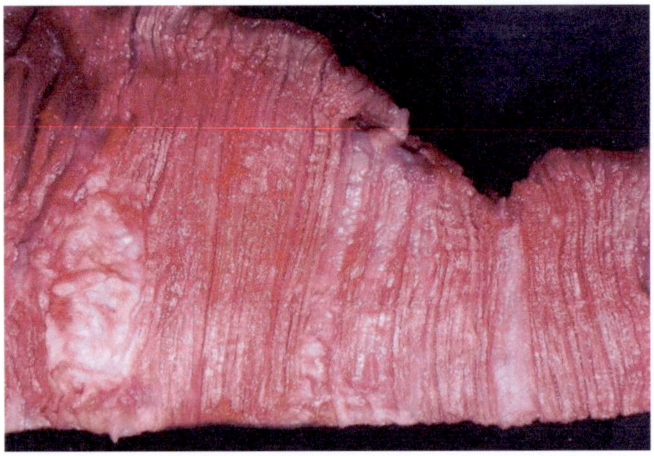

Fig. 1.82 Waxy necrosis of skeletal muscle. Bovine Theileriosis. In longitudinal sections of skeletal muscle, the striated or massed muscle fibers are necrotic, resulting in grayish-white, homogeneous, and wax-like appearance. (Chen Huaitao)

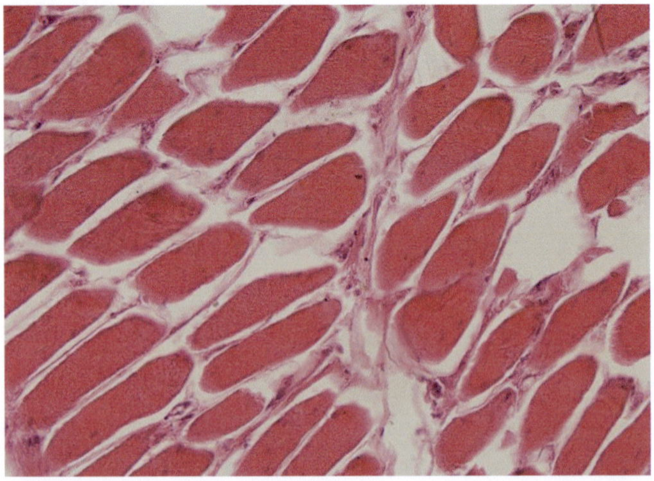

Fig. 1.83 Waxy necrosis of skeletal muscle. The striated muscle fibers are necrotized and coagulated resulting in the disappearance of horizontal stripe, deep-eosin-staining, and homogeneous glassy appearance. HE ×400. (Chen Huaitao)

3.2.3 Caseous Necrosis (Figs. 1.84, 1.85, and 1.86)

3.3 Liquefactive Necrosis (LN)

3.3.1 Abscess (Figs. 1.87 and 1.88)

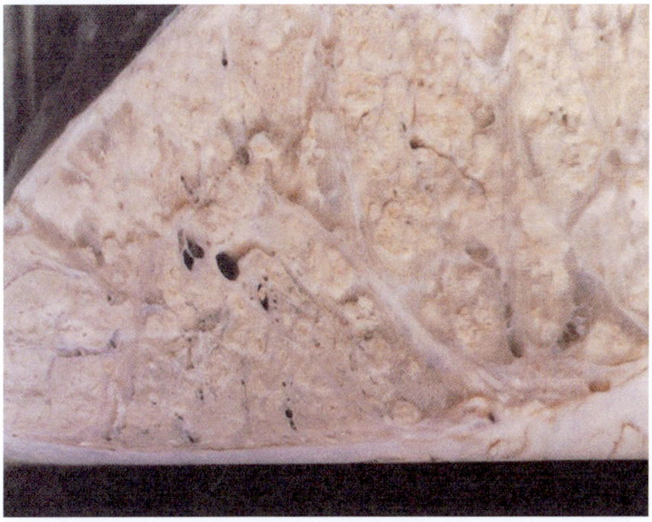

Fig. 1.84 Caseous necrosis. Bovine pulmonary tuberculosis. Caseous necrosis and calcification of tuberculosis nodules are present on lung section, which is yellowish-white in color. (Veterinary Pathology Unit, Gansu Agricultural University)

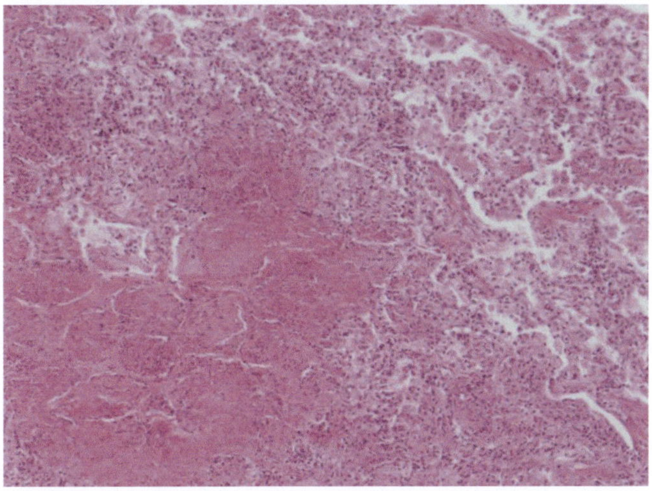

Fig. 1.85 Caseous necrosis. Bovine tuberculosis. The red-stained area in the tuberculosis nodules is the focus of caseous necrosis, which is clearly defined from the surrounding area. The outline of alveoli is still recognizable. HE ×100. (Wang Wenhui)

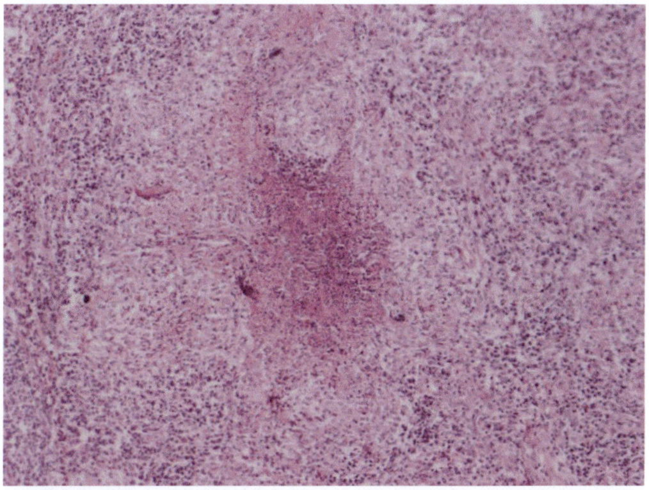

Fig. 1.86 Caseous necrosis. Bovine tuberculosis. Caseous necrosis begins from the center of a lymph node tuberculosis nodule with numerous epithelioid cells at the periphery. HE ×100. (Wang Wenhui)

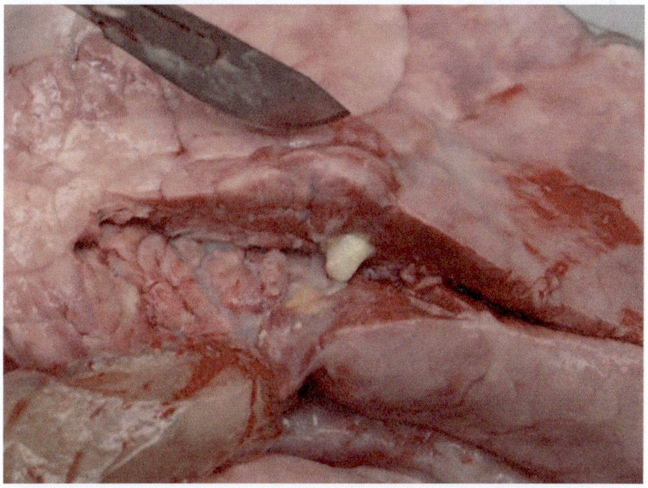

Fig. 1.87 Abscess. Lung abscess. The abscess was cut open and thick yellowish-white pus was seen coming out. (Gu Changqin)

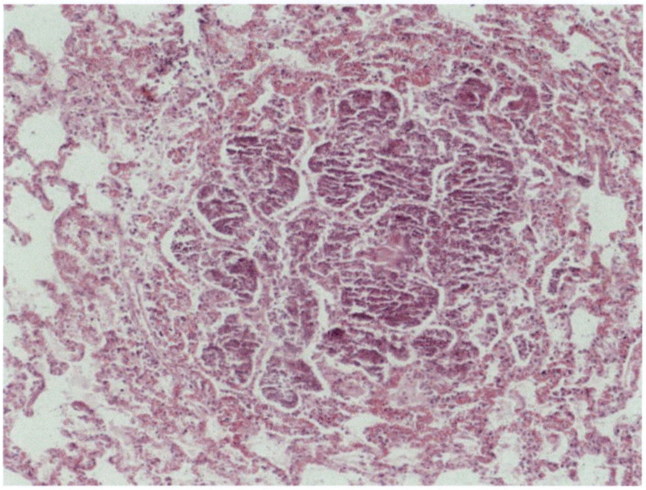

Fig. 1.88 Suppuration. A small purulent focus is present in the lung with alveoli filled with pus cells and lung tissue beginning to dissolve and necrotize. HE ×100. (Wang Wenhui)

3.3.2 Fat Necrosis (Figs. 1.89, 1.90, and 1.91)

3.3.3 Cerebral Softening (Encephalomalacia, Fig. 1.92)

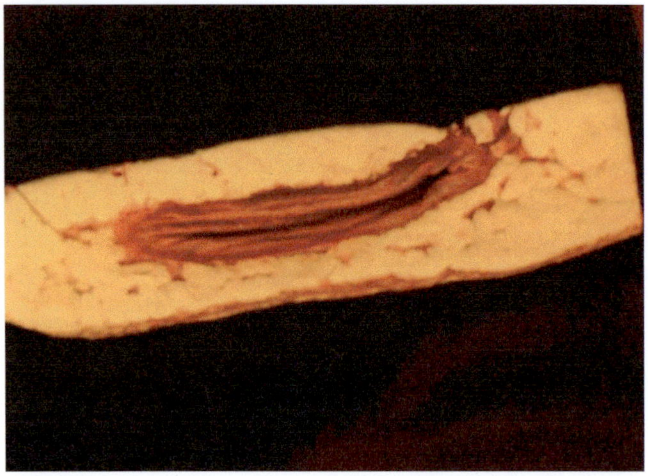

Fig. 1.89 Fat necrosis. Diffuse necrosis of the fatty tissue around the colon. The necrotic tissue was grayish white, hard in texture, and lost its original luster. (Veterinary Pathology Unit, Gansu Agricultural University)

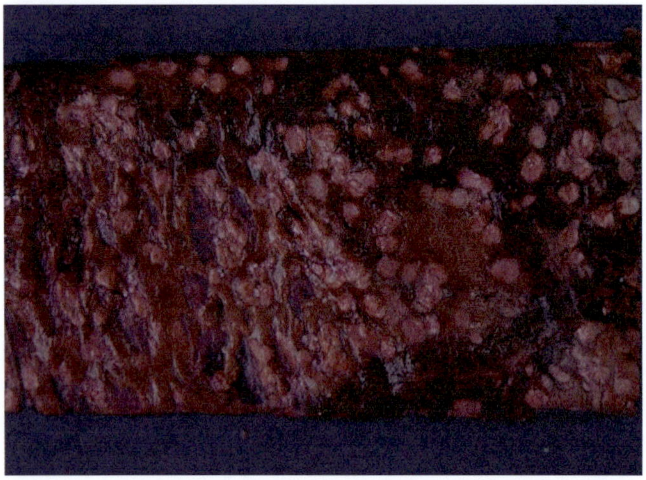

Fig. 1.90 Fat necrosis. Multiple foci of necrosis in the fat of the porcine greater omentum. The necrotic foci were round in shape, yellowish-white in color, and clearly bounded from the surrounding tissues. (Veterinary Pathology Unit, Gansu Agricultural University)

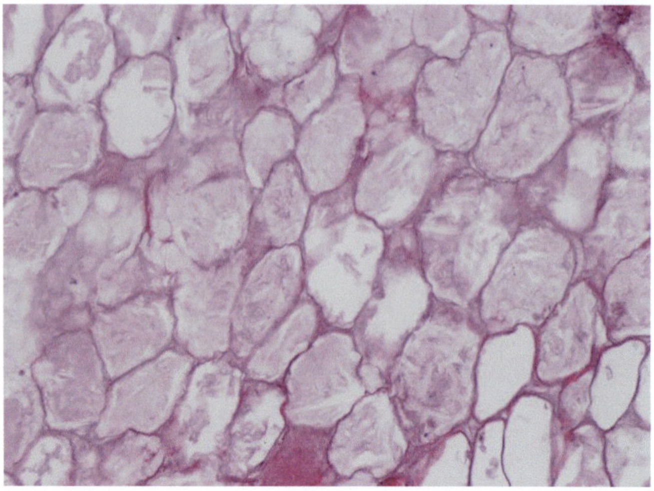

Fig. 1.91 Fat necrosis. Necrosis of subcutaneous adipose tissue. The inhomogeneous basophilic substances (calcium soap) are present in necrotic adipocytes, in which the gaps left from the dissolution of needle-like fatty acid crystals were barely visible. HE ×100. (Wang Wenhui)

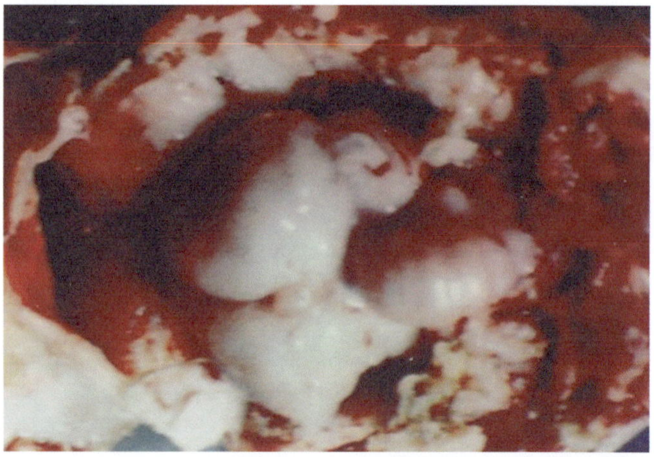

Fig. 1.92 Encephalomalacia. Encephalomalacia of chick. The cerebellum is atrophied in diseased chicks, with softened and damaged tissue in the posterior part of the brain. (Chen Jianhong)

4 Apoptosis (Figs. 1.93, 1.94, 1.95, 1.96, 1.97, 1.98, and 1.99)

Apoptosis is also known as programmed cell death (PCD).

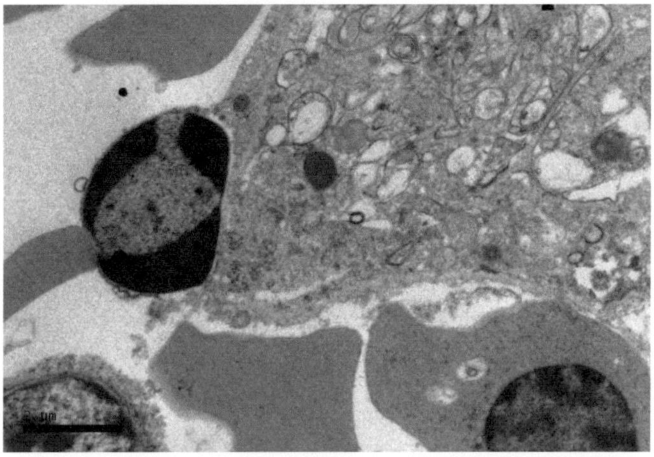

Fig. 1.93 Annular nuclei. Lung. Type II alveolar epithelial cells are in the early stages of apoptosis, with nuclear chromatin margination in an annular form. ×10,000. (Wang Wenhui)

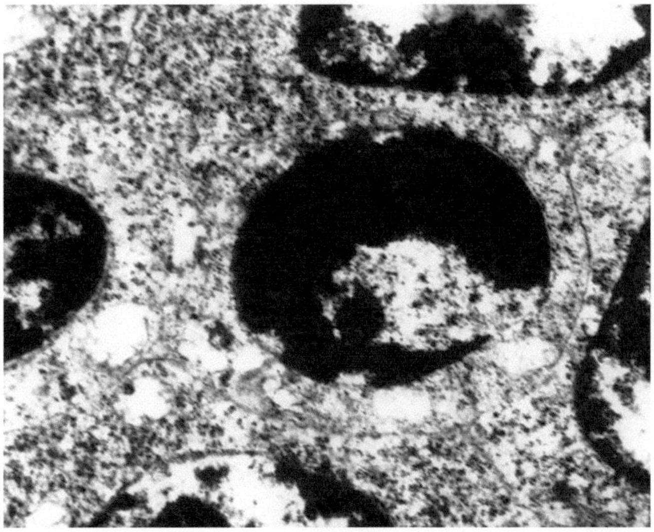

Fig. 1.94 C-shaped nucleus. Copper poisoning in ducklings. Thymic lymphocytes were apoptotic and their nuclear chromatin was cohesive and C-shaped. ×10,000. (Cui Hengmin)

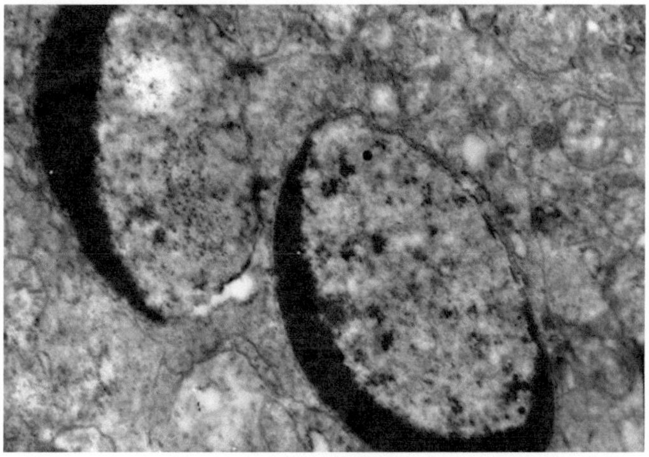

Fig. 1.95 Crescent-shaped nucleus. Copper poisoning in ducklings. The spleen lymphocytes are apoptotic with nuclear chromatin coalesced into a crescent shape. ×15,000. (Cui Hengmin)

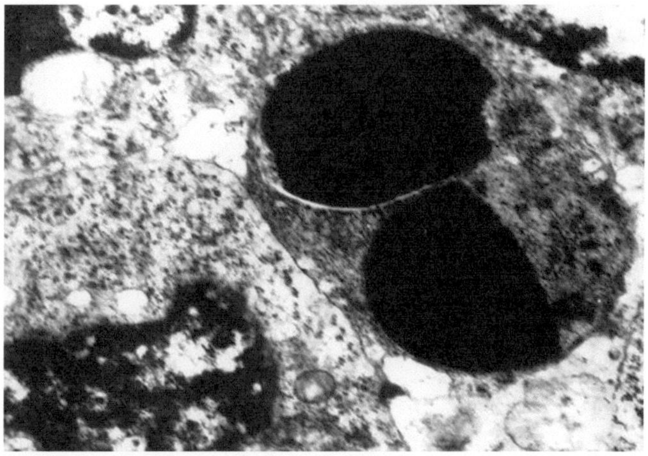

Fig. 1.96 Chromatin condensation. Copper poisoning in ducklings. The bursal of Fabricius lymphocytes are apoptotic with nuclear chromatin coalesced into two dense clumps. ×15,000. (Cui Hengmin)

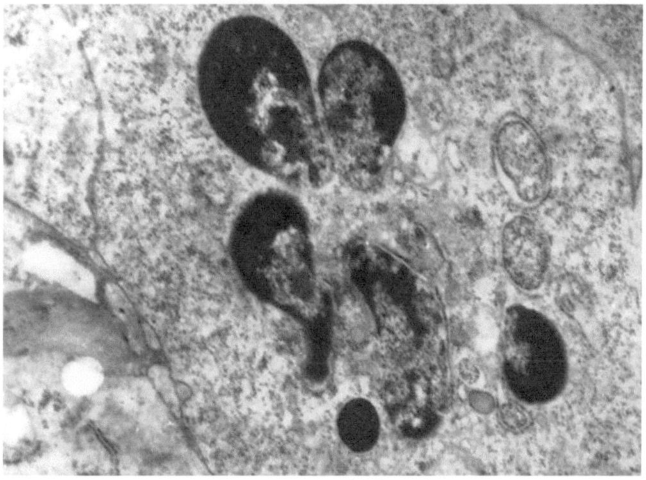

Fig. 1.97 Apoptotic body. Copper poisoning in ducklings. Apoptotic cells in the thymus began to form apoptotic bodies. ×15,000 (Cui Hengmin)

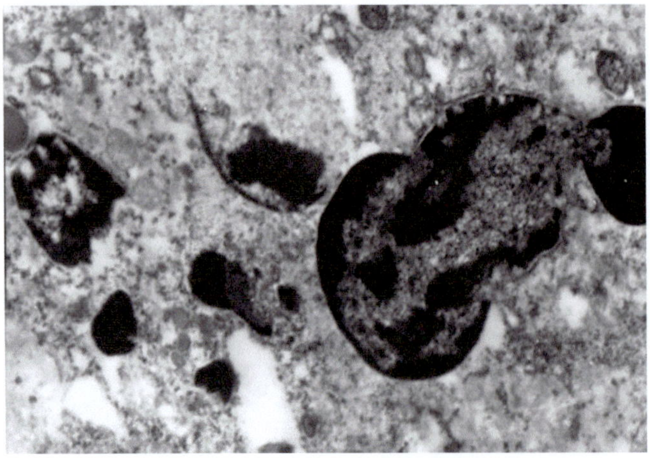

Fig. 1.98 Apoptotic body. Copper poisoning in ducklings. The apoptotic lymphocytes in the spleen have been lysed into apoptotic bodies. ×12,000. (Cui Hengmin)

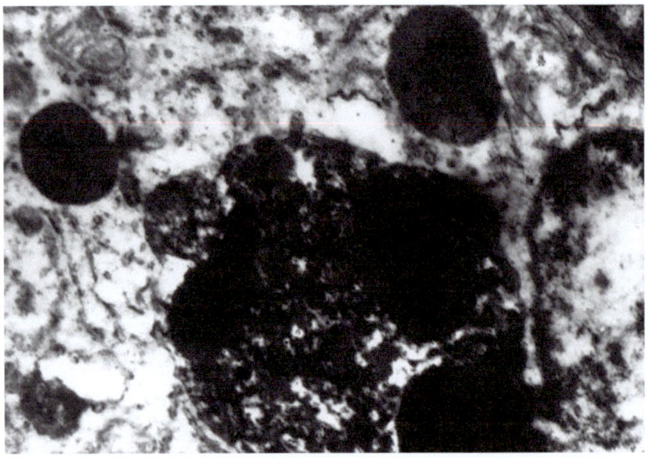

Fig. 1.99 Apoptotic body. Copper poisoning in ducklings. Apoptotic cells of the bursa of Fasciola have formed apoptotic vesicles. ×13,000. (Cui Hengmin)

5 Deposit of Pathological Substances

5.1 Pathological Calcification

5.1.1 Dystrophic Calcification (Figs. 1.100, 1.101, and 1.102)

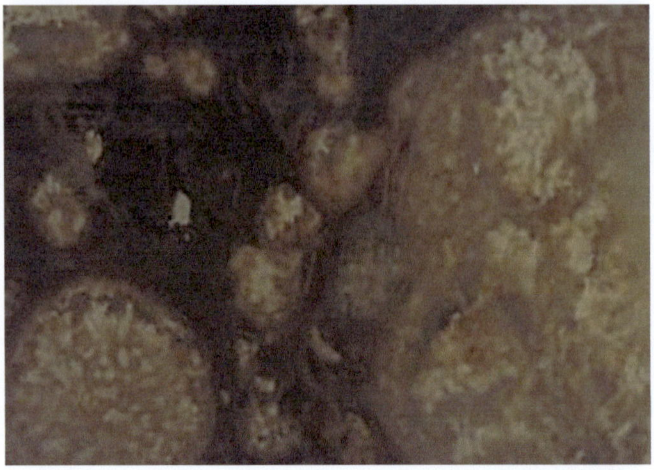

Fig. 1.100 Parasitic calcification. Calcification of dead echinococcus larvae in the spleen of a cow. The calcified foci are grayish-white granular and hard in texture. (Wang Wenhui)

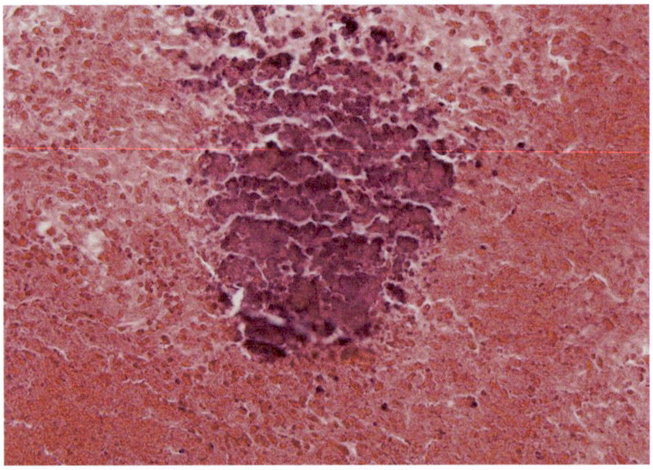

Fig. 1.101 Calcification of caseous necrotic material. Caseous necrosis (red-stained portion) occurs in tuberculous nodules, and the blue masses of granular calcium salt deposits are visible in the center of the necrotic material. HE ×400. (Chen Huaitao)

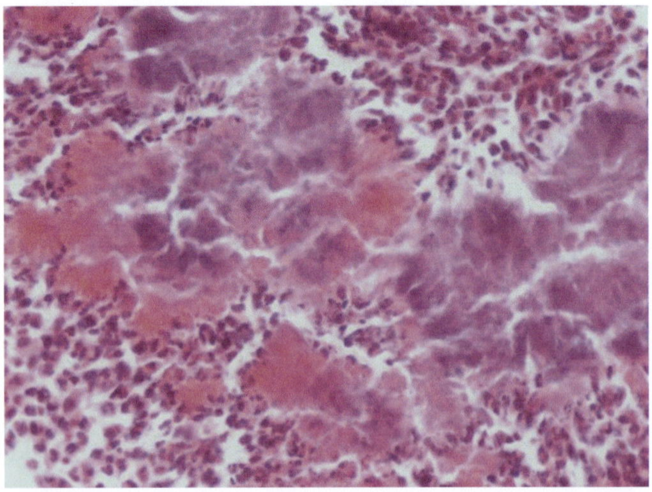

Fig. 1.102 Calcification of bacterial necrotic material. The figure shows the calcification of a dead bacterial clot in the center of a bovine actinomycete granuloma. The calcified foci are bluish-purple, but the bacteria without calcium salt deposits are red. HE ×400. (Wang Wenhui)

5.1.2 Metastatic Calcification (Figs. 1.103 and 1.104)

5.2 Uratosis (Figs. 1.105, 1.106, 1.107, and 1.108)

Uratosis, or gout, is a disorder of purine metabolism, which commonly occurs in poultry. It is characterized by the deposition of uric acid and urate crystals in internal organs and joints, among other areas.

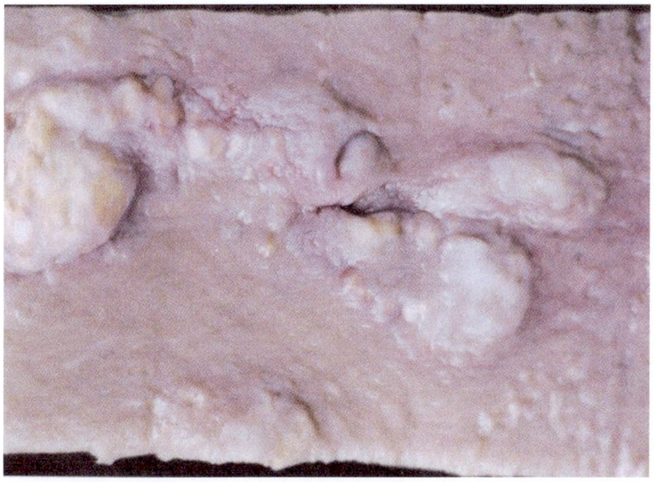

Fig. 1.103 Arterial wall calcification. Yellowish-white hard calcified nodules of variable sizes are observed on the wall of the aorta, protruding from the inner surface of the artery. (Chen Huaitao)

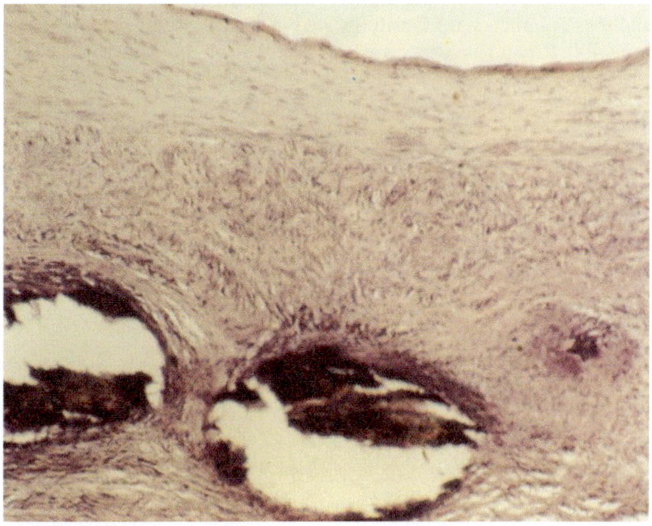

Fig. 1.104 Arterial wall calcification. There are two blue calcium-depositing foci in the mid-membrane of the arterial wall, some of which were dislodged at the time of section preparation. HE ×100. (Chen Huaitao)

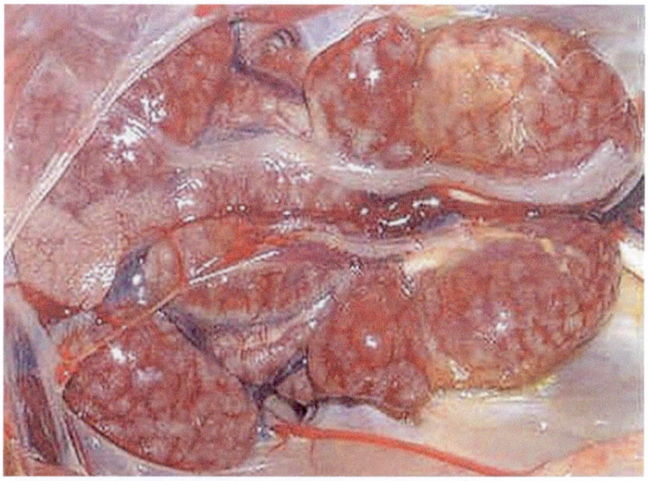

Fig. 1.105 Renal urate deposition. Gout in chickens. The uric acid deposits in kidneys, and the kidneys are enlarged with a pale color and a florid surface. (Yue hua)

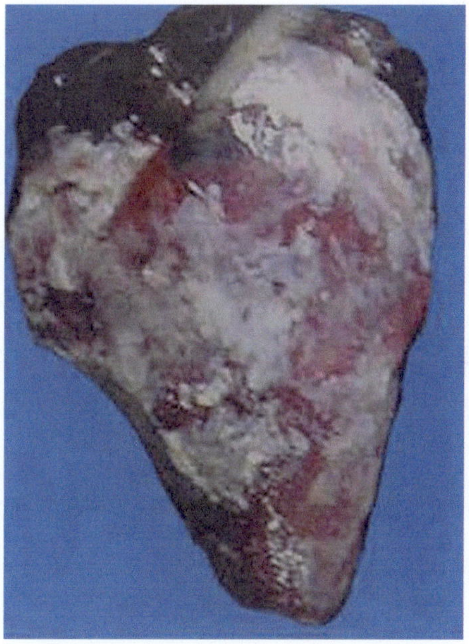

Fig. 1.106 Epicardial urate deposition. Gout in chickens. A white, dry, and lime-like deposit of urate is present on the epicardium. (Yue hua)

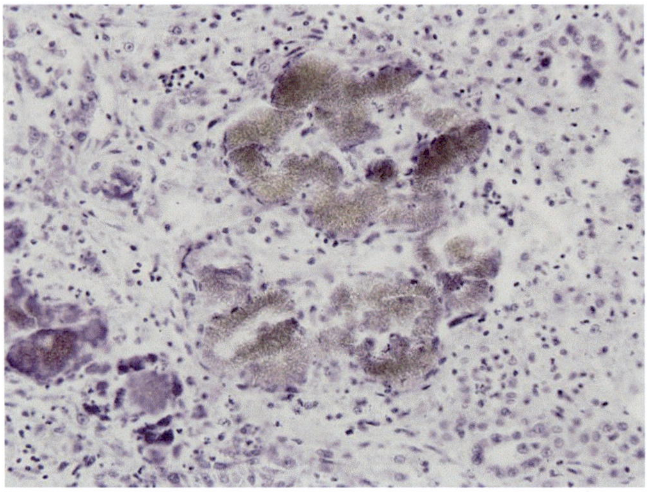

Fig. 1.107 Renal urate deposition. A large amount of pale greenish-yellow radiating urate crystals are present in the renal tubules of the chicken kidney. Uric acid stain ×400. (Chen Huaitao)

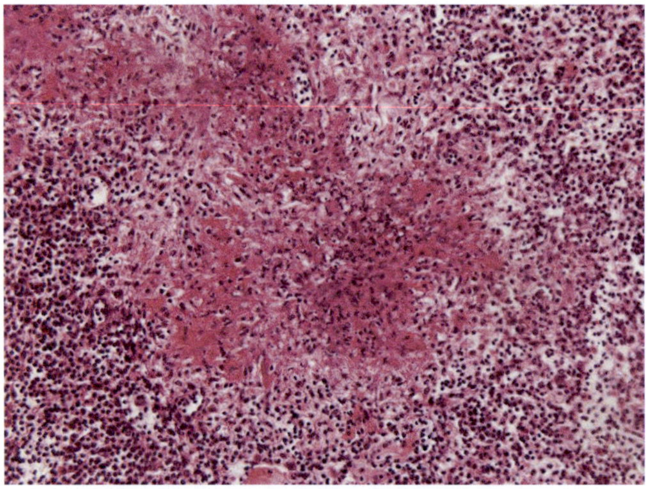

Fig. 1.108 Splenic urate deposition. Localized tissue necrosis in chicken spleen due to urate deposition, which is structureless red substance. HE ×400. (Chen Huaitao)

5.3 Pathological Pigmentation

Pathological pigmentation is an increase in pigmentation in tissues or pigmentation in tissues that were not pigmented previously, which are produced by the body or enter the body from outside via the respiratory and digestive tracts and the skin; the former is called endogenous pigmentation and the latter is exogenous pigmentation.

5.3.1 Endogenous Pigments (Figs. 1.109, 1.110, 1.111, 1.112, 1.113, 1.114, and 1.115)

It mainly includes melanin, hemosiderin, porphyrins, lipofuscin, and bilirubin.

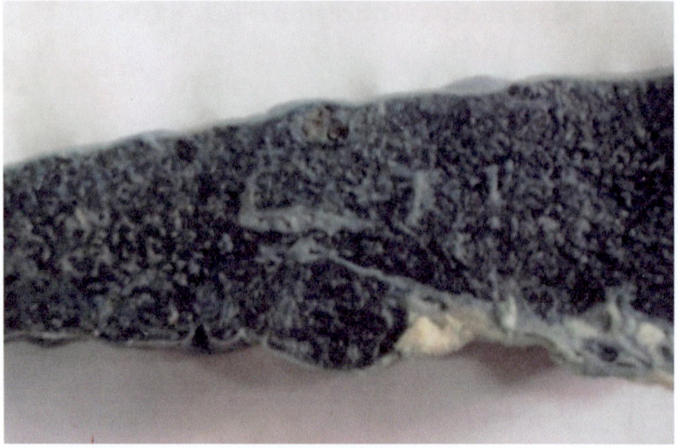

Fig. 1.109 Spleen hemosiderin deposition. Hemosiderin deposits in the spleen with a blue color after Prussian blue staining. (Chen Huaitao)

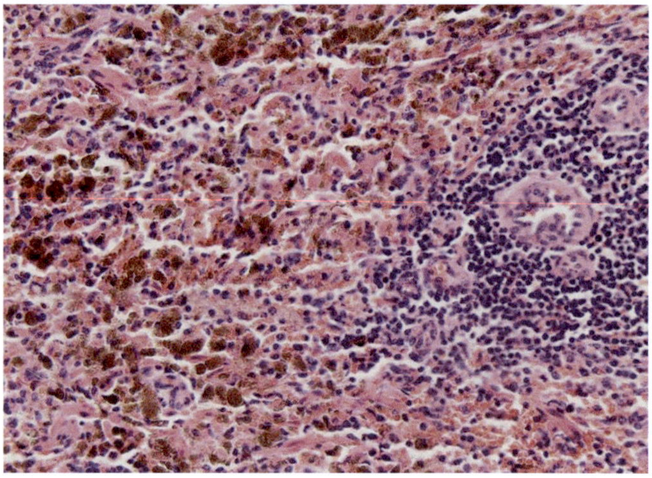

Fig. 1.110 Hemosiderin deposition. Many scattered golden yellow clumps or granules are present in spleen tissue, which is hemosiderin, and these pigments are mostly located in the plasma of macrophages. HE ×400. (Chen Huaitao)

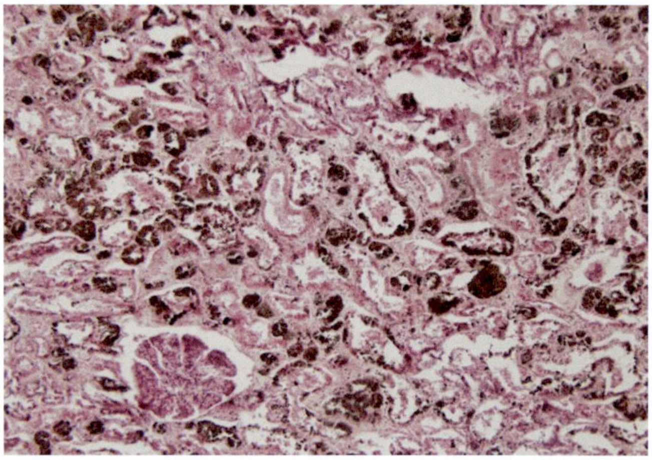

Fig. 1.111 Renal hemosiderin deposition. Yellow hemosiderin deposits in renal tubular epithelial cells. HE ×100. (Chen Huaitao)

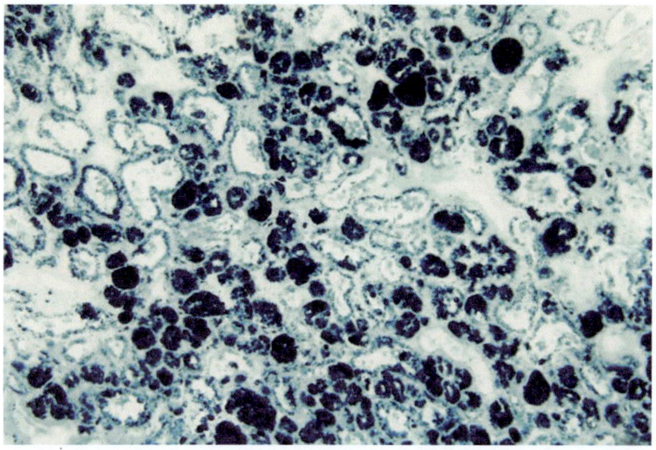

Fig. 1.112 Renal hemosiderin deposition. Hemosiderin in renal tubular epithelial cells is stained dark blue by Prussian blue. Prussian blue staining ×400. (Chen Huaitao)

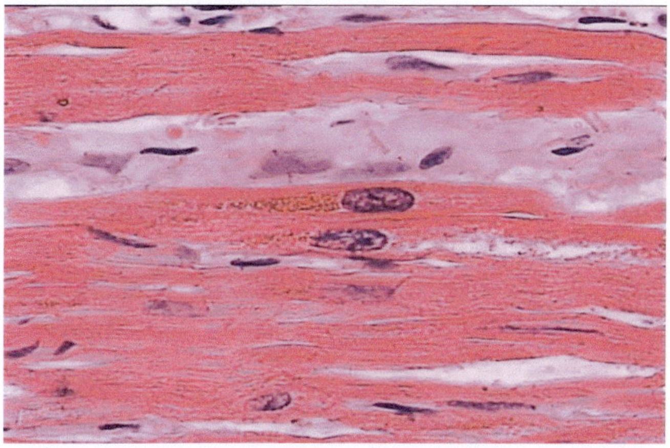

Fig. 1.113 Cardiac lipofuscin deposition. Myocardial lipofuscin is deposited, and lipofuscin granules are mostly deposited in the cytoplasm of muscle cells at both ends of the nucleus. HE ×400. (Kong Xiaoming)

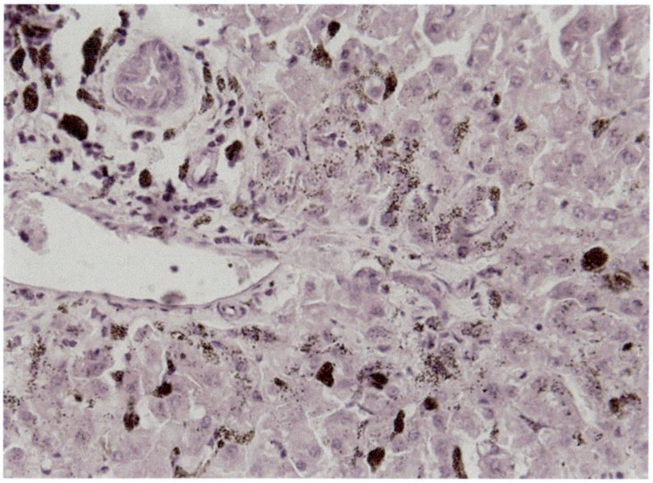

Fig. 1.114 Hepatic melanin deposition. Hepatic melanosis in sheep. A large amount of dark brown or black granules are present in the cells of the hepatic sinusoids and interstitium. HE ×400. (Chen Huaitao)

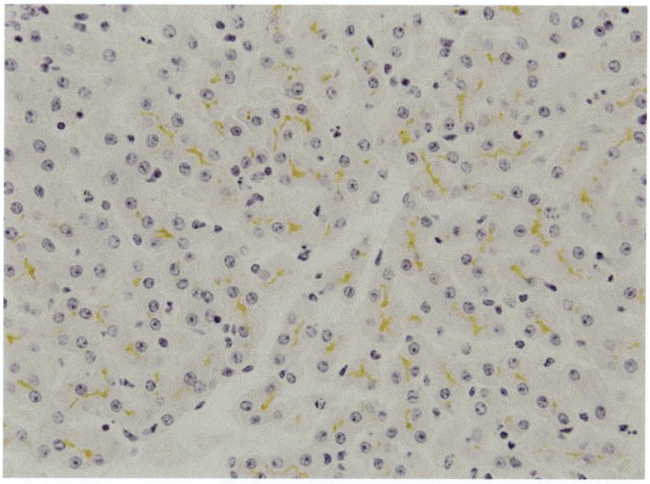

Fig. 1.115 Biliary pigmentation. Small strips of yellow material are present between the hepatocyte cords, which is the bile pigment accumulated in the capillary bile ducts. HE ×400. (Veterinary Pathology Laboratory, Gansu Agricultural University)

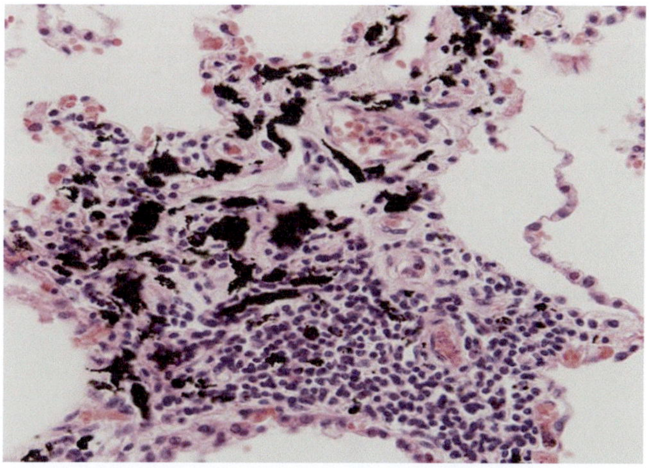

Fig. 1.116 Pulmonary charcoal particle sedimentation. Some black charcoal particles deposits in the peribronchial and other interstitial spaces of the lungs, with localized connective tissue hyperplasia, and lymphocytic infiltration. HE ×400. (Chen Huaitao)

5.3.2 Exogenous Pigments (Figs. 1.116, 1.117, and 1.118)

It mainly includes charcoal, silicon, iron, lead, and other inorganic and organic pigment substances.

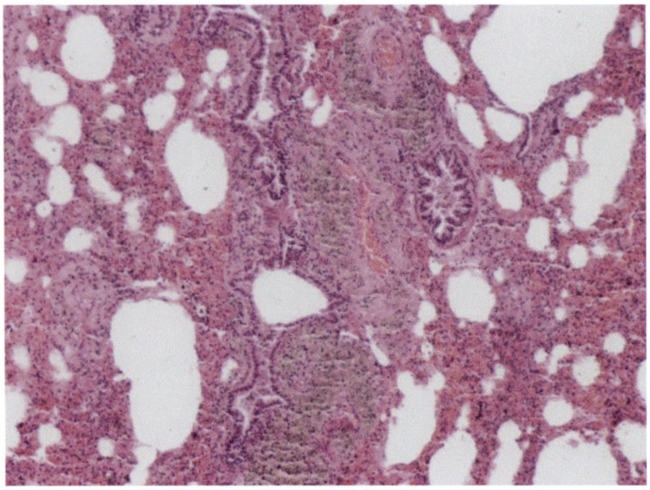

Fig. 1.117 Lung inorganic dust deposition. Equine lung (pneumoconiosis): brownish-yellow dust deposits in the interstitium around the fine bronchi, blood vessels and alveolar septa, which caused the thickening of the alveolar septa, connective tissue hyperplasia, and distortion of the fine bronchioles by compression. HE ×100. (Wang Wenhui)

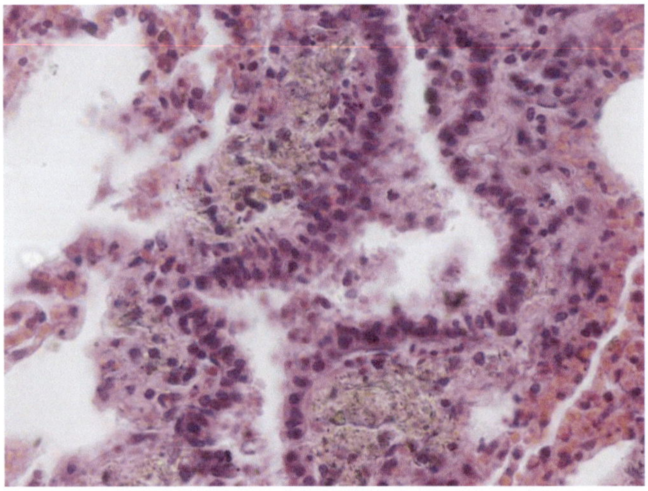

Fig. 1.118 Inorganic dust deposition. Equine lung (pneumoconiosis): The magnification of dust in Fig. 1.117, which is a brownish-yellow irregular crystalline substance, deposited mainly around the fine bronchi. HE ×400. (Wang Wenhui)

5.4 Concretion, Calculus (Figs. 1.119, 1.120, and 1.121)

There are various types of calculi, common ones include gallstones, intestinal stones, urinary stones, and salivary stones.

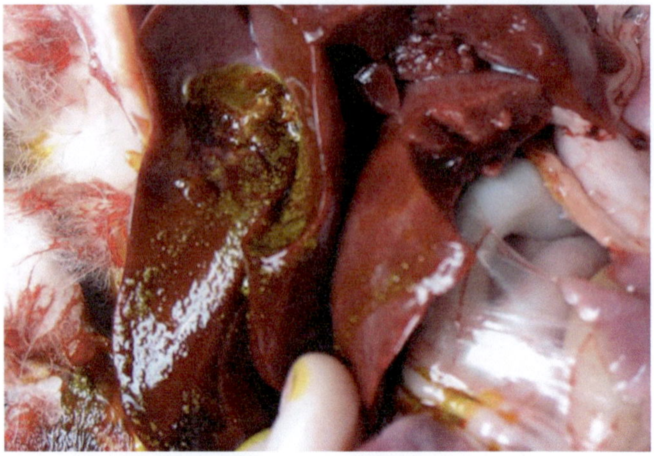

Fig. 1.119 Gallstones. Tiny yellow stones with a hard texture are present in the gallbladder of a sick dog. (Chen Huaitao)

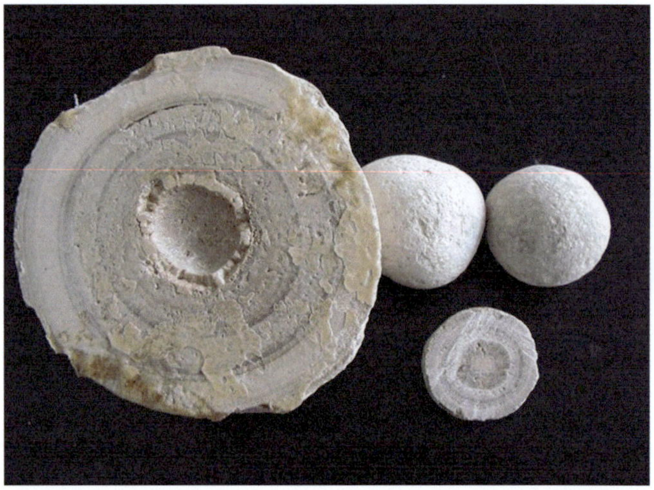

Fig. 1.120 Intestinal calculi. Intestinal calculi in horses. The calculi are hard with a smooth surface, and the cut surface is concentric laminae. (Wang Xinhua)

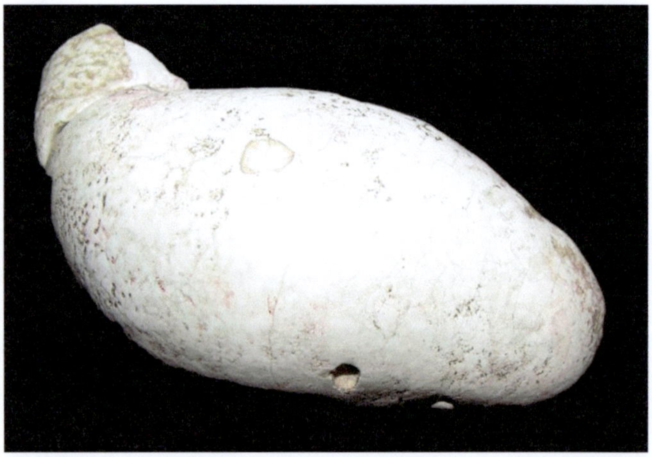

Fig. 1.121 Salivary stones. The illustration shows a large mango-like white salivary stone measuring 10.0 cm × 4.3 cm. This stone was removed from the salivary gland duct of a donkey. (Veterinary Pathology Unit, Gansu Agricultural University)

Bibliography

1. Huaitao C, Deming Z, editors. Veterinary pathology. Beijing: China Agricultural Press; 2013.
2. Cheville NF. Cell pathology. 2nd ed. Ames: Iowa State University Press; 1983.
3. Jones TC, Hunt RD, King NW. Veterinary pathology. 6th ed. Philadelphia: Lippincott Williams; 1997.
4. Mouwen JMVM, de Groot ECBM. A colour atlas of veterinary pathology. Utrecht: Wolfe Medical Publications Ltd; 1982.

2 Localized Disturbances of Blood Circulation

1 Hyperemia

1.1 Arterial Hyperemia (Figs. 2.1 and 2.2)

1.2 Venous Hyperemia (Figs. 2.3, 2.4, 2.5, 2.6, 2.7, 2.8, 2.9, 2.10, 2.11, 2.12, and 2.13)

Venous hyperemia is referred to as congestion.

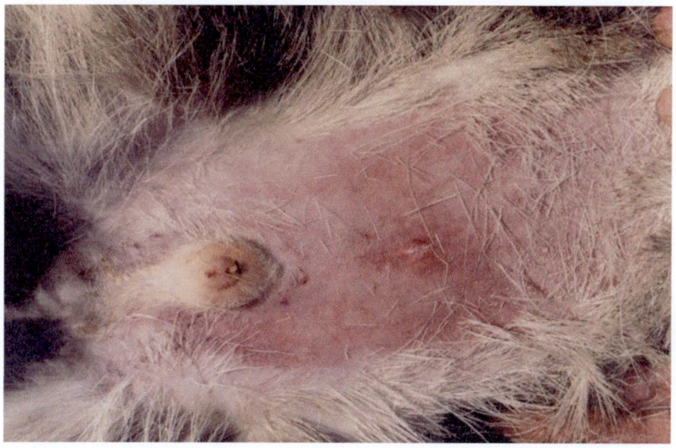

Fig. 2.1 Skin hyperemia. Abdominal skin hyperemia and flushing due to urethral calculi in male musk deer with subcutaneous edema. (Chen Huaitao)

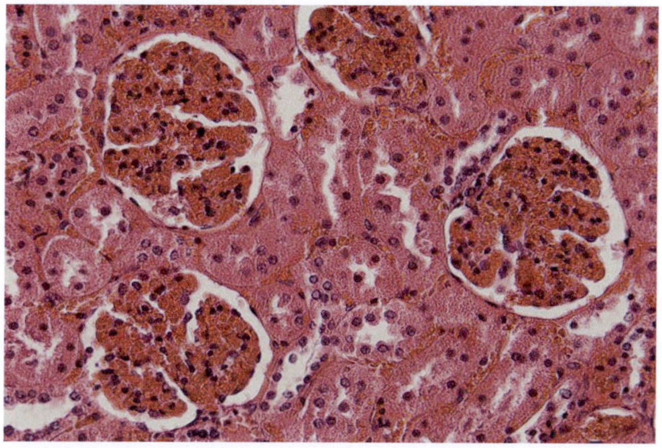

Fig. 2.2 Hyperemia. Small glomerular arteries and glomerular capillaries are dilated and the glomerulus is slightly enlarged. HE ×400. (Chen Huaitao)

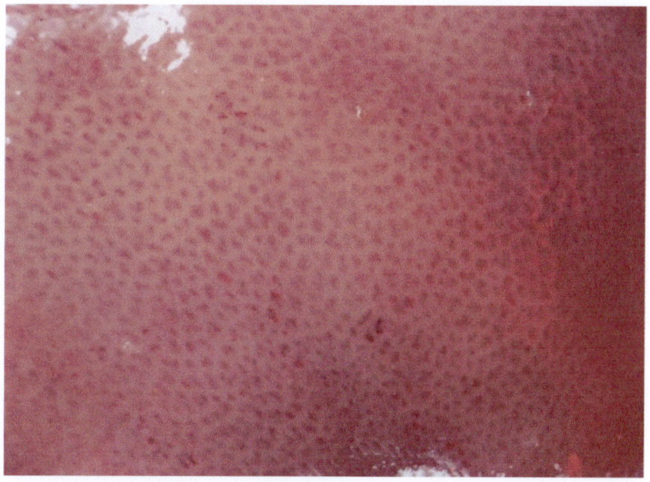

Fig. 2.3 Congestion. Pig liver is congested and degenerated, with a red and yellow pattern on the surface, similar to the sight of a cut surface of betel nut. (Chen Huaitao)

H. Chen, *Color Atlas of Veterinary Pathology*, https://doi.org/10.1007/978-981-96-7617-0_2

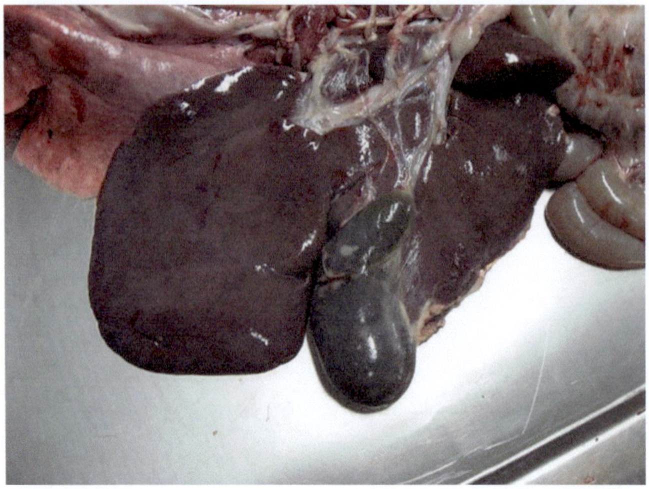

Fig. 2.4 Congestion. The liver of the affected goat was congested, enlarged, and dark grayish red, with distended gallbladder. (Wang Wenhui)

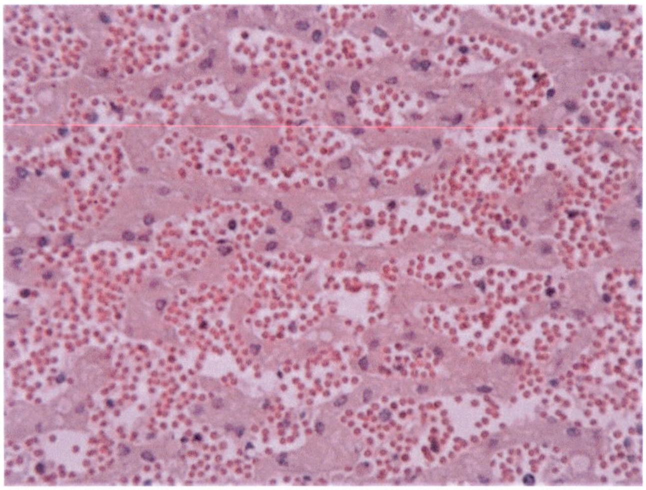

Fig. 2.5 Congestion. Liver. Liver sinuses are dilated, filled with red blood cells and other blood cells. Some hepatocytes are atrophied. HE ×200. (Liu Sidang)

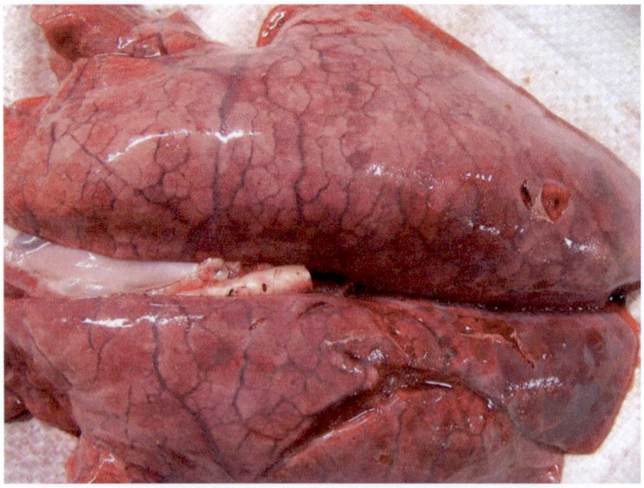

Fig. 2.6 Congestion. Porcine streptococcal disease. The lungs are congested and enlarged, with dark red color and widened interstitium. (Liu Andian)

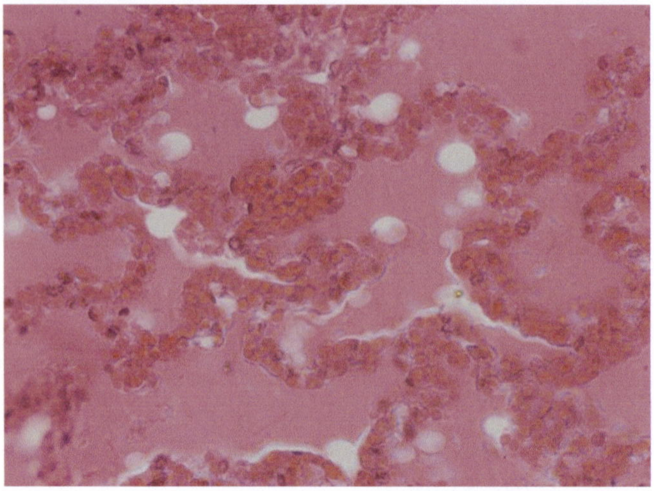

Fig. 2.7 Congestion. Alveolar septum capillaries are dilated and filled with red blood cells. A large amount of serum is present in alveolar cavity. HE ×400. (Wang Wenhui)

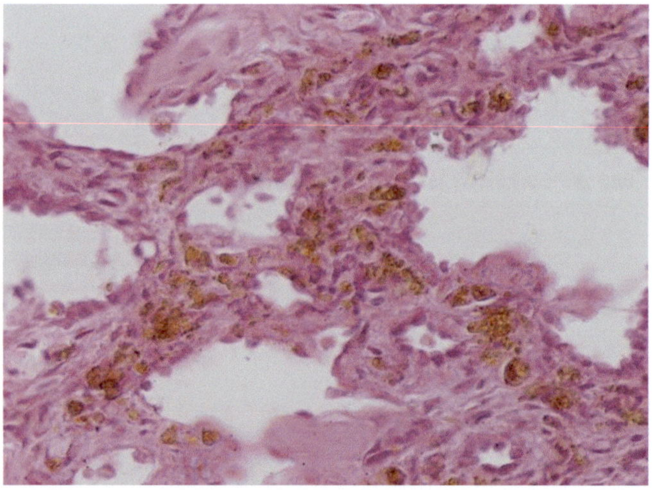

Fig. 2.8 Chronic pulmonary congestion. The alveolar septa are congested and hemorrhagic with the deposition of hemosiderin. The connective tissue is hyperplastic, and the alveolar septum is widened. HE ×400. (Chen Huaitao)

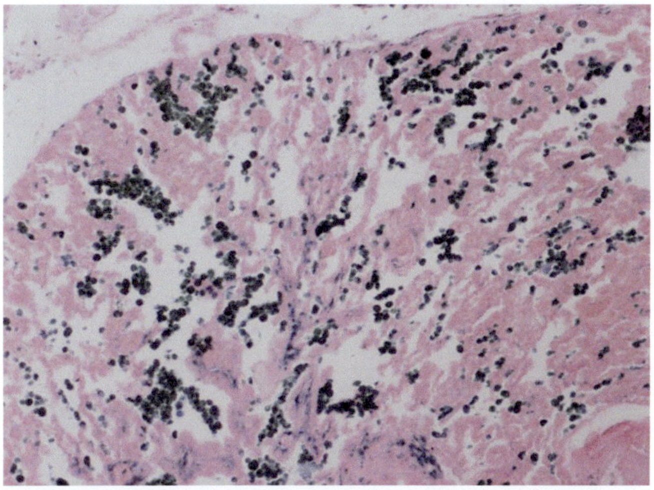

Fig. 2.9 Chronic pulmonary congestion. The alveolar septum is congested, the alveolar cavity is small, and many heart failure cells with hemosiderin inside are present. Prussian blue stain ×200. (Chen Huaitao)

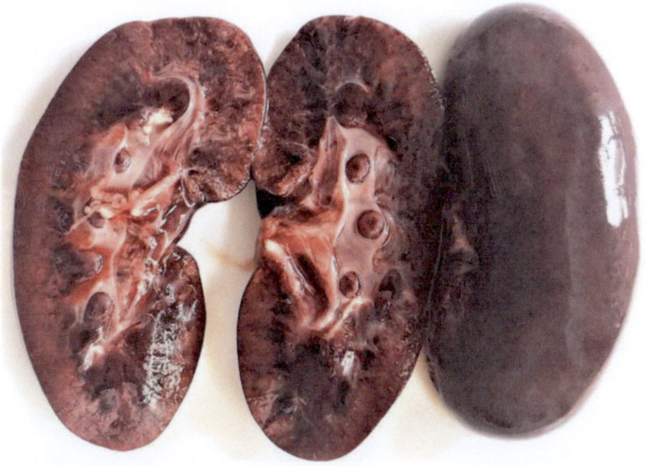

Fig. 2.10 Congestion. The kidney is congested and enlarged, with a dark purple color and a large amount of dark red blood flowing from the cut surface. (Liu Sidang)

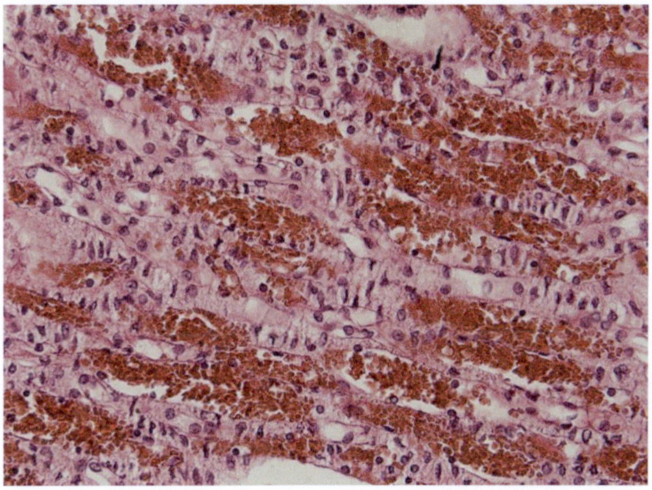

Fig. 2.11 Congestion. Small renal interstitial veins and capillaries are markedly dilated and filled with red blood cells. HE ×400. (Chen Huaitao)

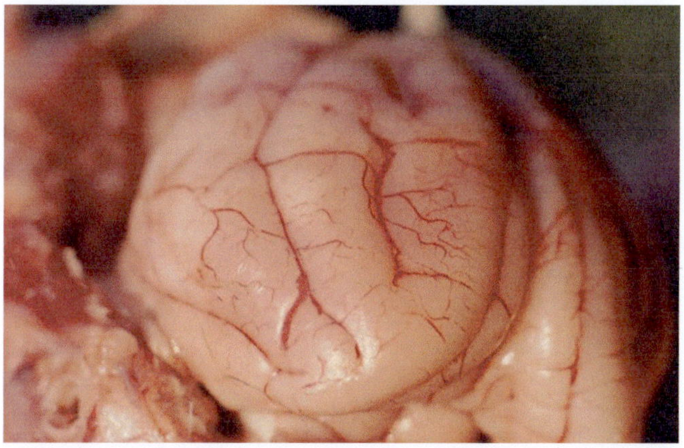

Fig. 2.12 Congestion. The soft meningeal vessels of the musk deer brain are engorged and congested with a presence of few hemorrhagic spots. (Chen Huaitao)

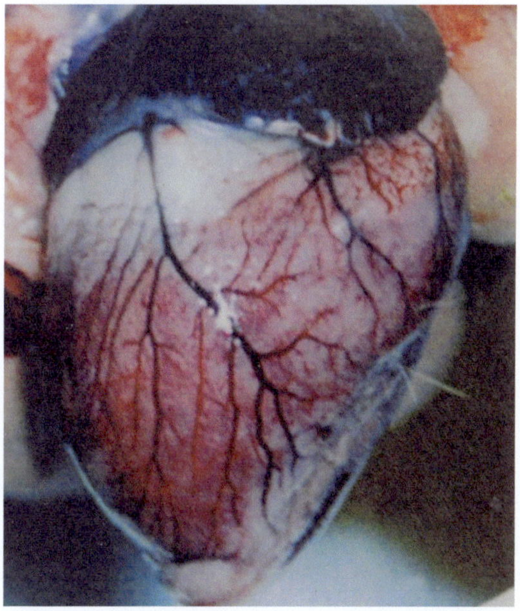

Fig. 2.13 Congestion. The epicardial veins of the sick rabbit are congested and engorged with dendritic appearance. (Ren Keliang)

2 Hemorrhage

2.1 Rupture Bleeding (Figs. 2.14, 2.15, 2.16, 2.17, 2.18, 2.19, 2.20, 2.21, and 2.22)

2.2 Exudative Hemorrhage (Fig. 2.15)

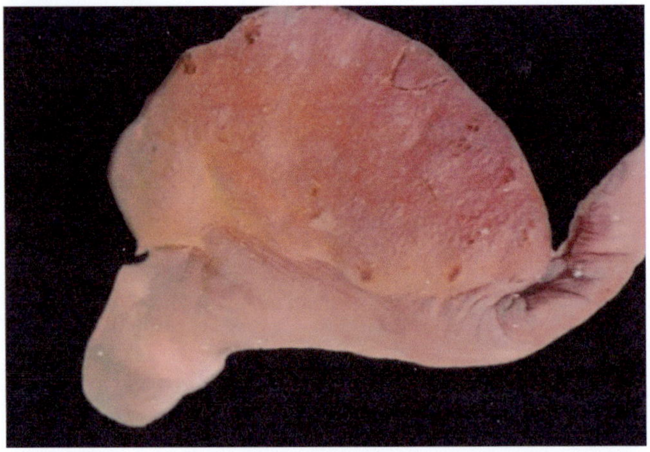

Fig. 2.14 Hematoma. Splenic hematoma. A large amount of blood accumulates under the capsule of the spleen, which appears as a mass-like elevation in dark red color. (Wang Wenhui)

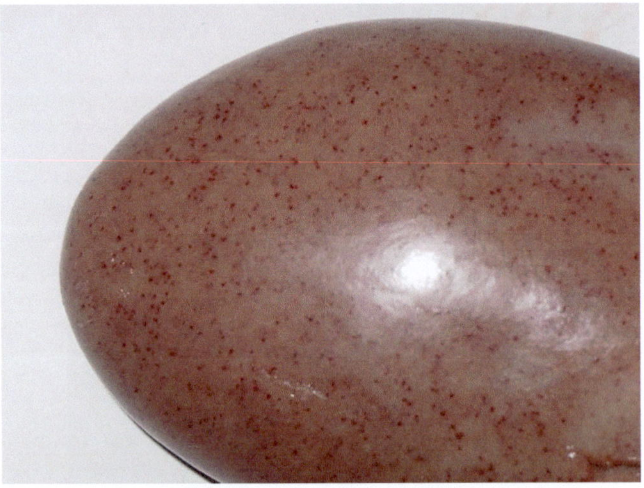

Fig. 2.15 Petechiae. A large amount of punctate hemorrhagic spots are present on the surface of the kidney of the affected pig; the kidney is enlarged and grayish-yellow in color. (Gu Changqin)

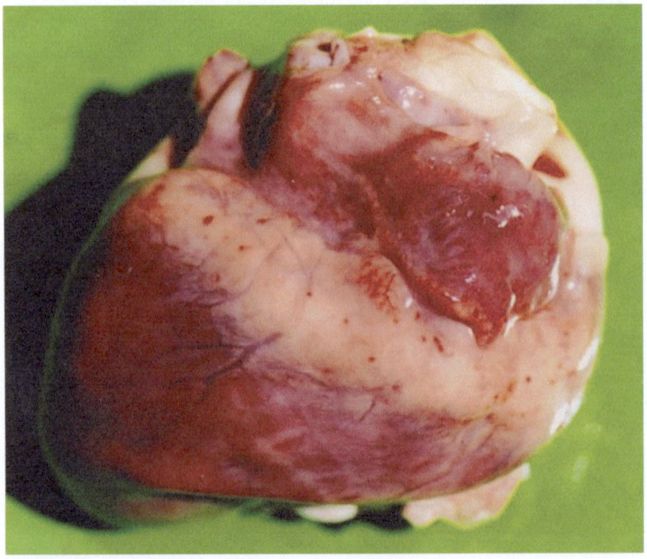

Fig. 2.16 Petechiae. Scattered punctate hemorrhages (bruises) are present in the coronary fat of the affected pig. (Yao Jinshui)

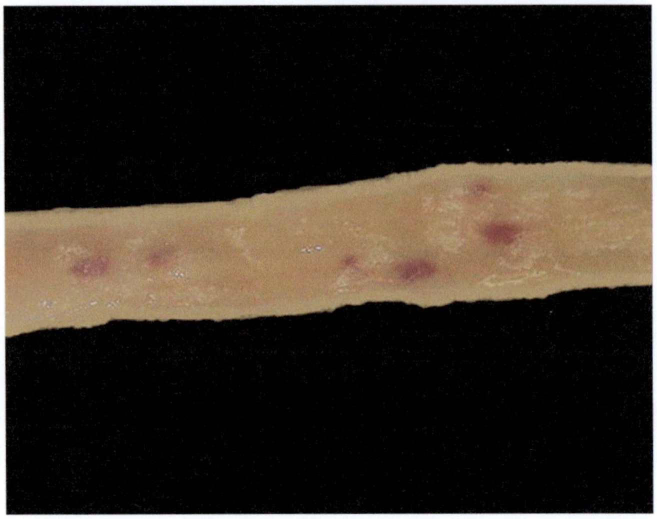

Fig. 2.17 Ecchymosis. Mottled hemorrhage (bruising) of the duodenal mucosa in chicks. (Wang Wenhui)

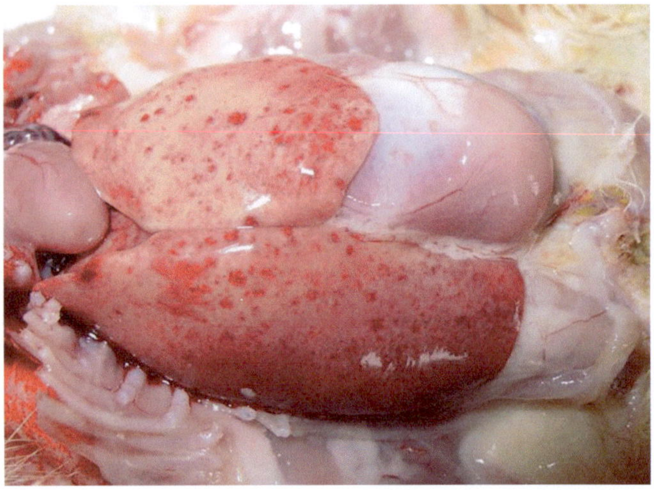

Fig. 2.18 Petechiae and ecchymosis. Viral hepatitis in ducks. A large number of hemorrhagic spots are present on the liver surface. (Hu Xueying)

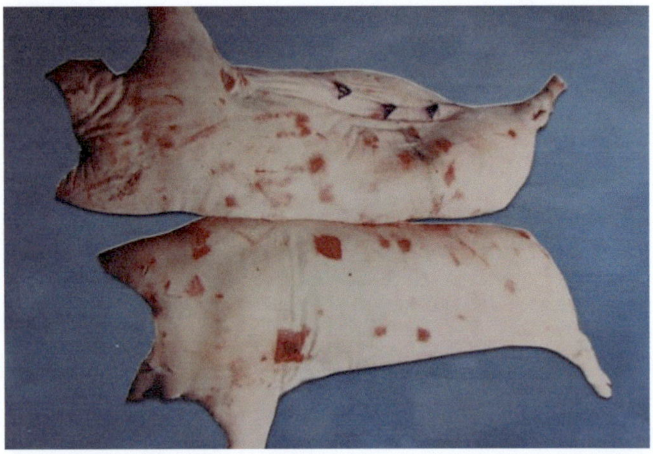

Fig. 2.19 Ecchymosis. Subacute swine erysipelas. Square and diamond-shaped hemorrhagic spots (bruises) are present on the dorsal and ventral skin of the sick pigs. (Zhou Shiqi)

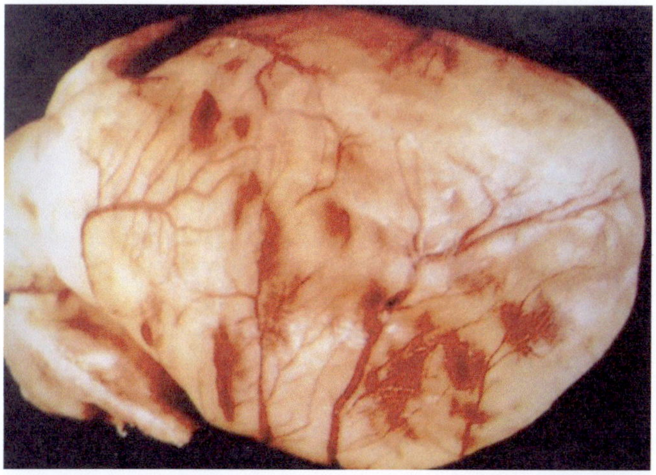

Fig. 2.20 Ecchymosis. Viral hemorrhagic disease in rabbits. Hemorrhagic spots (bruises) of the epicardium. (Feng Zeguang)

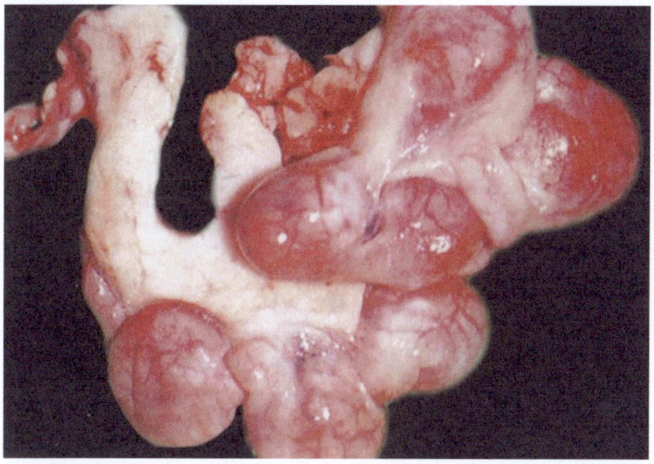

Fig. 2.21 Hemorrhagic infiltrationSalmonellosis in rabbits. The uterine serosa was markedly congested, edematous, and hemorrhagic, with large areas of hemorrhagic infiltration. (Wang Yongkun)

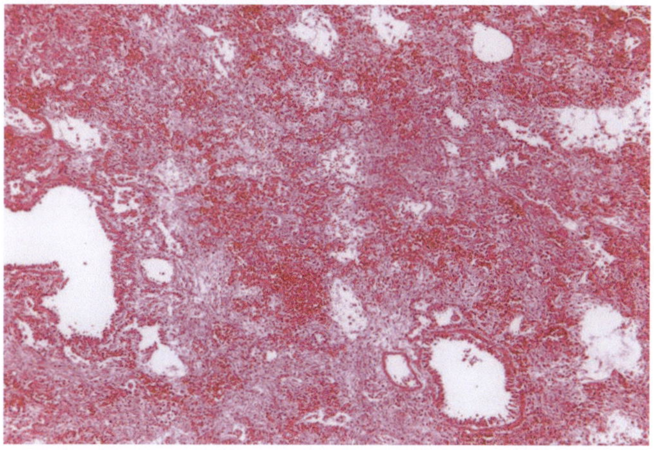

Fig. 2.22 Hemorrhage. Bovine moldy sweet potato poisoning. Alveolar septal capillaries are severely congested and hemorrhagic, and the alveolar cavity is mostly filled with red blood cells and serum with only a few alveoli being observed. HE ×100. (Yang Mingqi)

3 Thrombus

3.1 White Thrombus (Fig. 2.23)

3.2 Mixed Thrombus (Figs. 2.24 and 2.25)

3.3 Hyaline Thrombus (Fig. 2.26)

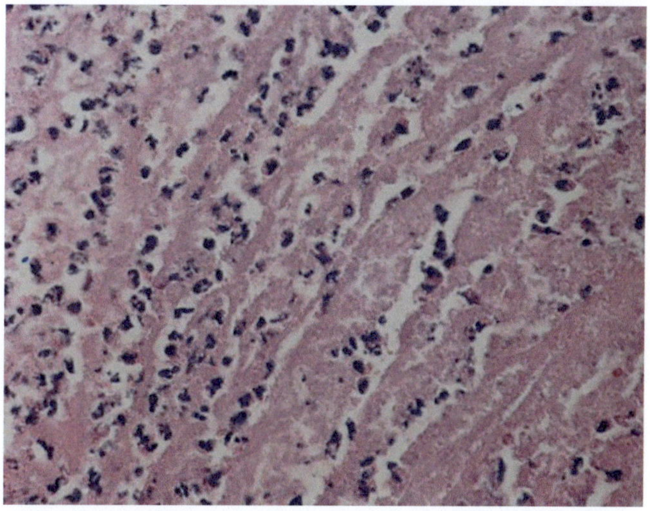

Fig. 2.23 White thrombus. Chronic swine erysipelas. White thrombus is present on the cardiac mitral valve, composed of platelets and neutrophils in a lamellar structure. HE ×400. (Liu Baoyan)

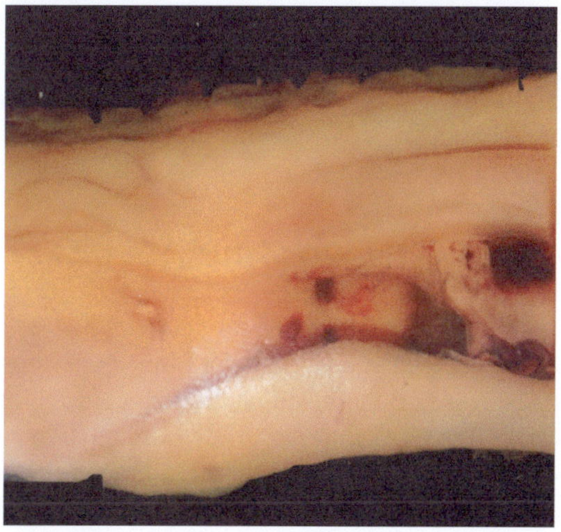

Fig. 2.24 Mixed thrombus. Mixed thrombus in the jugular vein of a horse. The thrombus is unevenly colored in red and white, with a rough surface. (Veterinary Pathology Unit, Gansu Agricultural University)

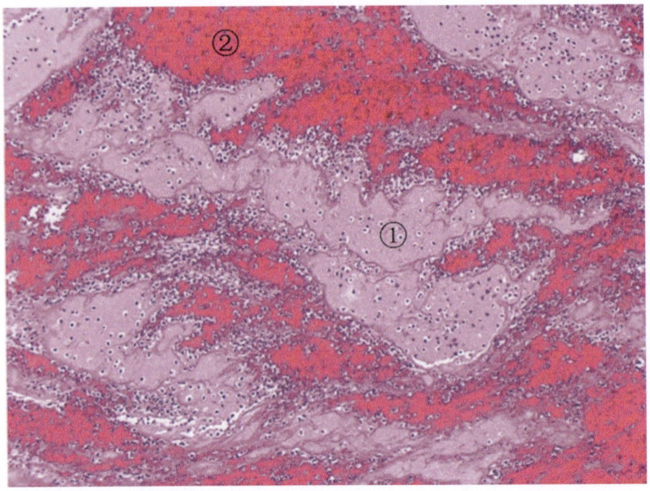

Fig. 2.25 Mixed thrombus. Histology of the mixed thrombus: the white thrombus (composed of platelets and leukocytes) is light-stained① and the red thrombus (composed of fibrin and red blood cells) is dark-stained②. HE ×200. (Pathological Anatomy Unit, Northeast Agricultural University)

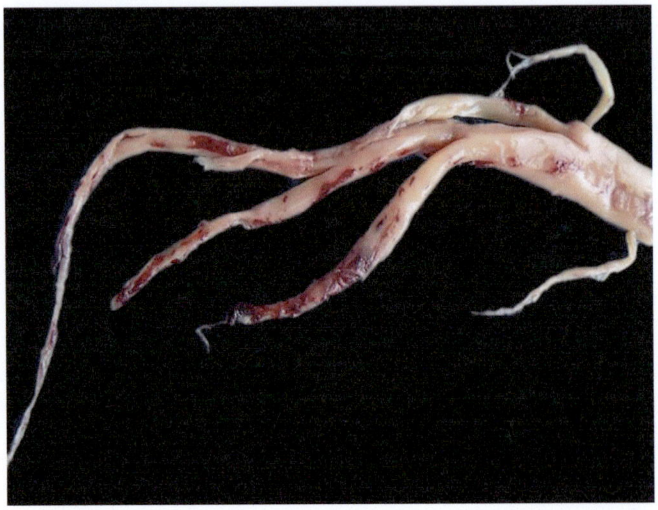

Fig. 2.27 Chicken fat-like clotting. A chicken fat-like clot removed from a large blood vessel, which is elastic, mainly yellowish and locally red (embolus). (Chen Huaitao)

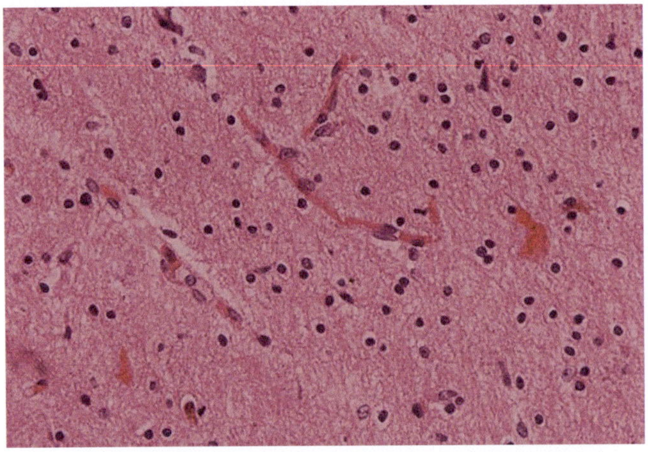

Fig. 2.26 Hyaline thrombus. The brain tissue is congested and there is microthrombosis in small blood vessels. HE ×400. (Chen Huaitao)

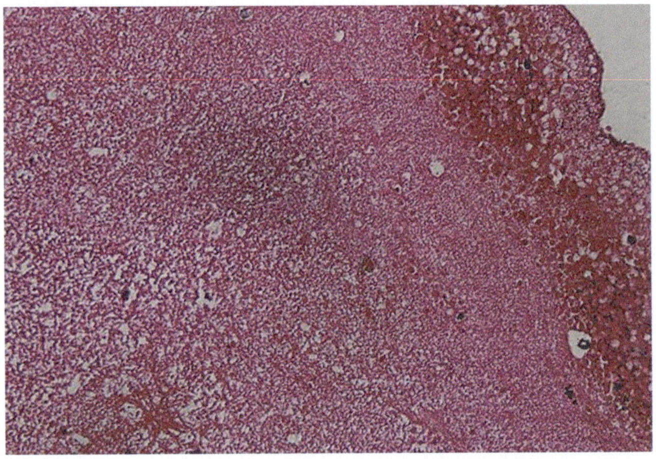

Fig. 2.28 Chicken fat-like clotting. Canine distemper. Chicken lipid-like clot consisting mainly of fibrin with a uniform structure and only a few red blood cells at the edges. HE ×100. (Chen Huaitao)

3.4 Chicken Fat-Like Clotting (Figs. 2.27 and 2.28)

Chicken fat-like clot is a kind of clot formed after the death of animals. Because the blood clotting process is slow, the red blood cells sink, and the clot is divided into two parts of yellowish and red, which resembles the fat of the chicken, so it is called chicken fat-like clot, which often appears in the heart and large blood vessels. Clinically it should be differentiated from thrombosis (Figs. 2.27 and 2.28).

4 Embolism (Figs. 2.29, 2.30, and 2.31)

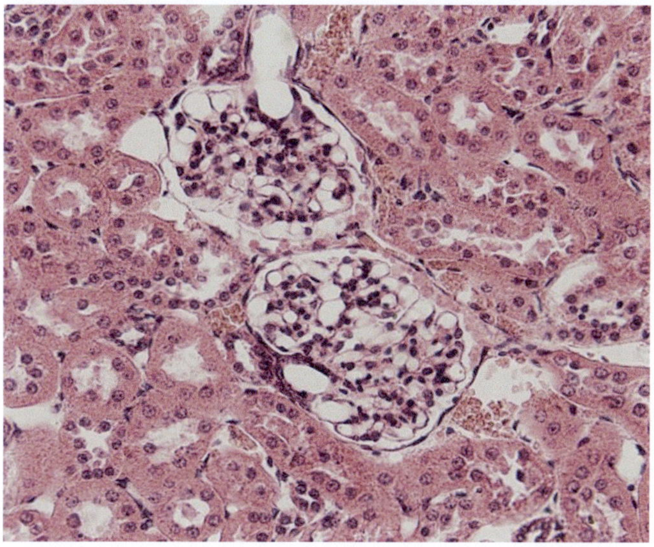

Fig. 2.29 Fatty embolism. Fatty embolism in rabbit kidney: the glomerular vessels are filled with plenty of vacuolated fat emboli. HE ×400. (Chen Huaitao)

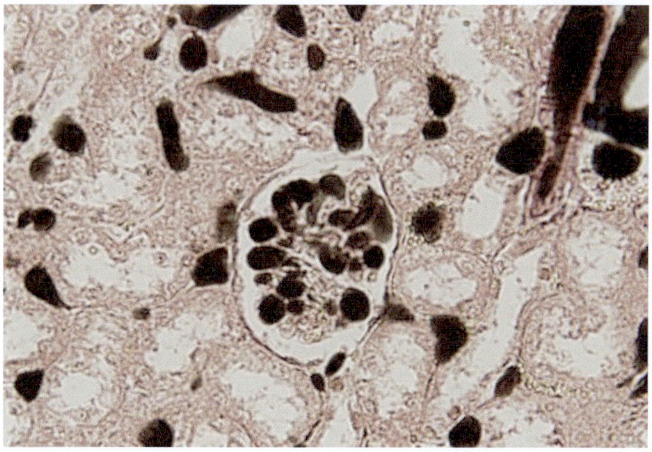

Fig. 2.30 Fatty embolism. Fatty embolism in rabbit kidney: the glomerular vessels and interstitial capillaries are occluded by a large number of blackish fat droplets. Osmium staining ×400. (Chen Huaitao)

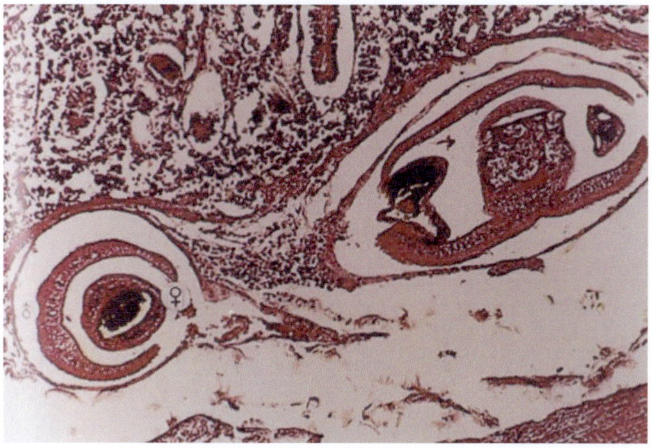

Fig. 2.31 Parasitic embolism. Orientobilharziasis in bovine. Embolism caused by orientobiharziasis is present in two vessels of the intestinal wall. HE ×100. (Liu Baoyan)

5 Infarct

5.1 Anemic Infarction (Figs. 2.32 and 2.33)

5.2 Hemorrhagic Infarction (Figs. 2.34 and 2.35)

6 Edema (Figs. 2.36, 2.37, 2.38, 2.39, 2.40, 2.41, and 2.42)

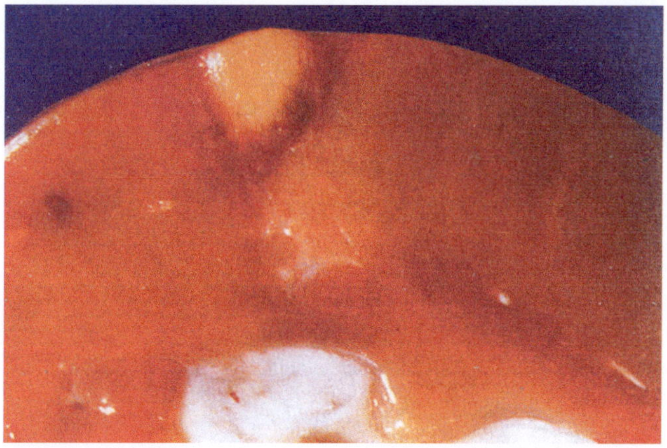

Fig. 2.32 Renal anemic infarction. The area of renal anemic infarction is often grayish-yellow in color, with a congested, hemorrhagic band visible around it. (Zhang Xujing)

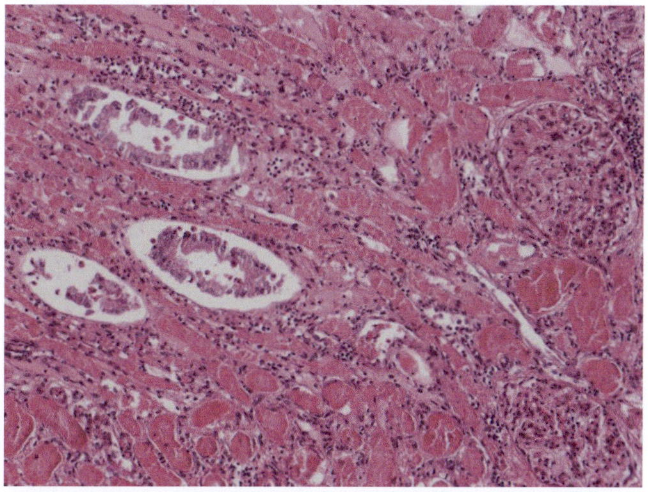

Fig. 2.33 Anemic infarction. Renal anemic infarction: tubules and glomeruli in the infarcted area were mostly necrotic and deeply eosin-stained; renal tubules were homogeneously coagulated, with indistinct lumen and disappearance of epithelial cell nuclei; some tubular epithelium was detached from the basement membrane; interstitial cells were mostly viable. HE ×100. (Wang Wenhui)

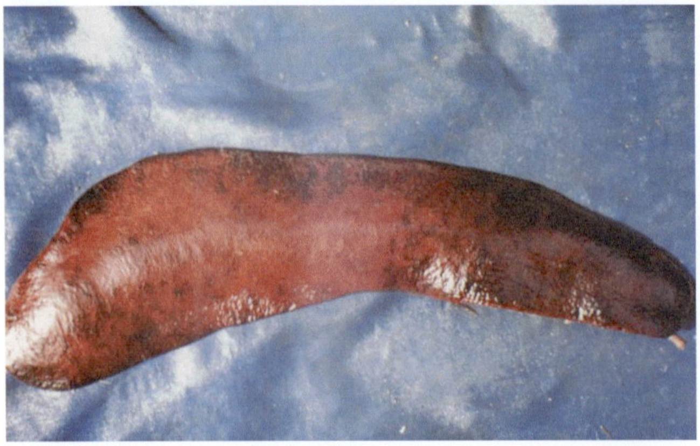

Fig. 2.34 Hemorrhagic infarction. Swine fever. The hemorrhagic infarction area is mainly located at the edge of the spleen in dark red color and often protruding from the surface of the spleen with relatively clear boundary from the surrounding tissue. (Chen Huaitao)

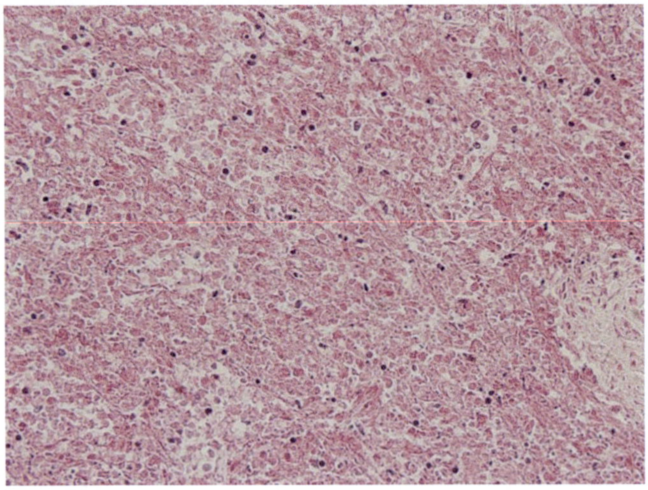

Fig. 2.35 Hemorrhagic infarction. Splenic hemorrhagic infarction: necrosis and disintegration of the lymphoid tissue with indistinct structure, but a large number of erythrocytes are densely present in the tissue. HE ×400. (Chen Huaitao)

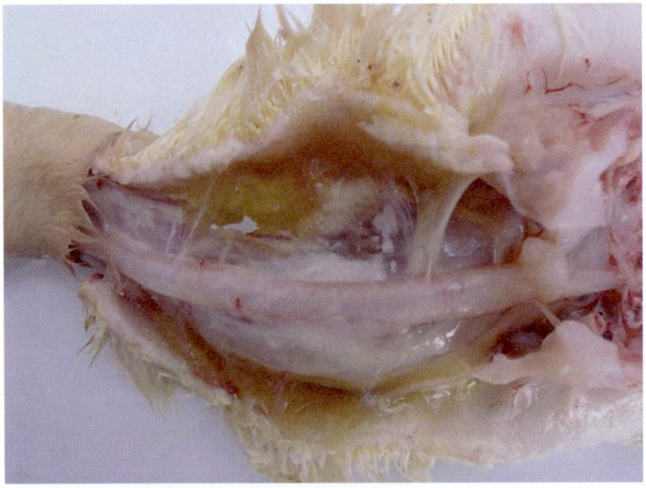

Fig. 2.36 Subcutaneous edema. Duck plague. Edema is present in the subcutaneous tissue of the sick duck with a yellow jelly-like appearance. (Hu Xueying)

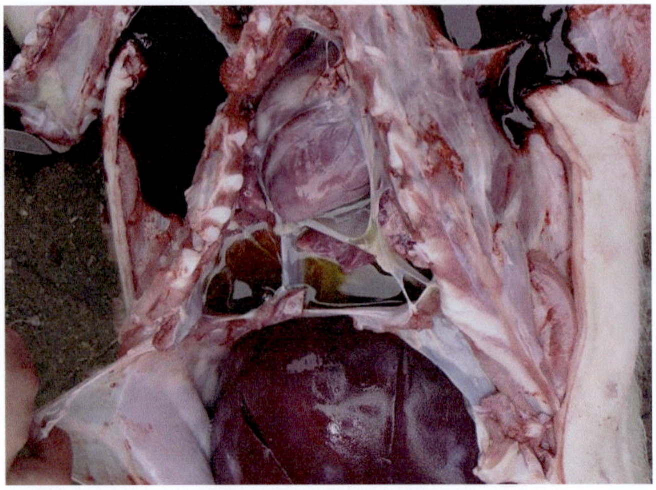

Fig. 2.37 Edema. Hemophilus parvum infection in pigs. A large amount of clear, yellowish fluid accumulates in the thoracic cavity (pleural effusion). (Wu Bin)

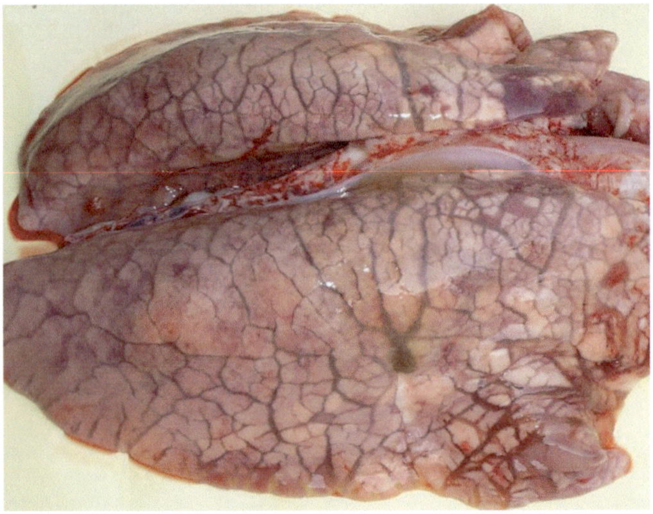

Fig. 2.38 Pulmonary edema. The size and weight of the affected porcine lungs are increased with a solider texture and markedly widened interstitium as well as a translucent jelly-like appearance. (Wu Bin)

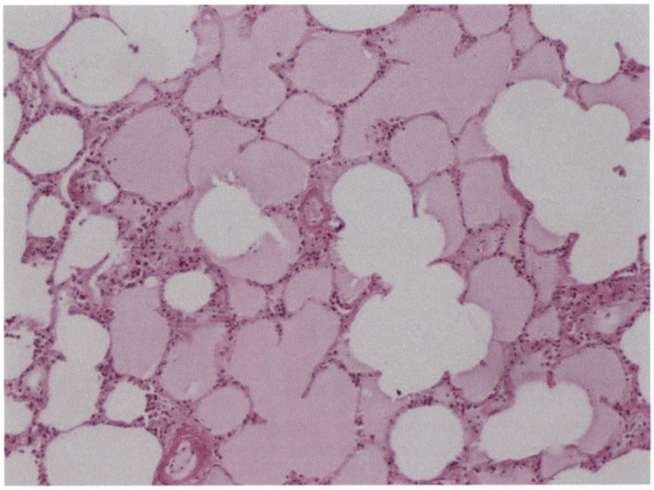

Fig. 2.39 Edema. Pulmonary edema: Most of the alveoli are dilated and filled with pale red serum; emphysema is present in a few alveoli. HE ×100. (Wang Wenhui)

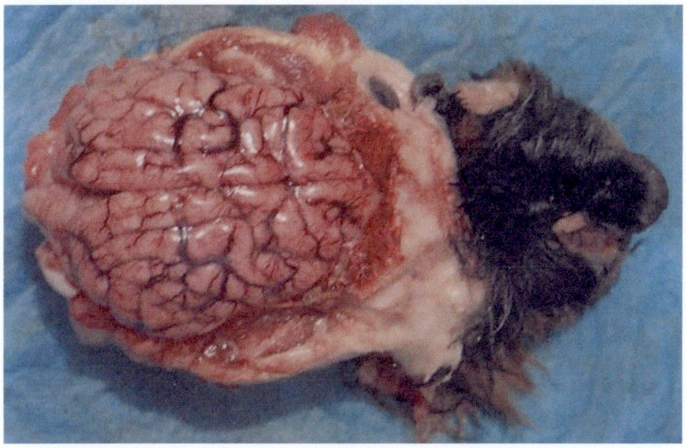

Fig. 2.40 Cerebral edema. Canine distemper. The meninges is congested, the cerebral mass is swollen, the cerebral sulcus is shallowed, and the surface of the cerebral gyrus is moist. (Chen Huaitao)

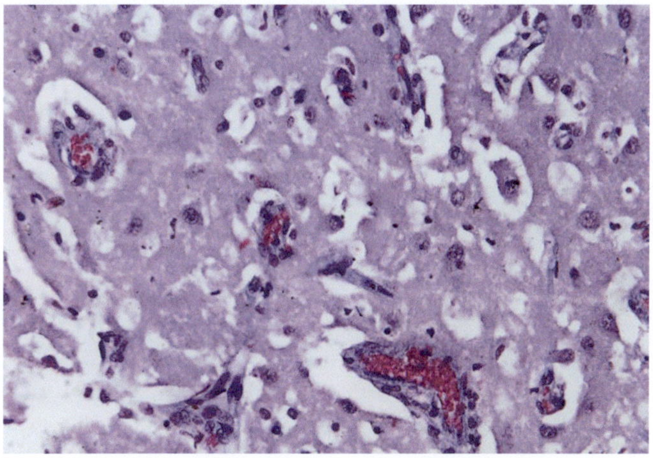

Fig. 2.41 Cerebral edema. Canine distemper. The cerebral vessels are congested, and the perivascular and pericellular gaps are widened with edema. HE ×400. (Chen Huaitao)

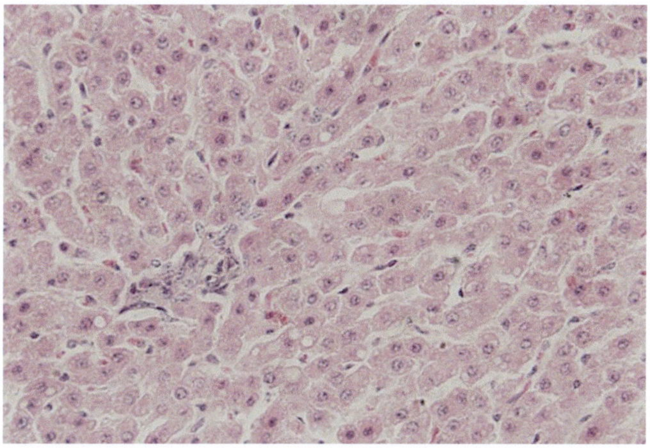

Fig. 2.42 Hepatic edema. The Dietrich's gap is significantly widened and the hepatic sinusoids are mildly congested. In addition, hepatocellular steatosis can also be observed. HE ×400. (Chen Huaitao)

Bibliography

1. Xuanren Z, editor. Pathological anatomy of domestic animals. Beijing: China Agricultural Press; 1988.
2. Kunxi Z, editor. Pathological anatomy of domestic animals (Second Edition). China Agricultural Press; 2000.

3 Adaptation and Repair of Tissues

1 Adaptation

1.1 Atrophy (Figs. 3.1, 3.2, 3.3, 3.4, 3.5, 3.6, and 3.7)

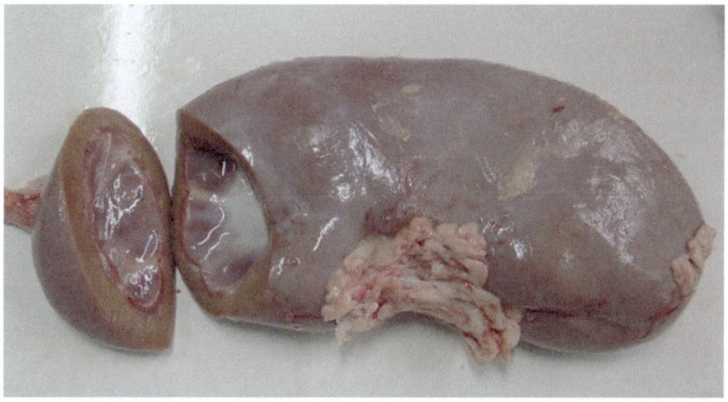

Fig. 3.1 Renal atrophy. The renal cortex is atrophic, thinning, and in earthy yellow color; the renal pelvis is dilated and filled with a yellowish mucus-like substance. (Hu Xueying)

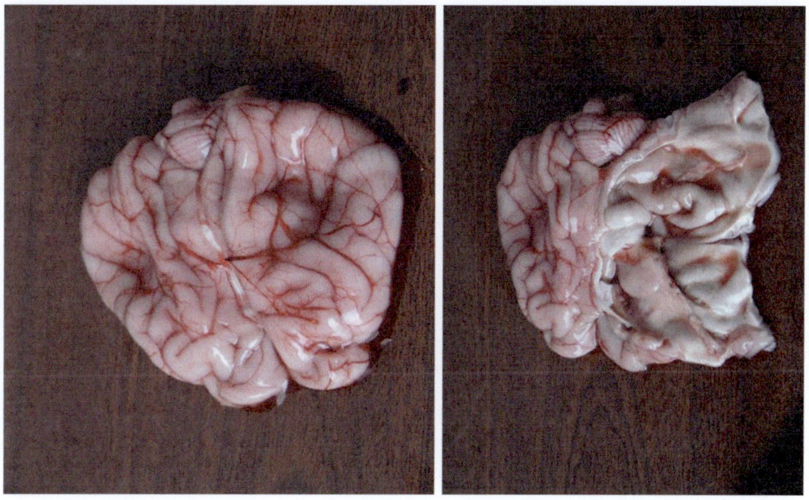

Fig. 3.2 Brain atrophy. Atrophy of the canine brain. There is a depression on the brain surface, the ventricular wall is markedly thinned, and pale red fluid accumulates in the ventricles. (Wang Xinhua)

H. Chen, *Color Atlas of Veterinary Pathology*, https://doi.org/10.1007/978-981-96-7617-0_3

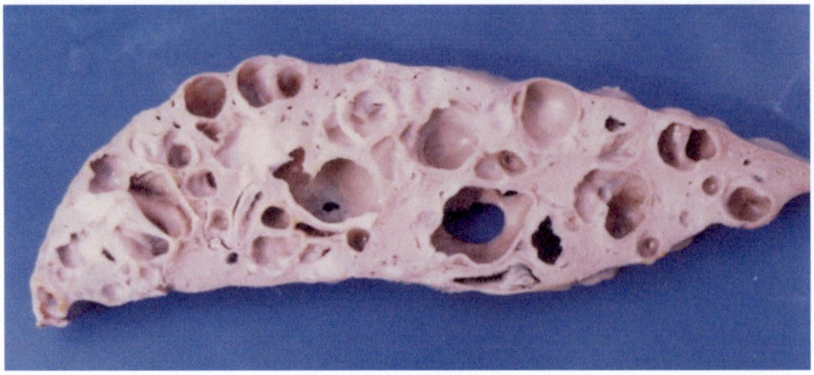

Fig. 3.3 Hepatic atrophy. A large number of echinococcal vesicles are present on the section surface of the affected ovine liver, and the liver parenchyma is obviously atrophied with a hardened texture. (Chen Huaitao)

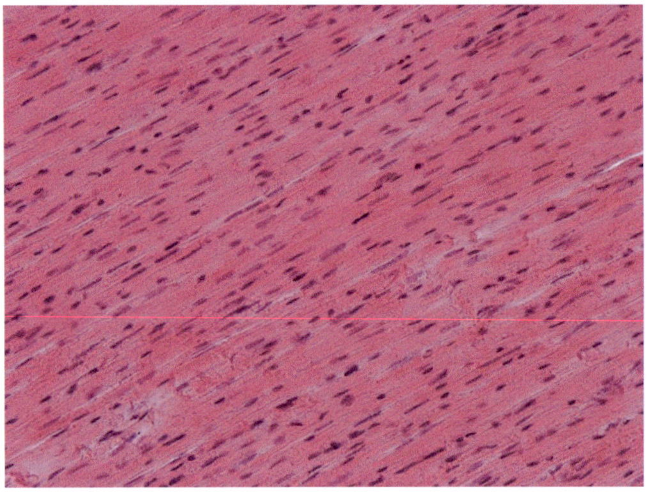

Fig. 3.4 Myocardial atrophy. Myocardial fiber atrophy: myocardial fibers are thinned and densely arranged with elongated, darkly stained nuclei. HE ×100. (Chen Huaitao)

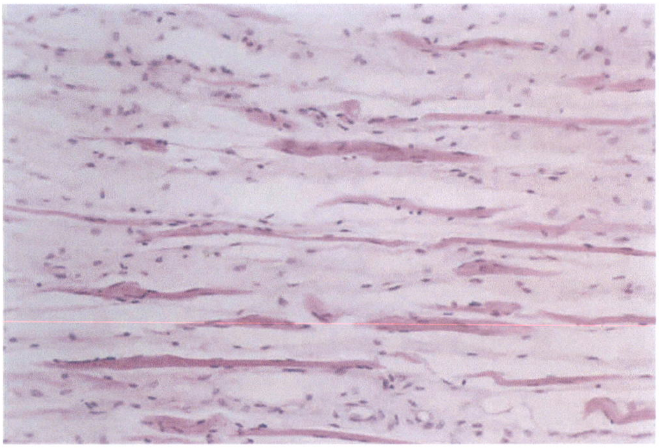

Fig. 3.6 Skeletal muscle atrophy. The muscle fibers are reduced, sparse with uneven thickness. The connective tissue between muscle fibers is hyperplastic. HE ×200. (Cui Hengmin)

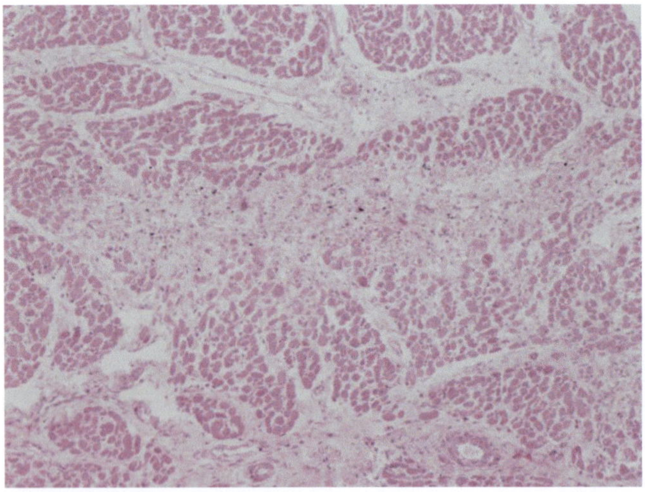

Fig. 3.5 Myocardial atrophy. Myocardial cross-section: the transverse diameter of the atrophied muscle fibers is reduced, and the gaps among myocardial fibers are widened with localized loss of muscle fibers. HE ×100. (Wang Wenhui)

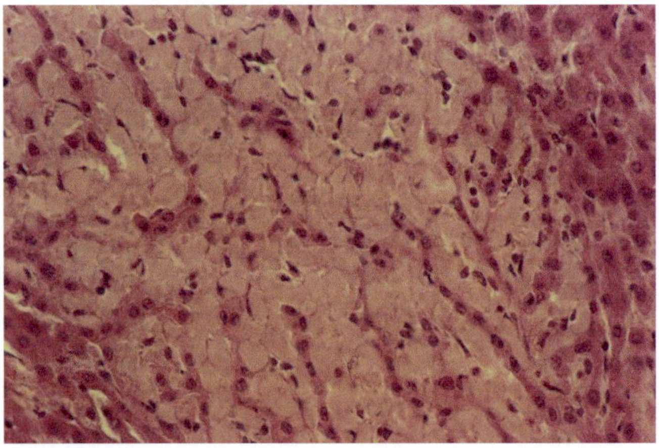

Fig. 3.7 Hepatocyte atrophy. Bovine tuberculosis. Hepatic amyloidosis: amyloid material deposits between the hepatic cords and the hepatic sinusoids, so the hepatic cords are compressed and atrophied in thin strips. HE ×400. (Chen Huaitao)

1.2 Hypertrophy (Fig. 3.8)

1.3 Hyperplasia (Fig. 3.9, 3.10, 3.11, 3.12, 3.13, and 3.14)

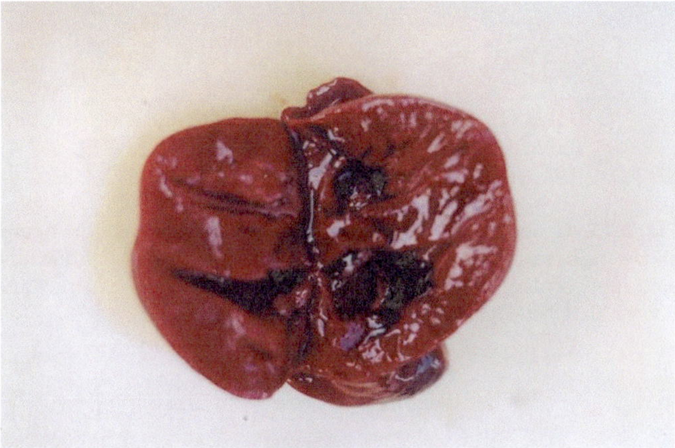

Fig. 3.8 Heart hypertrophy. In the transverse section of the porcine heart, both ventricular walls are thickened, especially the right ventricular wall. Both of the ventricles are smaller than normal ones. (Chen Huaitao)

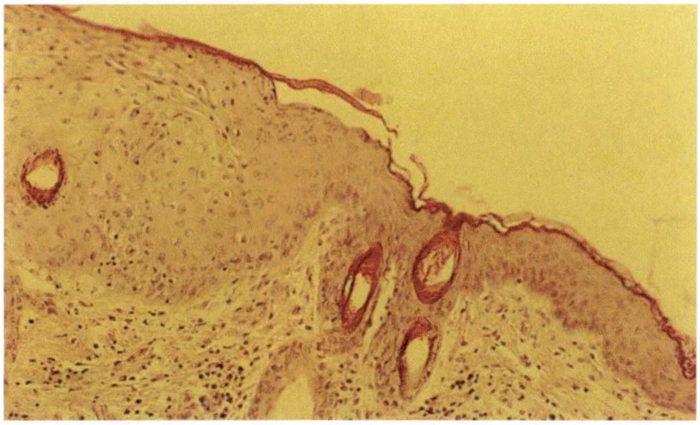

Fig. 3.9 Epidermal hyperplasia of the skin. Sheep pox skin. On the left, the epidermal cells are markedly hyperplastic and the epidermal layer is markedly thickened; on the right, the epidermal layer is normal. HE ×200. (Chen Huaitao)

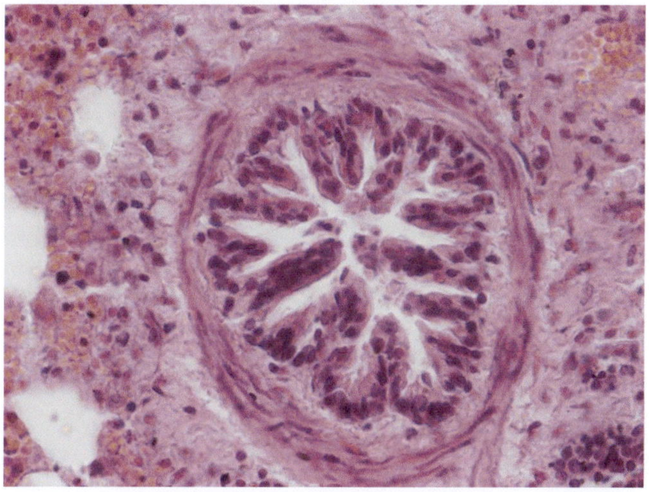

Fig. 3.10 Bronchial epithelial hyperplasia. Equine lungs. Epithelial cell hyperplasia of the fine bronchial mucosa is obvious with markedly increased mucosal folds. HE ×400. (Wang Wenhui)

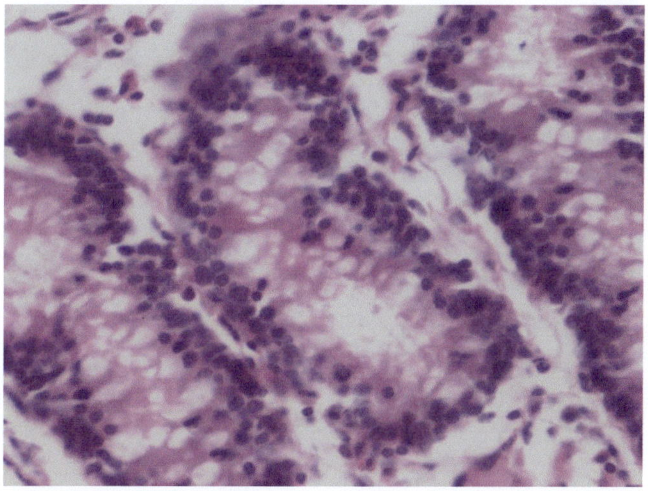

Fig. 3.11 Glandular epithelial hyperplasia of the intestine. Bovine paratuberculosis. Hyperplasia of intestinal glandular epithelium, which is in an irregular multilayered arrangement. HE ×400. (Wang Wenhui)

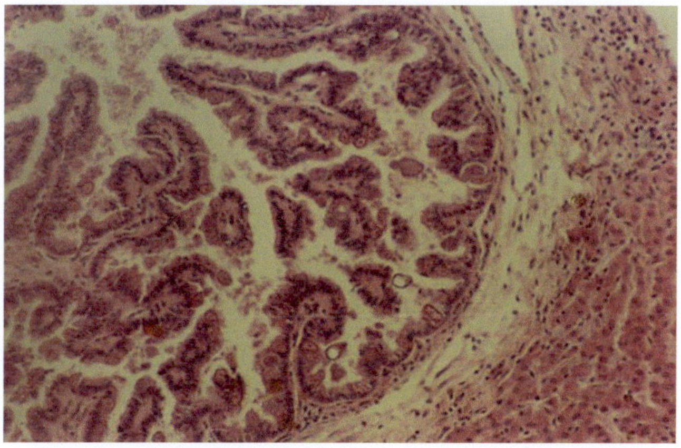

Fig. 3.12 Bile duct epithelial hyperplasia. Hepatic coccidiosis in rabbits. The epithelium of the hepatobiliary ducts is highly hyperplastic and protruded papilliform into the lumen; many coccidian oocysts are present in the epithelial cells and lumen. HE ×200. (Chen Huaitao)

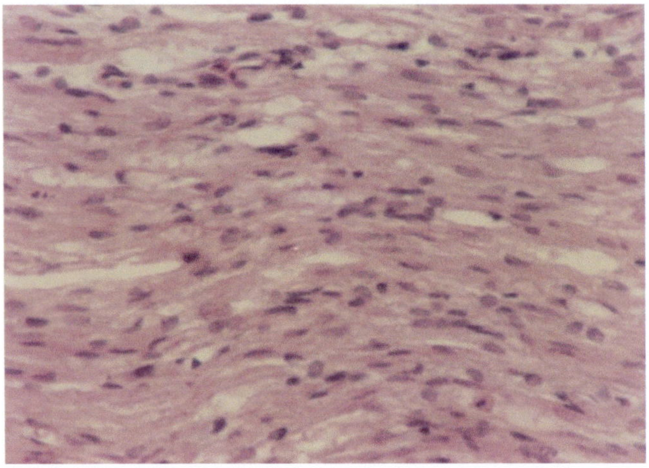

Fig. 3.13 Schwann's cell hyperplasia. Riboflavin deficiency in chicks. Proliferation of Schwann's cells is obvious and their number is increased markedly in the sciatic nerve. HE ×400. (Wang Wenhui)

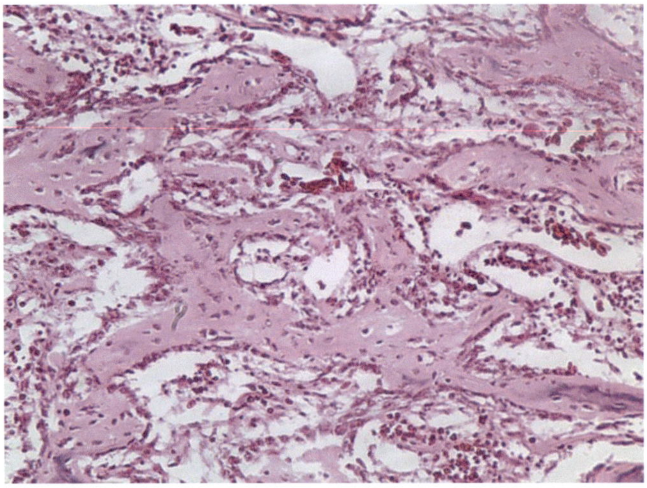

Fig. 3.14 Osteoid tissue hyperplasia. Calcium deficiency in chickens. The osteoid tissues in the long bone epiphysis are massively hyperplastic, forming osteoid trabeculae. HE ×400. (Cui Hengmin)

1.4 Metaplasia (Figs. 3.15, 3.16, and 3.17)

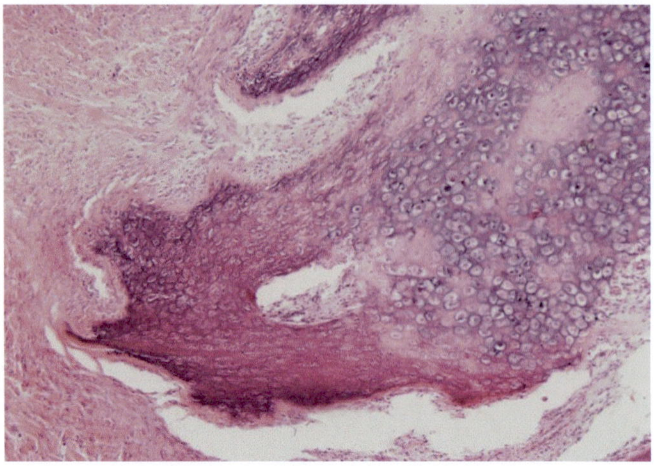

Fig. 3.15 Connective tissue metaplasia. The margin area of the figure shows the hyperplastic connective tissue, some of which has differentiated into cartilage tissue with a more typical cartilaginous structure. HE ×400. (Chen Huaitao)

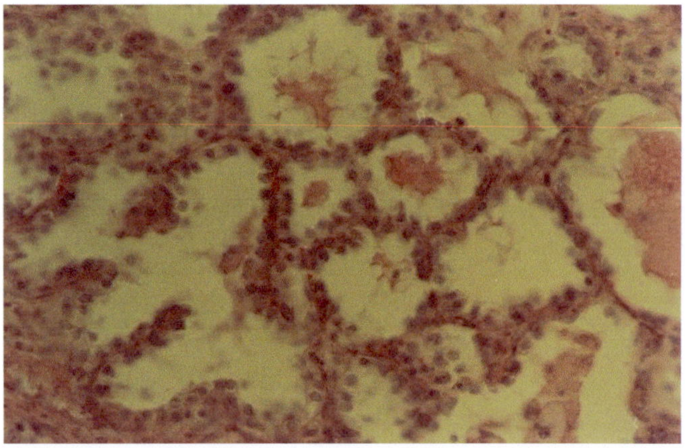

Fig. 3.16 Alveolar epithelial metaplasia. Sheep pox. Alveolar monolayer squamous epithelium has transited into monolayer cuboidal epithelium with alveoli resembling glandular acini. HE ×400. (Chen Huaitao)

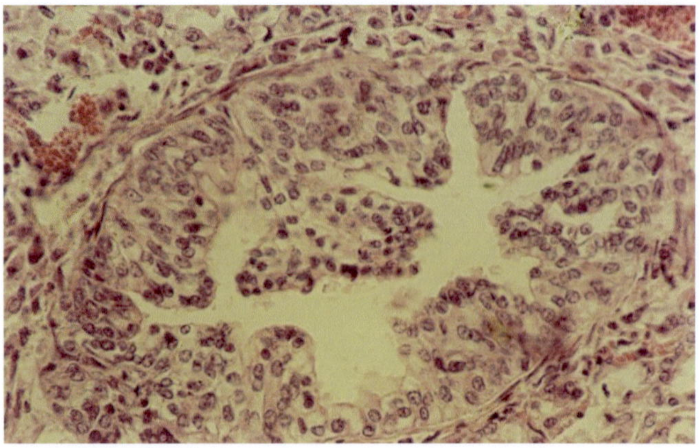

Fig. 3.17 Bronchiolar epithelial metaplasia. Metaplasia of the bronchiolar monolayer cuboidal epithelium into a stratified squamous epithelium. HE ×400. (Chen Huaitao)

2 Repair

2.1 Regeneration (Figs. 3.18, 3.19, and 3.20)

2.2 Granulation Tissue (Figs. 3.21, 3.22, 3.23, 3.24, and 3.25)

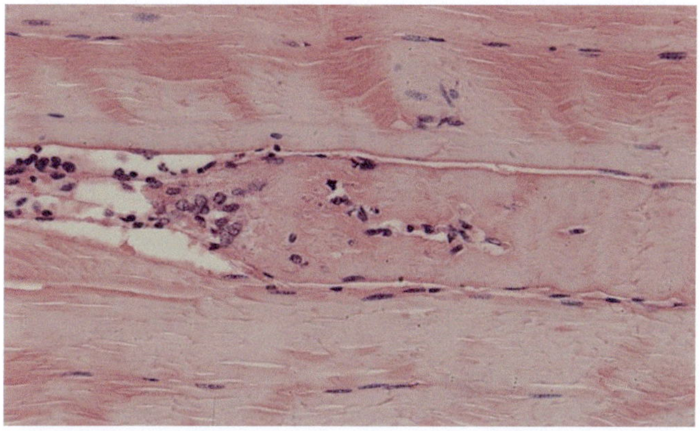

Fig. 3.18 Regeneration of muscle fibers. Regeneration of skeletal muscle: a regenerated muscle fiber is present in the middle of the figure, with multinucleated muscle buds visible at the broken ends of the fiber. HE ×400. (Chen Huaitao)

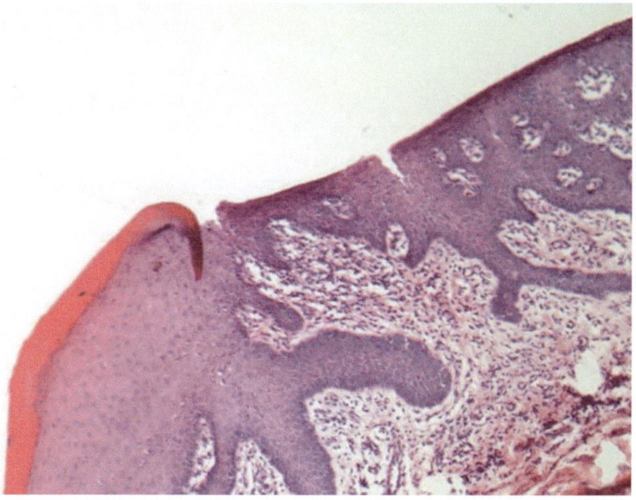

Fig. 3.19 Epithelial regeneration. Regeneration of stratified squamous epithelium: on the right, the regenerated epithelium is thinner with its surface unkeratinized yet; on the left, the normal skin epithelium is thicker and its surface layer is keratinized obviously. HE ×100. (Wang Wenhui)

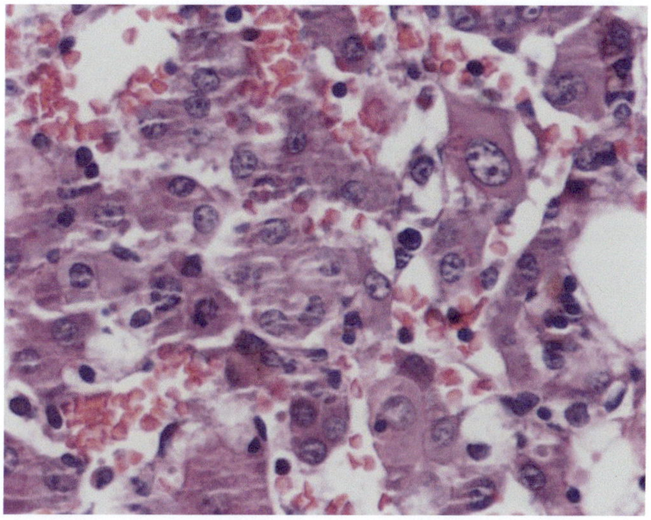

Fig. 3.20 Hepatocyte regeneration. In a foci of hepatic necrosis, some hepatocytes are regenerating. The regenerated hepatocytes are larger, with darker staining and larger nuclei, and mitotic figure can also be observed. HE ×400. (Chen Huaitao)

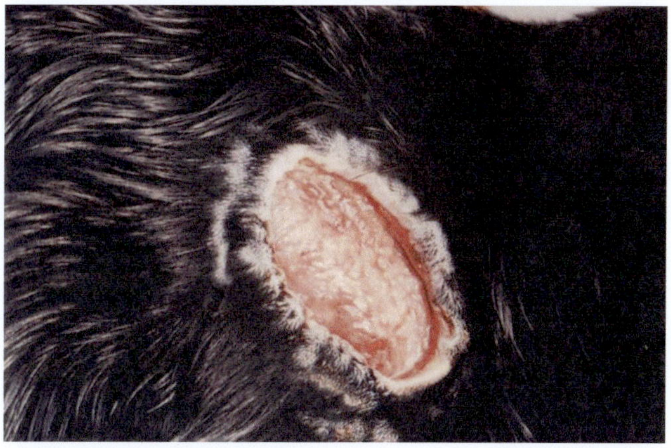

Fig. 3.21 Granulation tissue. Newly generated granulation tissue is present at canine skin trauma, which is bright red in color and tender in texture with uneven surface and a small amount of exudate. (Zhou Qingguo)

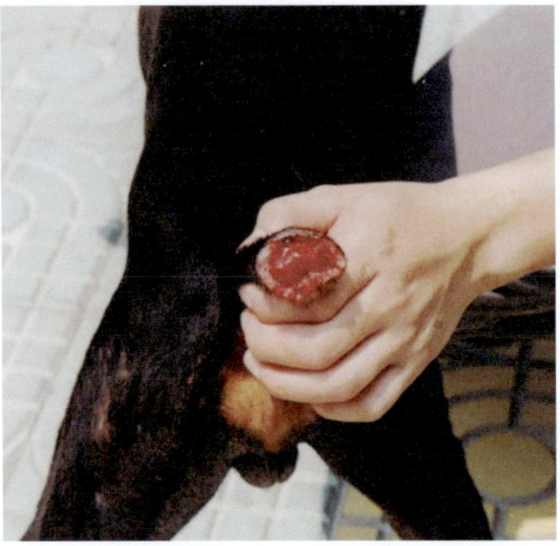

Fig. 3.22 Granulation tissue. The granulation tissue forms on the trauma surface of the dog tail after amputation, which is bright red, fragile, and highly vulnerable to bleeding. (Zhou Qingguo)

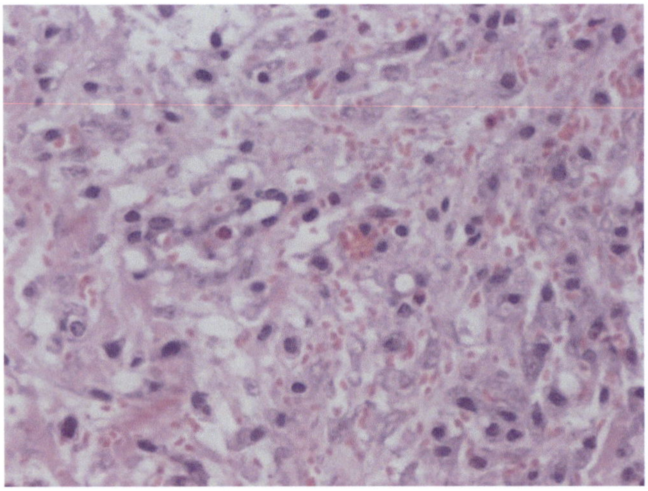

Fig. 3.23 Granulation tissue. The granulation tissue mainly consists of young fibroblasts, abundant nascent capillaries, a few collagen fibers, and inflammatory cells. HE ×400. (Wang Wenhui)

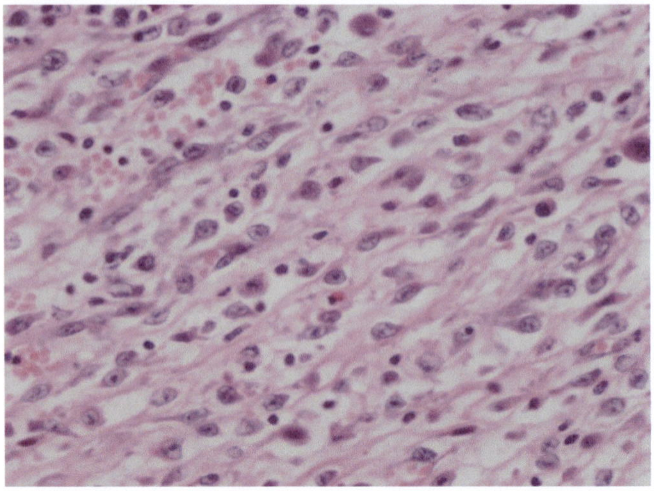

Fig. 3.24 Granulation tissue. Young fibroblasts in granulation tissue: they are large in size, spindle, irregular, or tadpole shaped, with mostly oval nuclei and distinct nucleoli, even two nucleoli for some cells. HE ×400. (Wang Wenhui)

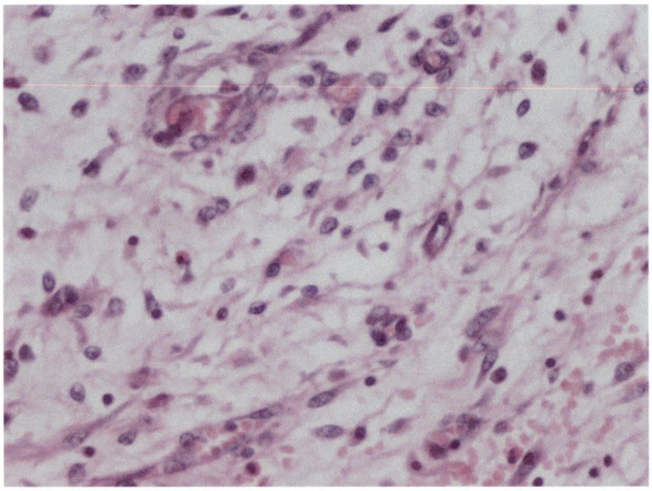

Fig. 3.25 Granulation tissue. Nascent capillaries are present in granulation tissue, some of which are congested, some are only lacunar. Fibroblasts, inflammatory cells, and erythrocytes are present among the vessels. HE ×400. (Wang Wenhui)

2.3 Organization (Figs. 3.26, 3.27, 3.28, and 3.29)

2.4 Wound Healing (Fig. 3.30)

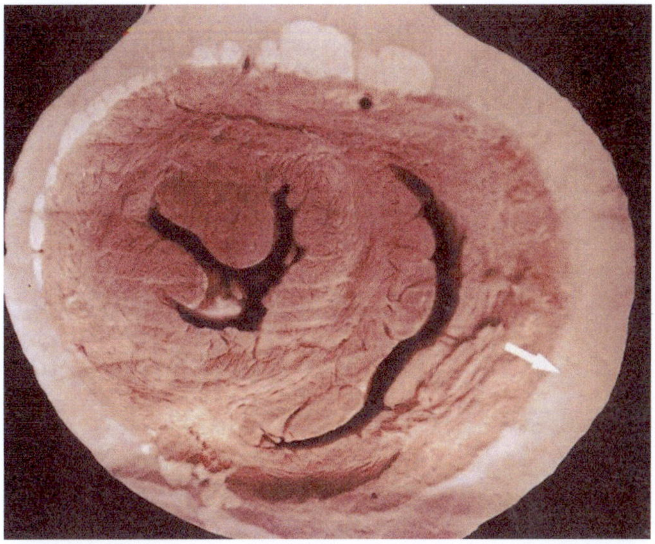

Fig. 3.26 Organization. Organization of bovine traumatic pericarditis (cross-section of the heart). Fibrin exuding from the epicardium is replaced by granulation tissue in pericarditis, forming a grayish, densely organized layer (↑). (Veterinary Pathology Unit, Gansu Agricultural University)

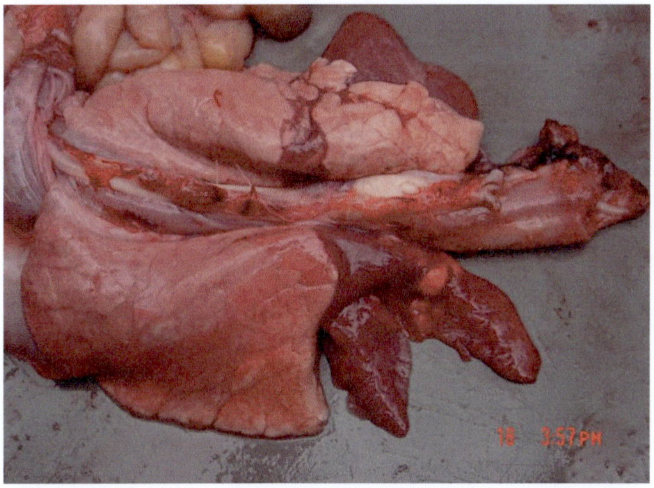

Fig. 3.27 Organization. Because of the inflammation, the apical and cardiac lobes of the pig lungs become organized and show carnification with grayish-red color, pliable texture, and thinning edges. (Hu Xueying)

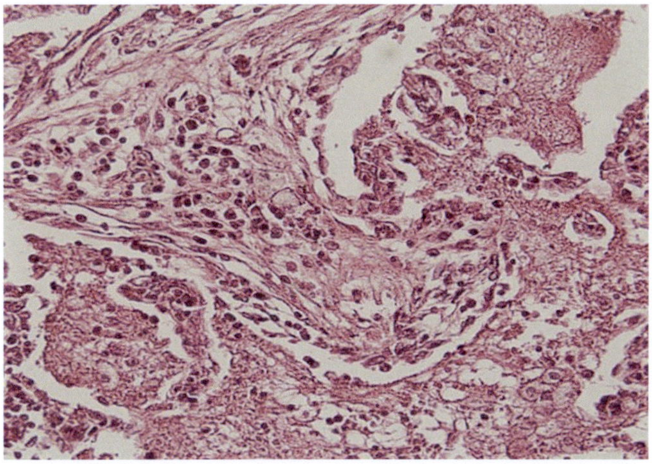

Fig. 3.28 Organization. Organization of pneumonia exudates: inflammatory exudates such as fibrin in the alveoli have been gradually replaced by granulation tissue. HE ×400. (Chen Huaitao)

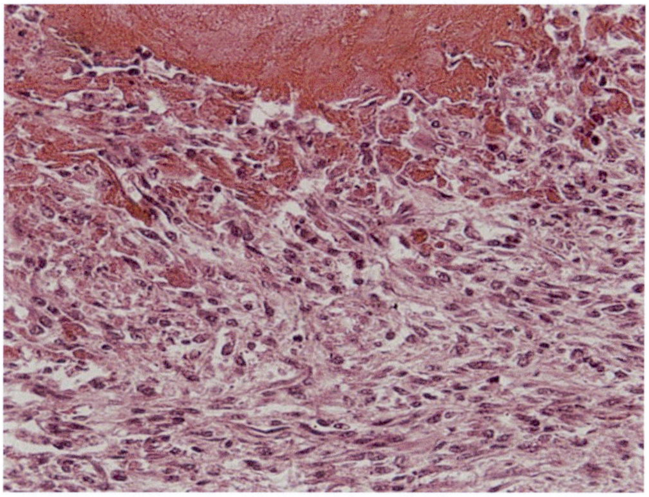

Fig. 3.29 Organization. Organization of endocardial thrombus: the endocardial thrombus (dark red -stained) material has been partially replaced by endocardial nascent granulation tissue. HE ×400. (Chen Huaitao)

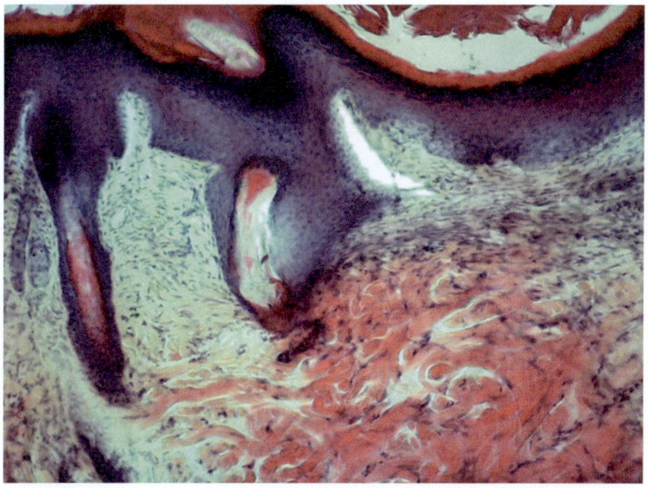

Fig. 3.30 Wound healing. Small wound healed: the regenerated skin epithelium is located in the upper right center of the figure, and there is proliferative connective tissue below it. HE ×100. (Veterinary Pathological Anatomy Unit, Northeast Agricultural University)

Bibliography

1. Huaitao C, editor. Pathological anatomy of domestic animals. 3rd ed. China Agricultural Press; 2006.

Inflammation

4

1 Inflammatory Cells

1.1 Neutrophil (Neutrophilic Granulocyte; Neutrophilic Leukocyte; Neutrophilic Cells) (Figs. 4.1, 4.2, 4.3, and 4.4)

1.1.1 Morphological Characteristics of Neutrophils

The morphology of neutrophils is characterized by a nucleus lobulating into two to five lobes (more lobed nuclei in sheep), usually two to three lobes. Reddish neutrophil granules are present in cytoplasm of neutrophils from domestic animals on HE sections, while coarse eosinophilic granules are present in neutrophils from poultry and rabbits, and hence they are named heterophilic granulocytes. Neutrophils are mostly present in acute inflammation, septic inflammation, and early inflammation.

1.1.2 Phagocytosis by Neutrophils

1.2 Eosinophilic Granulocytes (Eosinophilic Cells; Eosinophilic Leukocyte; Eosinophil) (Figs. 4.5 and 4.6)

The morphology of eosinophils is characterized by cytoplasm filled with coarse bright red eosinophilic granules, with less nuclear lobulation usually with two lobes for mature cells. Eosinophils are often observed in allergic inflammation, parasitic infections, salt poisoning, and eosinophil myositis.

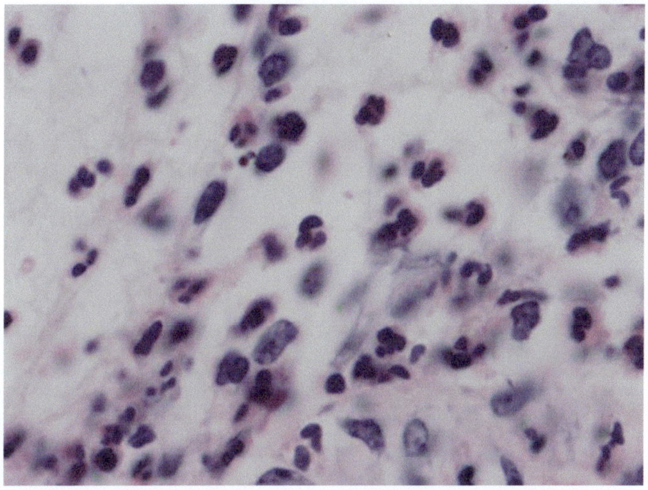

Fig. 4.1 Neutrophils. Neutrophils in inflammatory exudate (bovine): the cells are lightly eosin-stained with relatively abundant cytoplasm, and most of the nuclei lobulate into two to three lobes. HE ×1000. (Wang Wenhui)

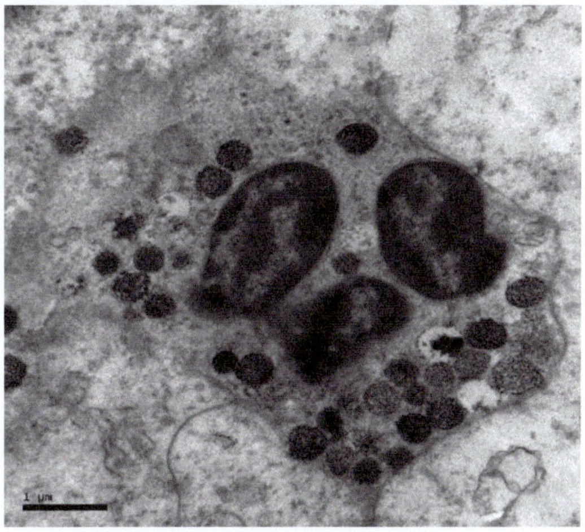

Fig. 4.2 Neutrophils. Ultrastructural features of a neutrophil: The diagram shows a neutrophil of a camel with a nucleus lobulating into three lobes, and granules of different electron density with boundary membranes are present in cytoplasm, which in turn contains densely packed fine granules. ×20,000. (Wang Wenhui)

H. Chen, *Color Atlas of Veterinary Pathology*, https://doi.org/10.1007/978-981-96-7617-0_4

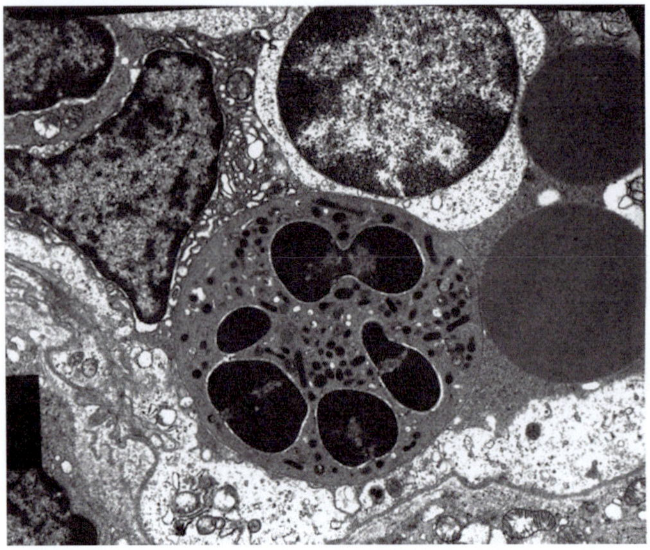

Fig. 4.3 Neutrophils. Chronic progressive pneumonia in sheep (natural case). Mastitis: a neutrophil in the interstitial capillaries of the mammary gland acinus, the nucleus of which lobulates into several lobes, and azurophilic as well as specific granules (in a round or dumbbell shape) are present in cytoplasm. (Deng Puhui)

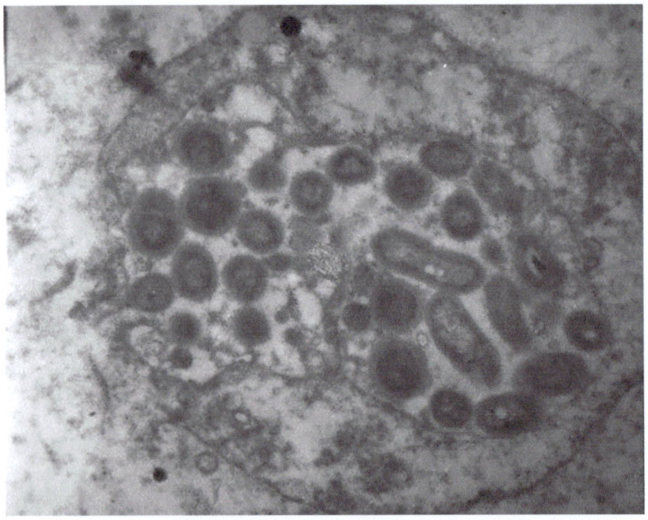

Fig. 4.4 Neutrophils. Bovine endometritis. Neutrophils are filled with large phagosomes containing bacteria. (Lv Xunxian)

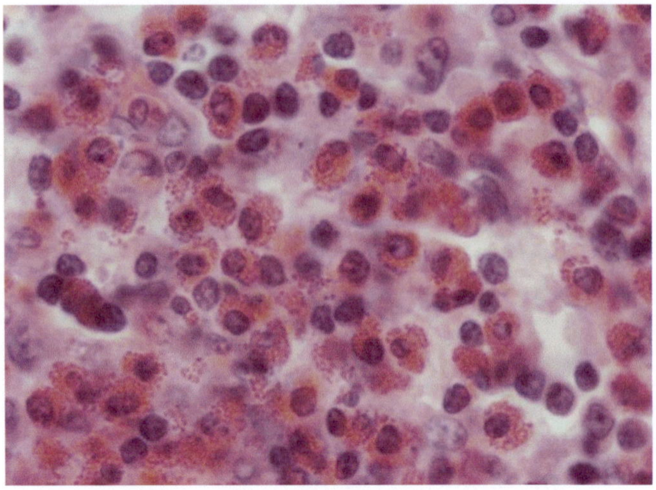

Fig. 4.5 Eosinophils. Eosinophils in porcine tissues: eosinophils are slightly larger than neutrophils and contain a large number of eosinophilic (red) granules in the cytoplasm. HE ×1000. (Wang Wenhui)

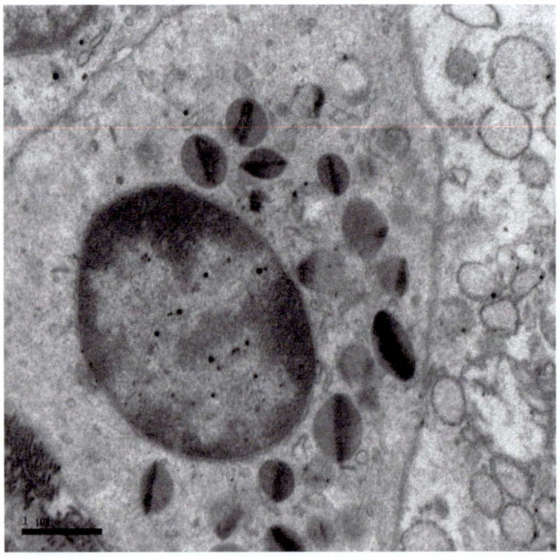

Fig. 4.6 Eosinophils. Ultrastructural features of eosinophils: the figure shows an eosinophil of camel with many spindle-shaped granules in the cytoplasm. The protein crystalline materials in the granules generally are located in the center of the longitudinal axis, with some located in the outer part. ×20,000. (Wang Wenhui)

1.3 Macrophages (Figs. 4.7, 4.8, 4.9, 4.10, 4.11, and 4.12)

Macrophages are a group of cells with powerful phagocytic capacity, including monocytes from the blood. Macrophages in tissues vary greatly in their morphology and size, generally having large bodies, round or oval shapes, light staining with abundant cytoplasm, and often containing phagocytic material; the nuclei are round, relatively small, and vesicular with many distinct nucleoli. Macrophages are commonly observed in late acute inflammation, chronic inflammation, encephalitis, certain nonsuppurative inflammatory conditions, and viral as well as parasitic infections.

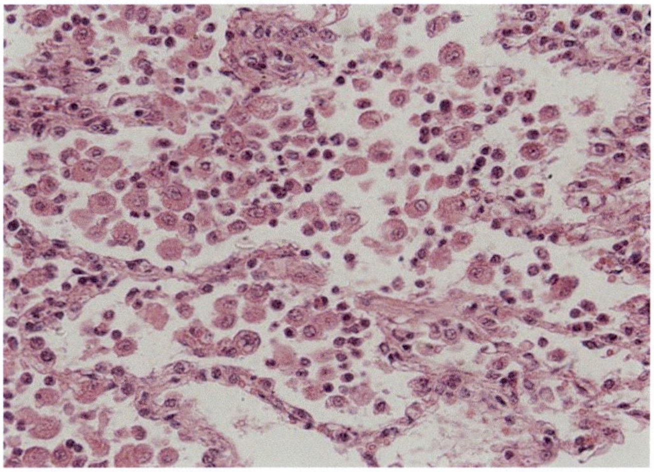

Fig. 4.7 Macrophages. Macrophages in the alveolar cavity in pneumonia: they are large but vary in size, with abundant reddish cytoplasm; the nuclei are relatively small, lightly stained, and vesicular, with distinct nucleoli. In addition, inflammatory cells such as plasma cells and lymphocytes are present in the alveoli. HE ×400. (Chen Huaitao)

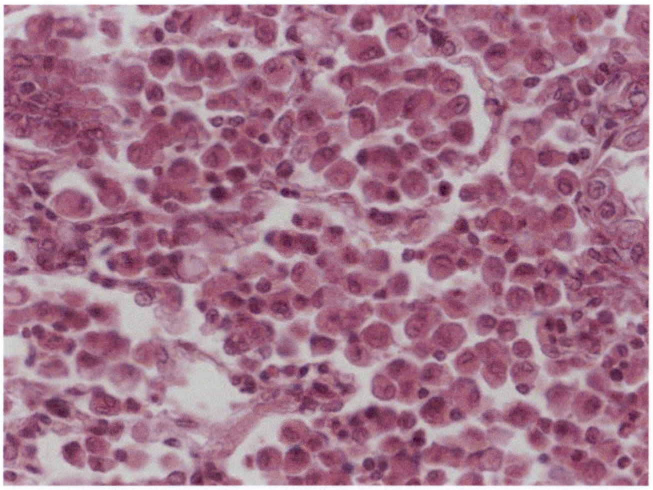

Fig. 4.8 Macrophages. Macrophages in the alveolar cavity: macrophages are dense and generally large in size, with phagocytosed nuclei or their fragments visible in the cytoplasm of some cells. HE ×400. (Wang Wenhui)

1.3.1 Morphological Characteristics of Macrophages

1.3.2 Phagocytosis by Macrophages

Macrophages show a very powerful phagocytic function and various phagocytic substances are often observed in their cytoplasm.

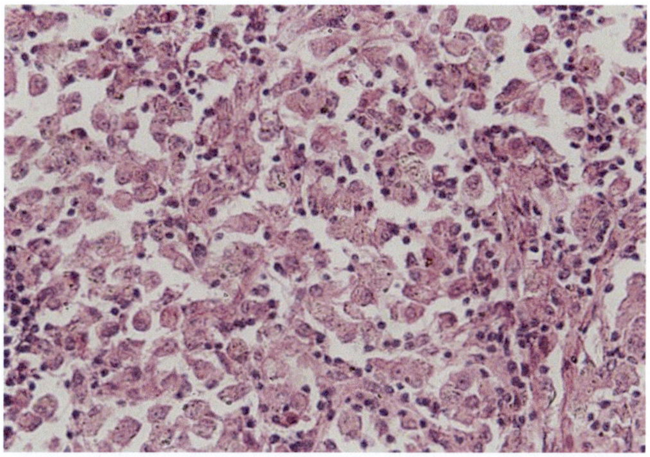

Fig. 4.9 Macrophages. Equine pneumoconiosis. Macrophages in bronchial lymph nodes: macrophages are numerous, large, and a large amount of engulfed brownish-yellow inorganic dust crystals and particles are present in the cell plasma, so this type of macrophages is called dust cells. HE ×400. (Chen Huaitao)

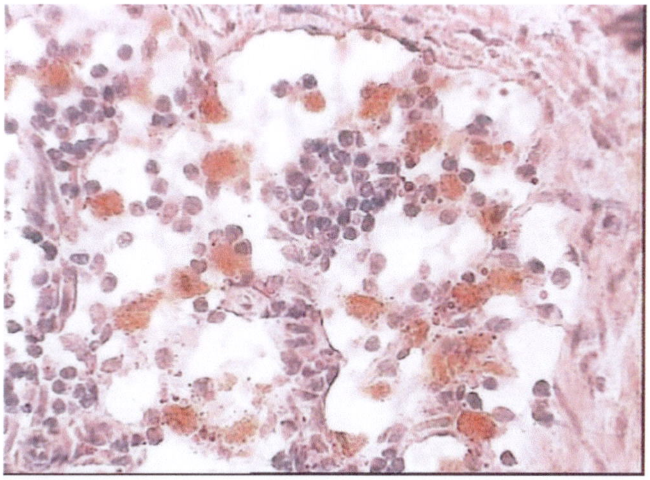

Fig. 4.10 Macrophages. Lymph nodes. Macrophages in lymphatic sinus: the engulfed fat (orange color) is present in cytoplasma. Sudan III staining ×400. (Hu Xueying)

1.4 Epithelioid Cell and Multiple Nuclear Giant Cell (Figs. 4.13, 4.14, 4.15, 4.16, 4.17, and 4.18)

Epithelioid cells are transformed from cells of the mononuclear macrophage system in response to some pathogenic factors and are so named because they are large, often con-

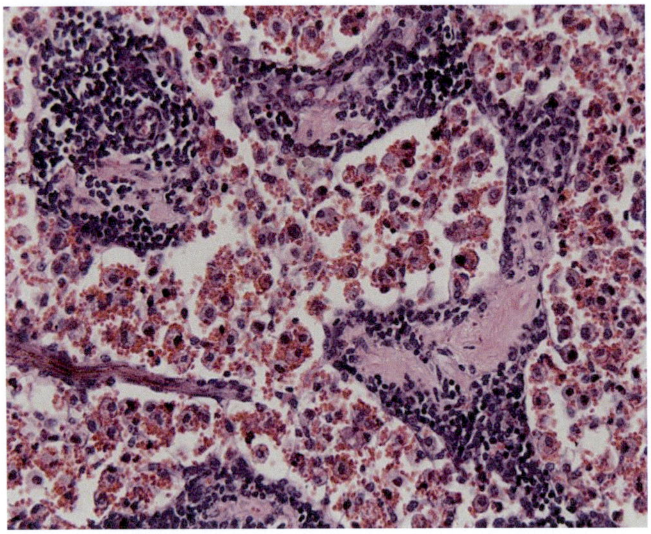

Fig. 4.11 Macrophages. Lymph nodes of red deer. Macrophages in the lymphatic sinus: there are plenty of macrophages and erythrocytes in the lymphatic sinus and some erythrocytes are engulfed by macrophages. HE ×400. (Meng Qingling)

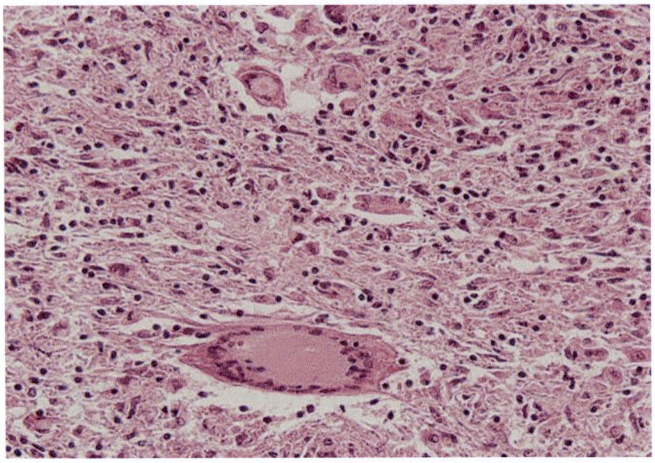

Fig. 4.13 Giant cells. A Langhans giant cell and a large number of epithelioid cells are in a tuberculous nodule. The former is large, rich in cytoplasm and with ring-shaped nuclei; the latter is with oval or spindle-shaped nuclei and lighter staining, while many lymphocytes can be observed. HE ×400. (Chen Huitao)

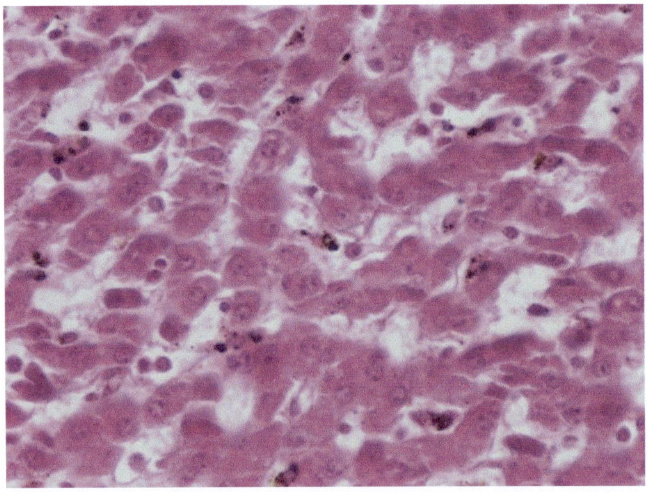

Fig. 4.12 Macrophages. Pig liver. There are macrophages containing yellowish-brown hemosiderin (Kupffer cell) in liver sinusoids. HE ×400. (Wang Wenhui)

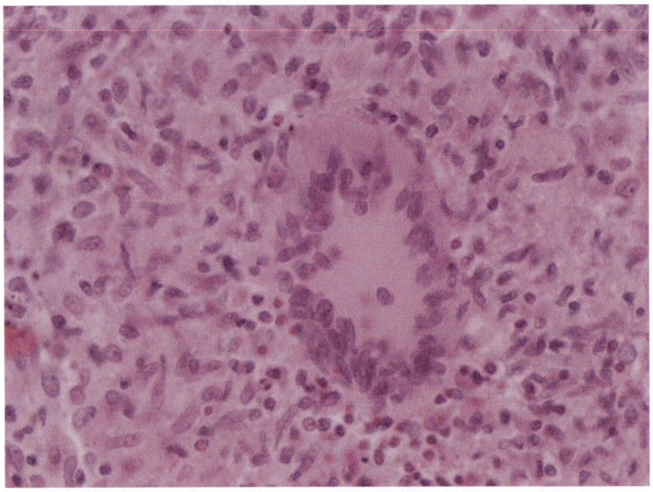

Fig. 4.14 Epithelioid cells and giant cells. This image shows a Langhans giant cell and a large number of surrounding epithelioid cells in a bovine tuberculous nodules. The Langhans giant cell is oval with many nuclei arranged in a ring; the epithelioid cell is indistinct with lightly stained nuclei; note that the nuclei of both cells are similar in size, shape, and staining. HE ×400. (Wang Wenhui)

tiguous, with indistinct cell boundaries and a flat epithelial appearance. Epithelioid cells with giant cells are seen in granulomatous inflammatory diseases. Multinucleated giant cells (giant cells) are large, rich in cytoplasm, and often contain several to dozens of nuclei of similar morphological size in a single cell body. Based on the arrangement of the nuclei, giant cells can be divided into two types: Langhans giant cells and foreign body giant cells. The nuclei of Langhans giant cells are generally distributed in the peripheral part of the cytoplasm in a horseshoe or ring shape, while the nuclei of foreign body giant cells are more irregularly scattered in the cytoplasm.

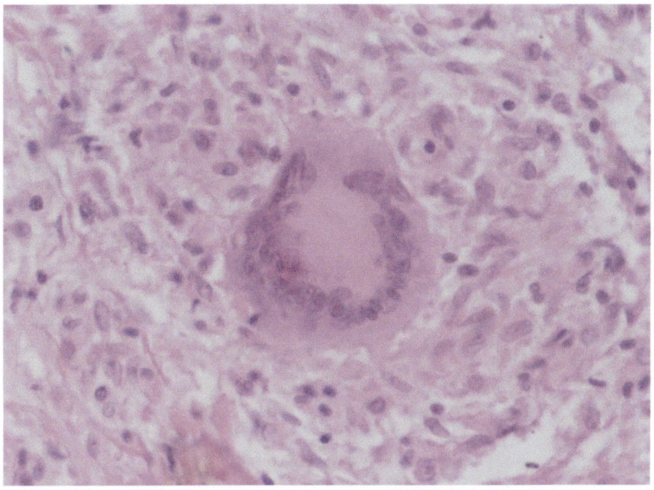

Fig. 4.15 Epithelioid cells and giant cells. Bovine tuberculosis nodule. There is a Langhans giant cell in the middle of the figure with nuclei arranged in a horseshoe shape, surrounded by some sparsely distributed epithelioid cells with lightly stained nuclei. HE ×400. (Wang Wenhui)

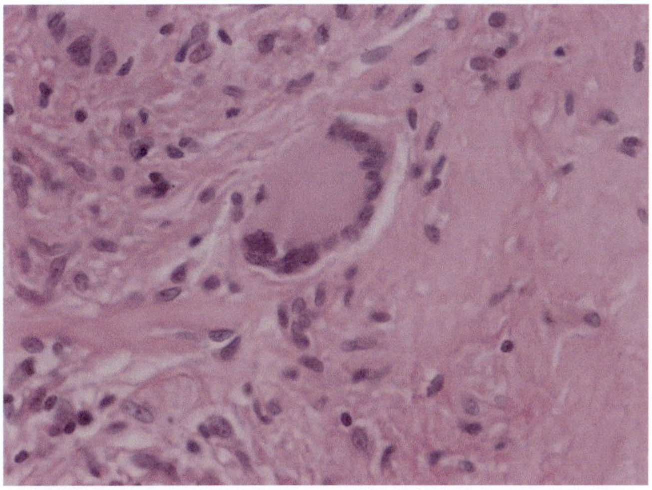

Fig. 4.16 Epithelioid cells and giant cells. The figure shows a Langhans giant cell and some epithelioid cells next to a caseous necrosis of a bovine nodule (lower right). The nuclei of the Langhans giant cells are arranged in a C-shape. HE ×400. (Wang Wenhui)

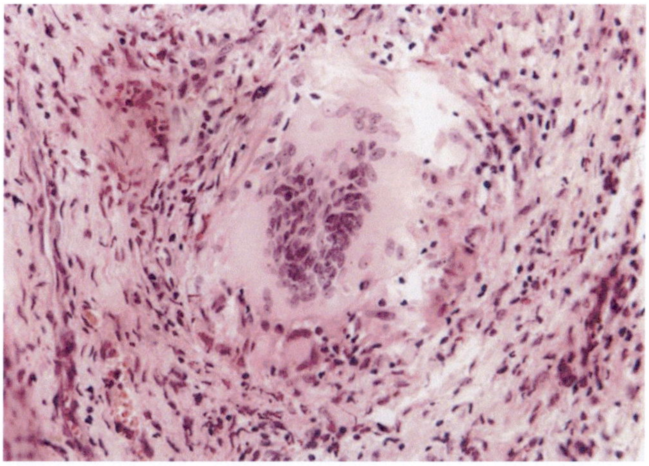

Fig. 4.17 Epithelioid cells and giant cells. An oversized giant cell is in the center of the image. The giant cell is irregularly shaped, with hundreds of nuclei accumulating disorderly in the cytoplasm. HE ×400. (Wang Wenhui)

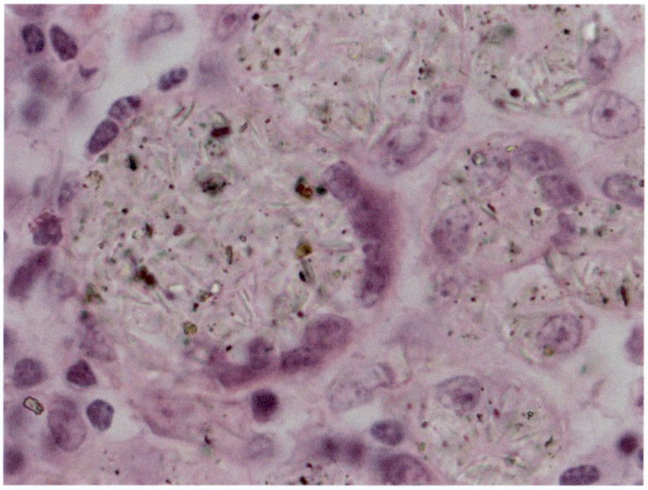

Fig. 4.18 Giant cells. Bovine lymph node. A large amount of brownish-yellow inorganic crystalline dust are engulfed in the cytoplasm of macrophages, and the nuclei are distributed along the cell border. The nearby macrophages also engulfed inorganic dust. HE ×1000. (Wang Wenhui)

1.5 Lymphocytes (Figs. 4.19 and 4.20)

Morphologically lymphocytes are classified into three categories: the large, the medium, and the small ones. Small lymphocytes are mature lymphocytes. Small lymphocytes are small in size with round, dark-stained nuclei and little cytoplasm. Lymphocytes are associated with the immune response of the body and are commonly found in chronic inflammatory conditions.

1.6 Plasma Cells (Fig. 4.21)

Plasma cells are important immune cells and often present along with lymphocytes in foci of chronic inflammation. Plasma cells are derived from B lymphocytes, slightly larger than small lymphocytes, ovoid, large at one end and small at the other, or pointed at one end and rounded at the other; the cytoplasm is grayish, but the perinuclear cytoplasm is pale; the nucleus is often located at one side, and the chromatin is

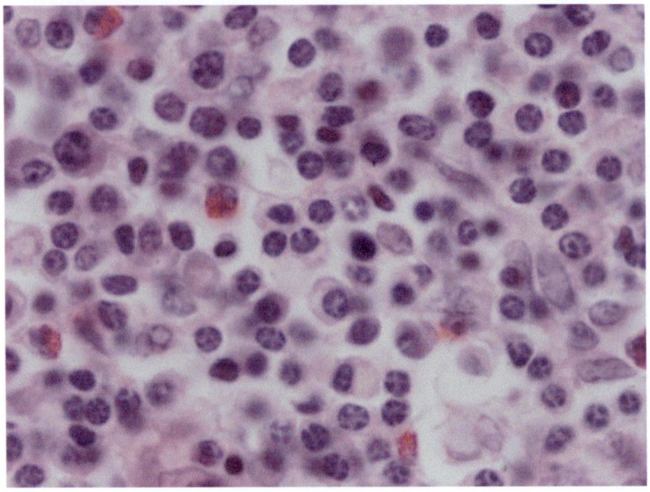

Fig. 4.19 Lymphocytes. Small lymphocytes in tissues: they are small, round in shape, with little cytoplasm; the nucleus is round and deeply stained, and the chromatin is coarsely granular often distributed along the nuclear membrane. ×1000. (Wang Wenhui)

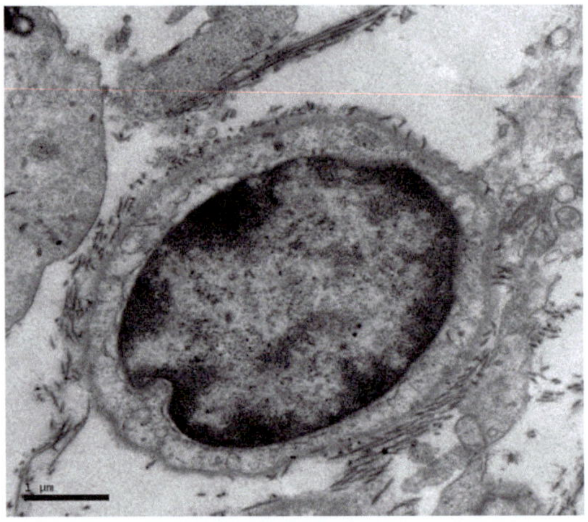

Fig. 4.20 Lymphocytes. Electron microscopy of a small lymphocyte: it contains little cytoplasm and organelles, and most of its chromatin is distributed along the nuclear membrane with a small defect at one end of the nucleus. ×20,000. (Wang Wenhui)

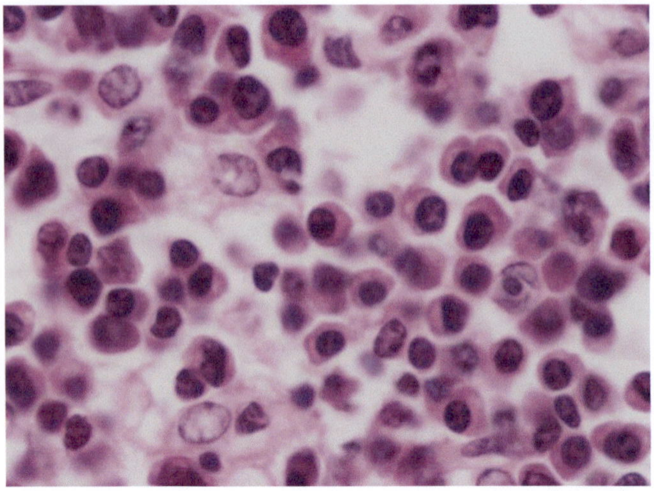

Fig. 4.21 Plasma cells. Plasma cells in tissues: most of the cells are ovoid or oval with abundant cytoplasm. The nucleus is often located at one end of the cell, and the chromatin is thick and distributed along the nuclear membrane, so the nucleus resembles a wheel. HE ×1000. (Wang Wenhui)

in lump and mostly distributed along the nuclear membrane, so the outer shape of the nucleus resembles the surface of a clock or a wheel. The cytoplasm is filled with coarse endoplasmic reticulum when observed under electron microscope.

2 Inflammatory Types

2.1 Alterative Inflammation (Fig. 4.22)

2.2 Exudative Inflammation

2.2.1 Serous Inflammation (Fig. 4.23)

2.2.2 Suppurative Inflammation (Purulent Inflammation) (Figs. 4.24, 4.25, 4.26, and 4.27)

2.2.3 Catarrhal Inflammation (Figs. 4.28 and 4.29)

2.2.4 Fibrinous Inflammation (Figs. 4.30 and 4.31)

2.2.5 Hemorrhagic Inflammation (Figs. 4.32 and 4.33)

2.3 Hyperplastic Inflammation

2.3.1 General Proliferative Inflammatory

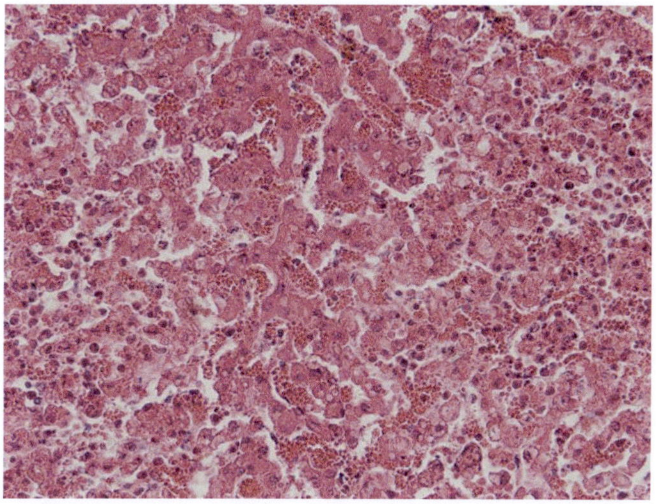

Fig. 4.22 Alterative inflammation. Alterative hepatitis: degeneration and necrosis of hepatocytes are obvious with congestion of the hepatic sinusoids and a lot of neutrophil infiltration among them. HE ×400. (Chen Huaitao)

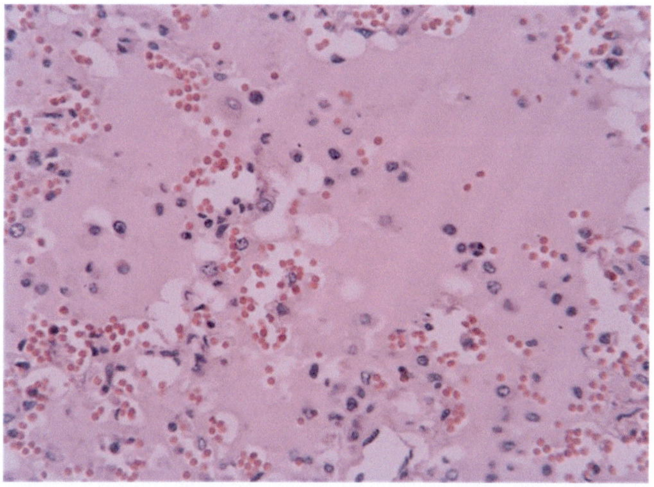

Fig. 4.23 Serous inflammation. Serous pneumonia: the capillary of alveolar septum is congested, the alveolar cavity is filled with serous fluid, and neutrophils and other inflammatory cells infiltrate. HE ×400. (Liu Sidang)

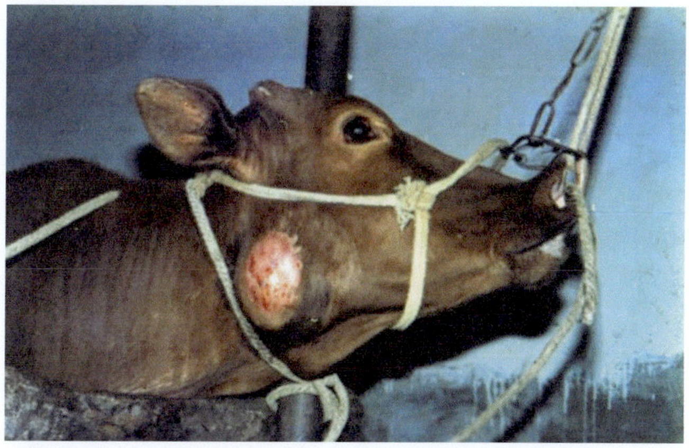

Fig. 4.24 Suppurative inflammation. Subcutaneous abscess: the lesion is at the right side of the neck of a yellow cow, which is swelling with hair loss, hemorrhage on the surface, fluctuating upon touching, and pus inside. (Zhou Qingguo)

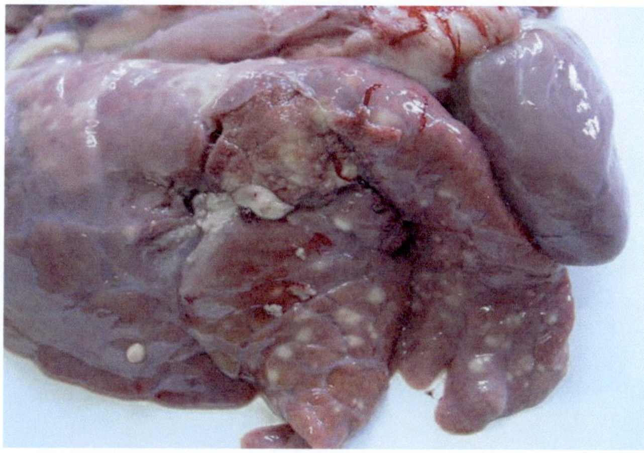

Fig. 4.25 Suppurative inflammation. Pulmonary abscess: scattered multiple abscesses are present on the surface of the lungs, grayish in color and clearly demarcated from the surrounding tissue. (Wu Bin)

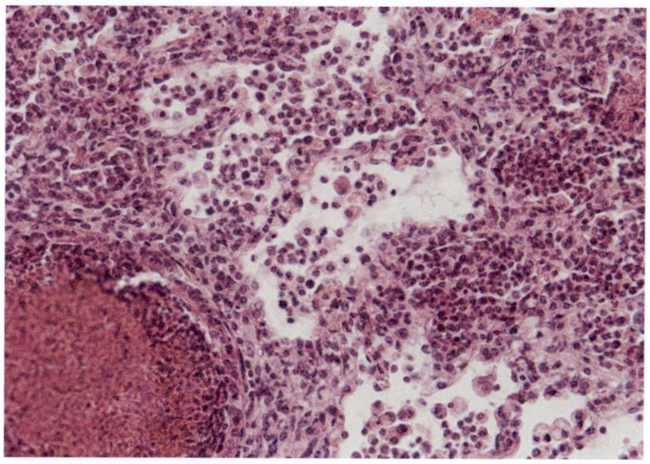

Fig. 4.26 Suppurative inflammation. Purulent bronchopneumonia: the bronchiolar lumen (only the part of it is shown) is filled with degenerated and necrotic neutrophils (pus cells), and there are also a number of neutrophils and pus cells in the alveoli and interstitium. HE ×400. (Chen Huaitao)

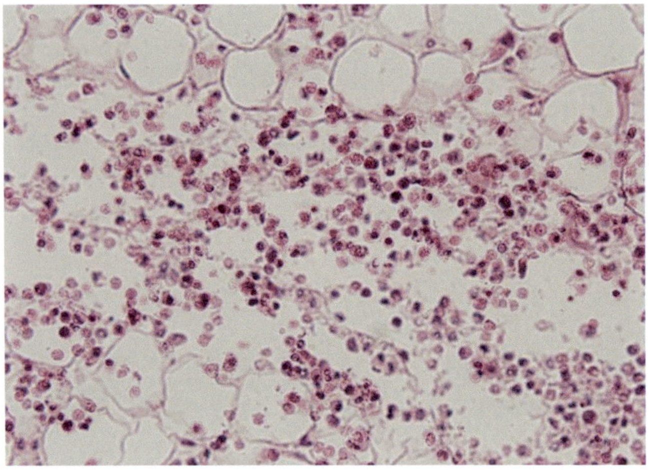

Fig. 4.27 Suppurative inflammation. Cellulitis (phlegmonous inflammation): A large number of neutrophils and pus cells diffusely infiltrate in loose connective tissue, resulting in histolysis and loose structure. HE ×400. (Chen Huaitao)

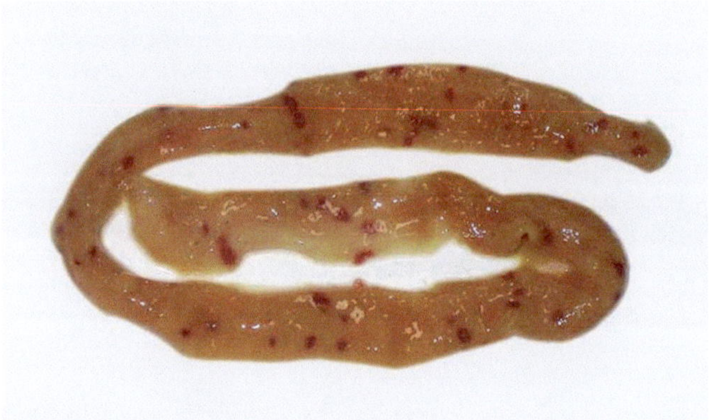

Fig. 4.28 Catarrhal inflammation. Catarrhal enteritis: The duodenal mucosa is covered with mucus with punctate hemorrhage. (Wang Wenhui)

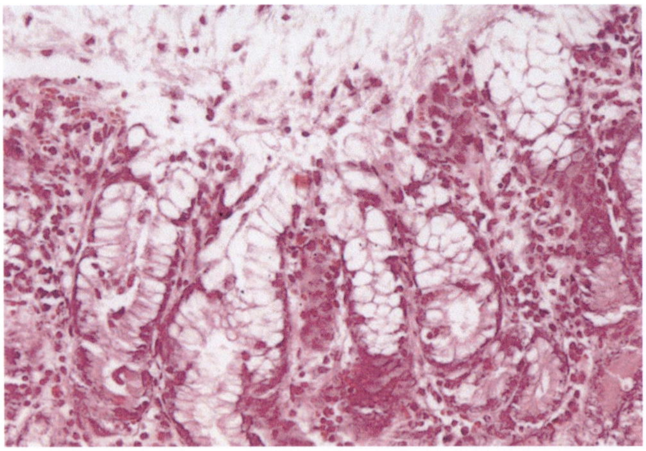

Fig. 4.29 Catarrhal inflammation. Catarrhal gastritis: The gastric mucosa is covered with a large amount of reddish mucus and broken epithelial cells. Gastric glandular goblet cells are increased, the lamina propria is congested and infiltrated with inflammatory cells. HE ×400. (Chen Huaitao)

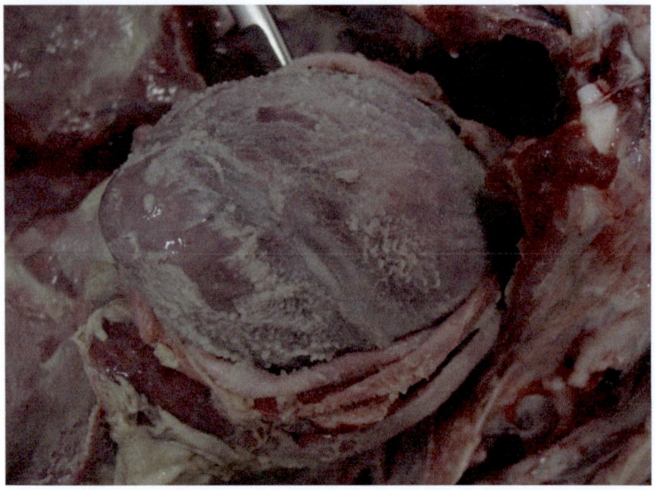

Fig. 4.30 Fibrinoid inflammation. Fibrinous pericarditis: massive fibrin exudates and adheres to the epicardium in a grayish, fuzzy fashion ("cor villosum"). (Wu Bin)

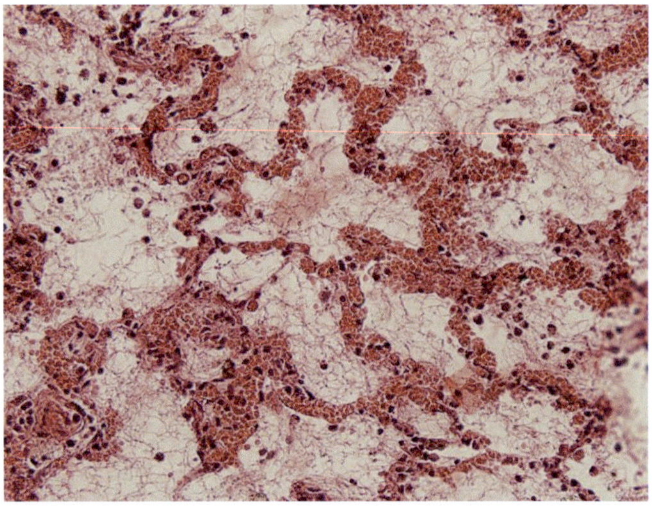

Fig. 4.31 Fibrinous inflammation. Fibrinous pneumonia: a large amount of fibrin and inflammatory cells exuded to the alveolar cavity. Capillaries in the alveolar septum are dilated and filled with red blood cells. HE ×400. (Chen Huaitao)

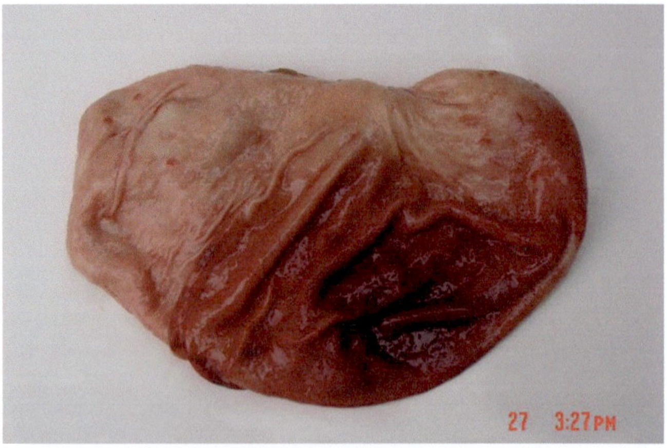

Fig. 4.32 Hemorrhagic inflammation. Hemorrhagic gastritis: extensive congestion and hemorrhage are present on the mucosa at the base of the stomach. The mucosal surface is covered with a small amount of mucus. (Hu Xueying)

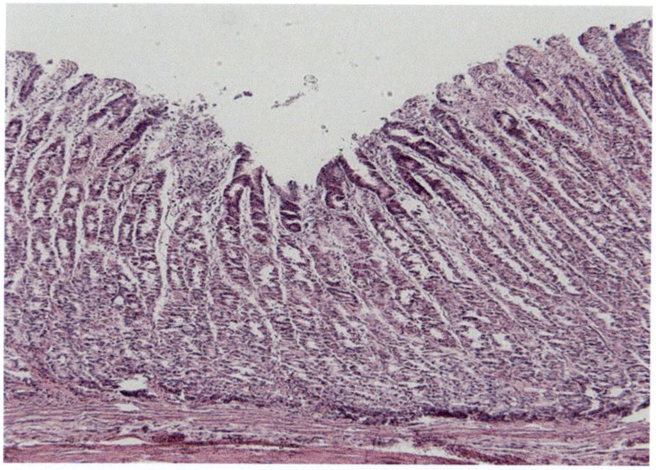

Fig. 4.33 Hemorrhagic inflammation. Hemorrhagic gastritis: The mucosal epithelium is exfoliated, and a large number of erythrocytes are present on the mucosal surface and superficial layer of the lamina propria with infiltration of inflammatory cells. HE ×100. (Chen Huaitao)

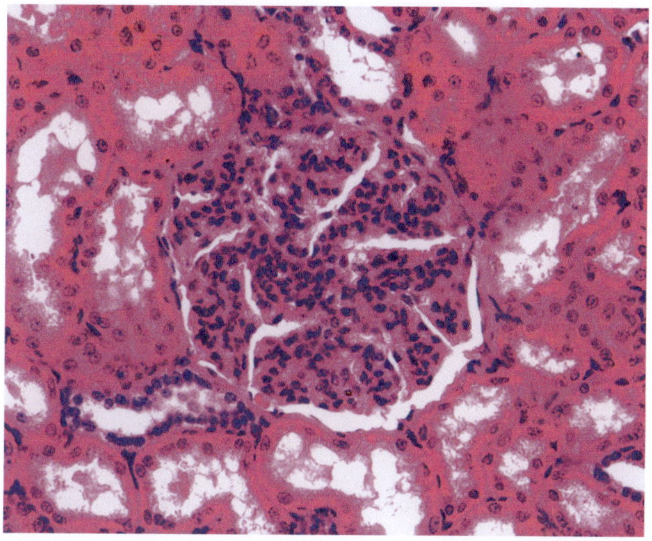

Fig. 4.34 Acute proliferative inflammatory. Acute proliferative glomerulonephritis: proliferation of glomerular capillary endothelial cells and mesangial cells that increases the number of cells in the glomerulus. HE ×400. (Wang Wenhui)

2.3.1.1 Acute Proliferative Inflammatory (Fig. 4.34)

2.3.1.2 Chronic Proliferative Inflammation (Fig. 4.35)

2.3.2 Granulomatous Inflammation (Figs. 4.36, 4.37, 4.38, and 4.39)

Granulomatous inflammation, or inflammatory granuloma, is a specific proliferative inflammatory disease with a chronic course. It is characterized by the proliferation of macrophages and the formation of granulomatous structures dominated by epithelioid cells and multinucleated giant cells.

Granulomatous inflammation can be classified into infective granulomas and foreign body granulomas. Infective granuloma is caused by biological inflammatory factors such as bacteria and mold such as *Mycobacterium tuberculosis*, *Mycobacterium nidulans*, and *Actinomyces*. It is also known as an atopic granuloma because of its specific structure. A typical granuloma consists mainly of epithelioid cells and giant cells with pathogenic bacteria or pathological products at its center.

Foreign body granuloma is caused by foreign bodies such as parasites, parasitic eggs, surgical sutures, silica dust, talcum powder, and certain insoluble metabolites (e.g., urate crystals, lipid-like substances). The basic structure is similar to that of infectious granuloma, i.e., both consist of cells such as epithelioid cells and giant cells, but have a foreign body at their center.

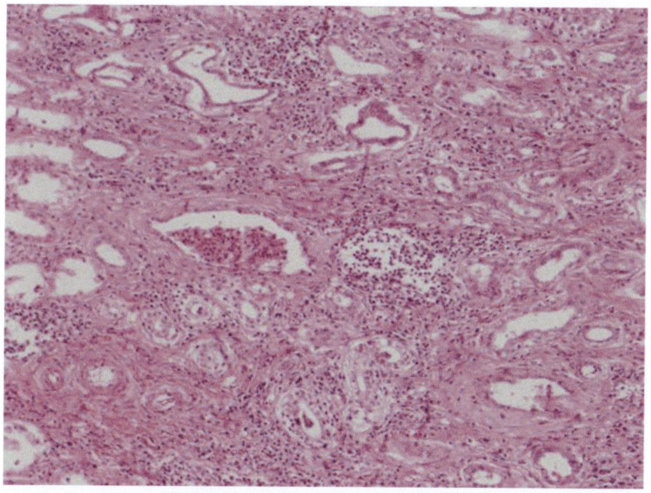

Fig. 4.35 Chronic proliferative inflammation. Chronic interstitial nephritis: interstitial fibrinous connective tissue is massively proliferated with varying degrees of infiltration with lymphocytes, plasma cells, and macrophages. Glomerular and tubular atrophy is present with dilatation of a few tubules. HE ×100. (Wang Wenhui)

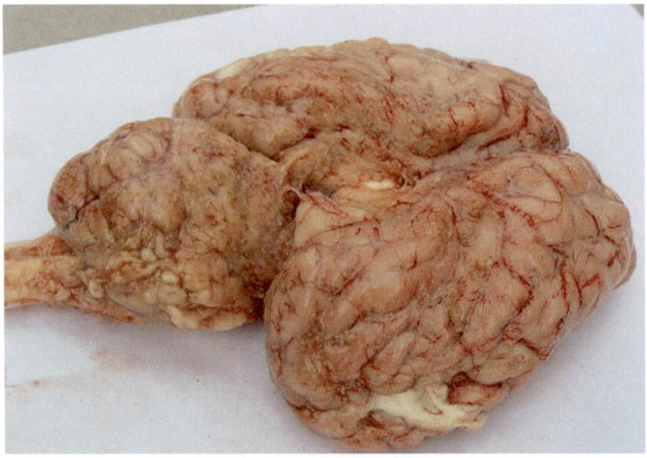

Fig. 4.36 Granulomatous inflammation. Nodules of tuberculosis in the soft meninges of dairy cows, which is miliary and grayish. (Liu Andian)

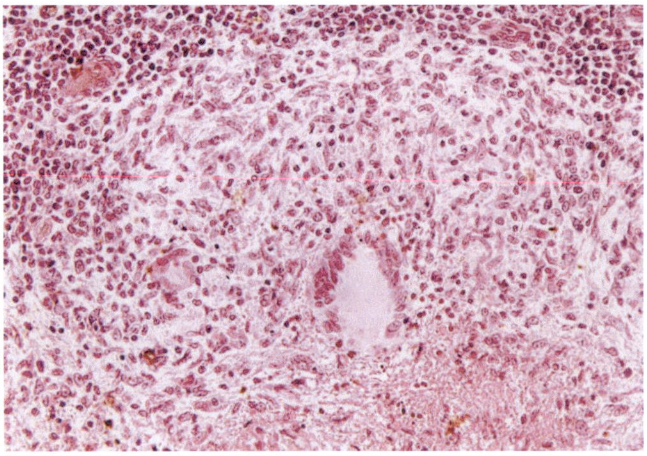

Fig. 4.37 Granulomatous inflammation. Bovine tuberculous granuloma (tuberculous nodule): the granuloma consists of a large number of epithelioid cells and a few giant cells. This figure shows only the upper part of the granuloma, and the center of the granuloma (lower part of the figure) is mild caseous necrosis. HE ×400. (Wang Wenhui)

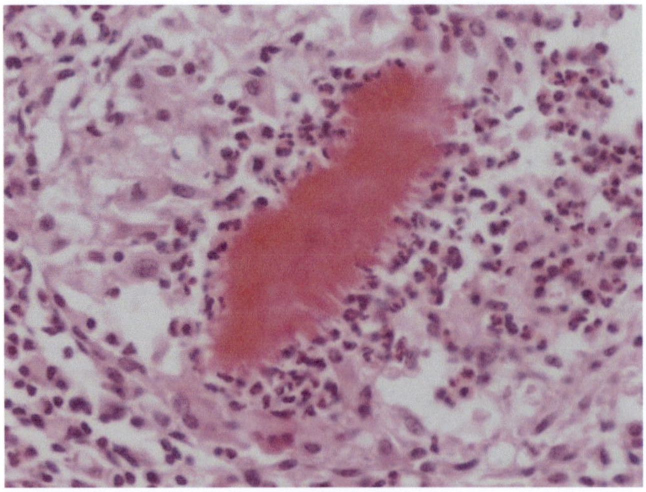

Fig. 4.38 Granulomatous inflammation. Bovine actinomycete granuloma: actinomycete mass and numerous neutrophils are present at the center of the lesion with epithelioid cells and individual giant cells at the periphery. HE ×400. (Wang Wenhui)

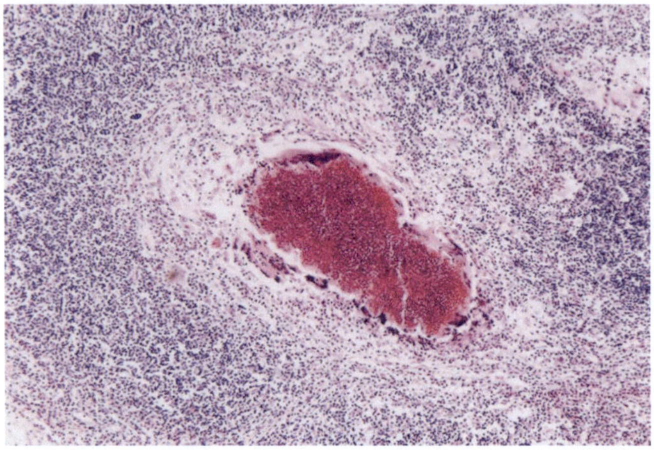

Fig. 4.39 Granulomatous inflammation. Parasitic granuloma (foreign-body granuloma): granuloma on the colon wall of the sick sheep caused by oesophagostomum. The oesophagostomum larvae remain at the center of the lesion, surrounded by foreign-body giant cells and lightly stained epithelioid cells, numerous lymphocytes and eosinophils in the outermost part. HE ×100. (Chen Huaitao)

Bibliography

1. Pulin L, editor. Animal pathology. Changchun: Jilin Science and Technology Press; 1994.
2. Puhui D, editor. Animal cytopathology. Beijing: China Agricultural Press; 1997.

5 Tumors

1 Tumors of Mesenchymal Tissue

1.1 Fibroma (Figs. 5.1, 5.2, 5.3, 5.4, 5.5, 5.6, 5.7, and 5.8)

Fibromata are benign tumors that occur in fibrinous connective tissue and are composed primarily of dense, mature fibroblasts, and collagen fibers. They are similar in morphology and stainability with normal fibroblasts and collagen fibers, but different in number and arrangement. Fibromata are more common in domestic animals and poultry, and it can occur wherever connective tissue is present, mostly in the subcutaneous, submucosal, intermuscular, fascial, and periosteal areas. Fibromata are more common in equines.

1.2 Fibrosarcoma (Figs. 5.9, 5.10, and 5.11)

Fibrosarcoma is a bounded or infiltrative malignant tumor of fibrous connective tissue, consisting of collagenous fibers, reticular fibers, and tumor cells. Its structure is similar to that

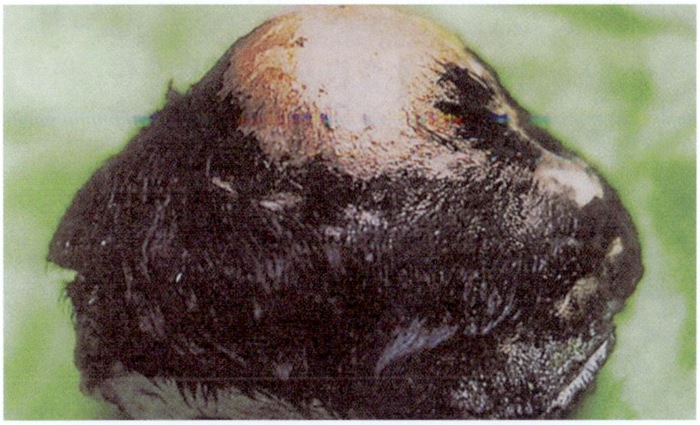

Fig. 5.1 Fibroma. Subcutaneous fibroma: a solitary large fibroma, which is protruding from the skin with no hair on the surface due to friction. (Chen Huaitao)

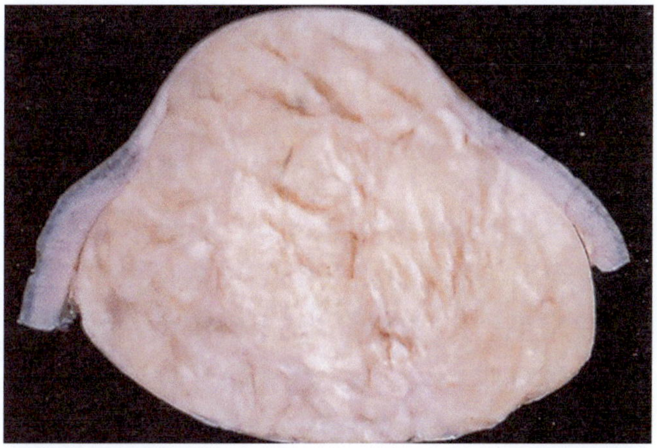

Fig. 5.2 Fibroma. Section of bovine subcutaneous fibroma, which is grayish with hard texture and filiform structure. The skin at the protruding area is thinned due to the pressure. (Chen Huaitao)

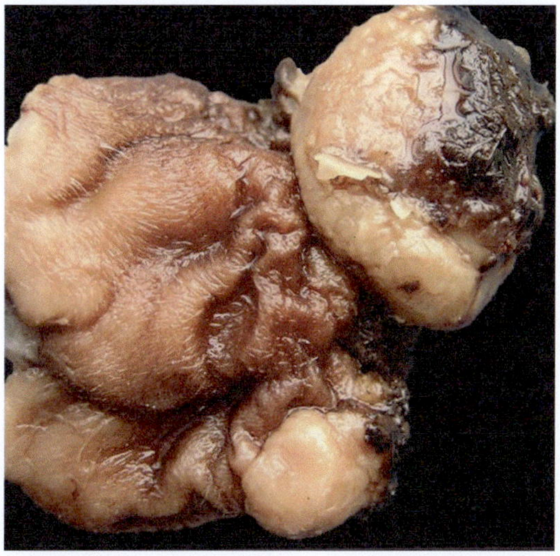

Fig. 5.3 Fibroma. Porcine subcutaneous fibroma: The tumor is nodular and hard, protruding from the skin surface, with localized skin hemorrhage and necrosis. (Chen Huaitao)

H. Chen, *Color Atlas of Veterinary Pathology*, https://doi.org/10.1007/978-981-96-7617-0_5

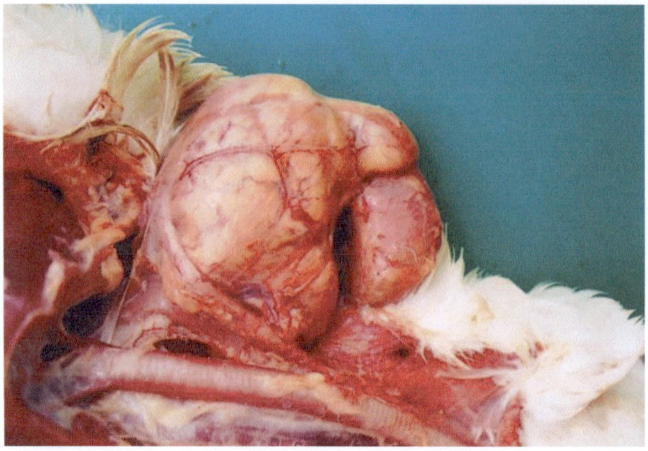

Fig. 5.4 Fibroma. Subcutaneous fibroma on the neck of the Muscovy duck: the tumor is large with lobulation. (Yao Jinshui)

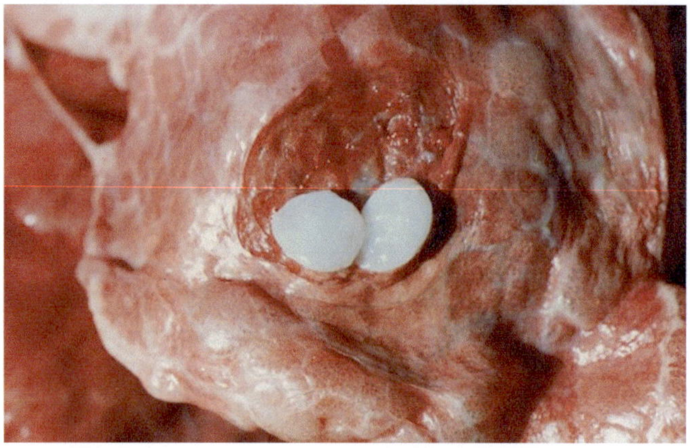

Fig. 5.5 Fibroma. Lung fibroma of Bactrian camel: the tumor is nodular, hard, grayish, and moist on the cut surface. (Chen Huaitao, Jia Ning)

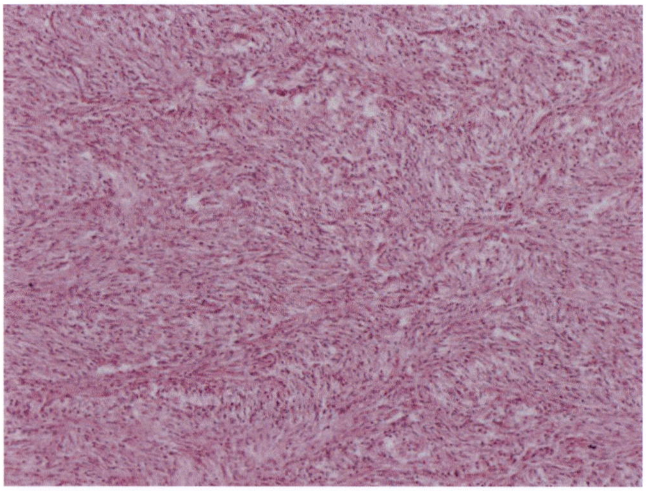

Fig. 5.6 Fibroma. The histology of fibroma is similar to that of fibrous connective tissue, but the arrangement of tumor cells and collagen fibers is irregular, which is either in a fascicle-like arrangement extending in one direction or in a swirling arrangement. A few small blood vessels are distributed in the interstitium. HE ×100. (Wang Wenhui)

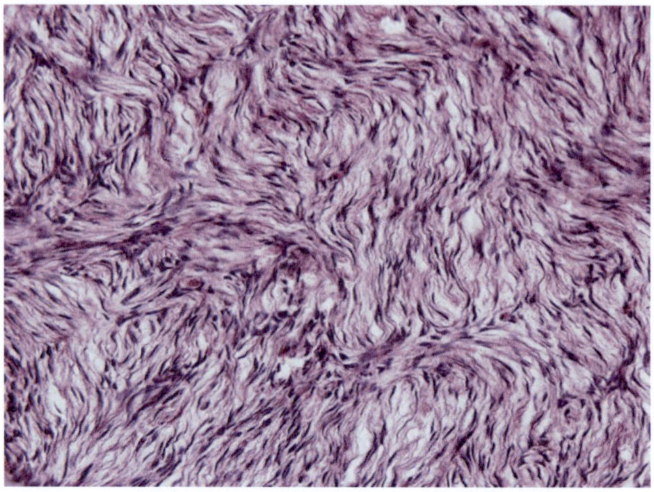

Fig. 5.7 Fibroma. Subcutaneous fibroma of the external genitalia of a male donkey: the collagen fibers are abundant. The fibers and tumor cells interlaced in bundles or arranged in a whirlpool pattern, and the tumor tissue is dense. HE ×400. (Chen Huaitao)

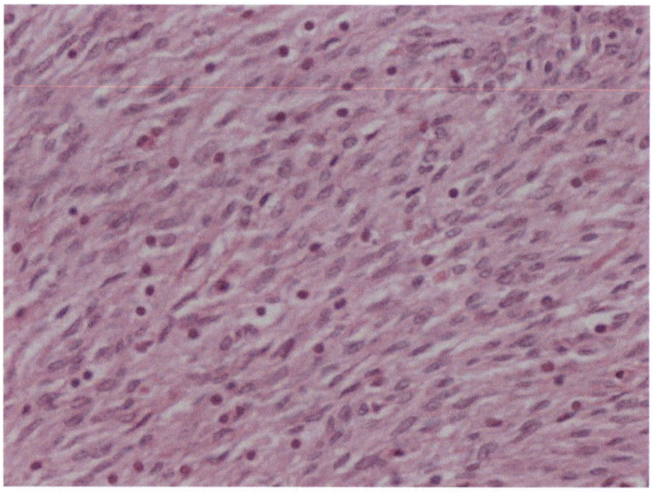

Fig. 5.8 Fibroma. Tumor cells are numerous, large in size and spindle-shaped, with few collagen fibers; lymphocytes are scattered among the tumor tissues. HE ×400. (Wang Wenhui)

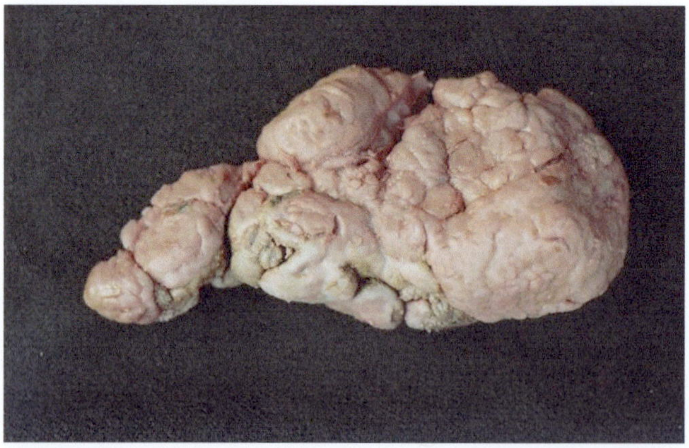

Fig. 5.9 Fibrosarcoma. Mule fibrosarcoma: it usually presents in multiple growth with marked surface hemorrhage and necrosis. (Chen Huaitao)

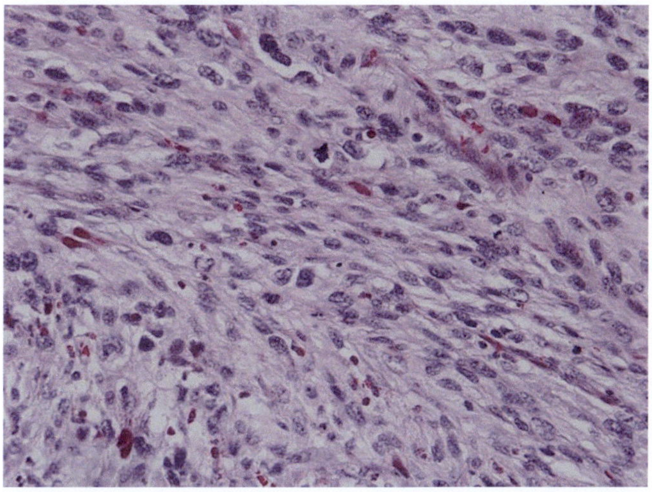

Fig. 5.10 Fibrosarcoma. Histology of fibrosarcoma: the histology is similar to fibroma, but the tumor cells are predominantly spindle-shaped with greater heterogeneity and more mitotic figs. HE ×400. (Chen Huaitao)

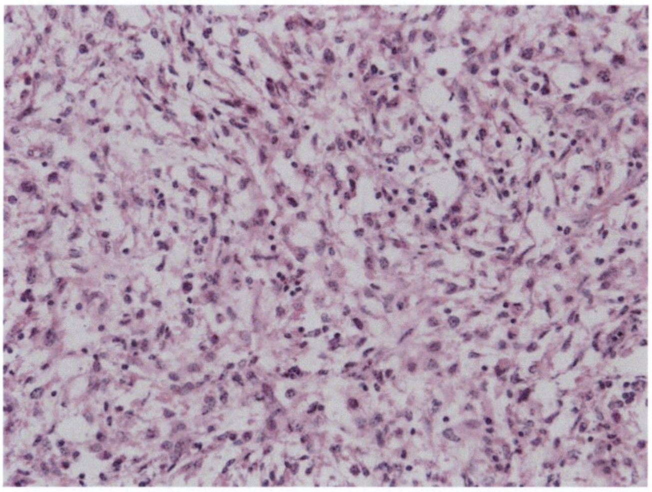

Fig. 5.11 Fibrosarcoma. Fibrosarcoma of the bovine bladder: tumor cells vary in size, but most of them are spindle-shaped, with more mitotic figures and inflammatory cell infiltration. HE ×400. (Chen Keyi)

of fibroma, but with a predominance of spindle-shaped cells. The close relationship of the cells to the reticular fibers is an important characteristics. Fibrosarcomas in domestic animals are generally less malignant.

1.3 Sarcomatoid (Sarcoid) (Figs. 5.12, 5.13, and 5.14)

Sarcoid is fibrosarcoma-like tumor that may be cause by viral infection. It often affects the skin of horses and cattle at the base of the ear or elsewhere, mostly in multiple, being like papilloma. There are usually ulcers on the surface. They

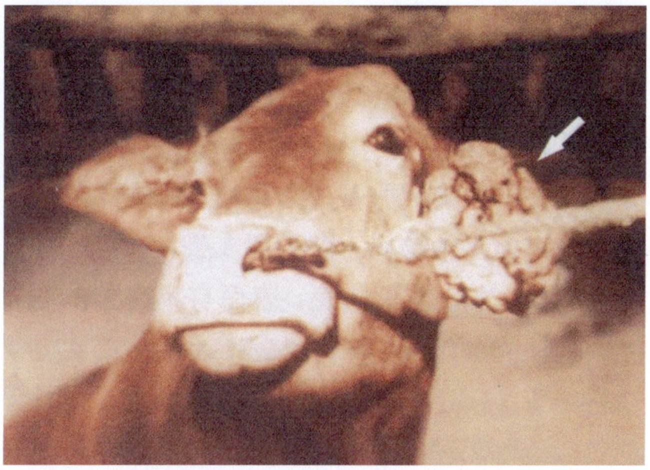

Fig. 5.12 Sarcomatoid tumor. Dermal sarcoid at the bovine ear root: dermal sarcoid is present on the ventral surface of both ears in the yellow cattle, with a large nodular mass in clusters on the left ear. (Chen Keyi)

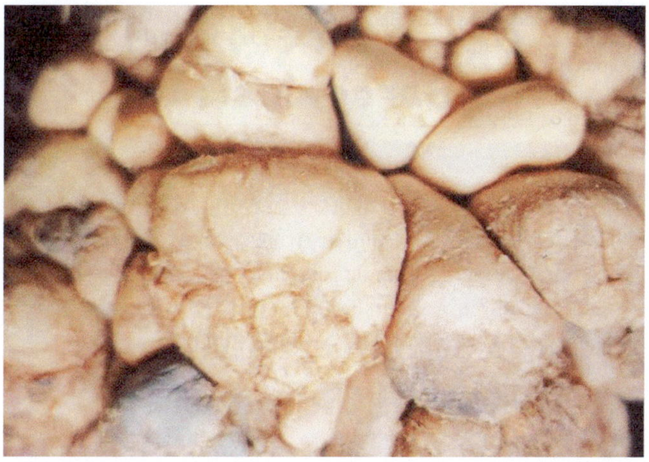

Fig. 5.13 Sarcomatoid tumor. Bovine cutaneous sarcoid: large, multiple tumors are present on the skin of a yellow cow, weighing up to 1325 g with a thick gray-brown keratinous "crust." (Chen Keyi)

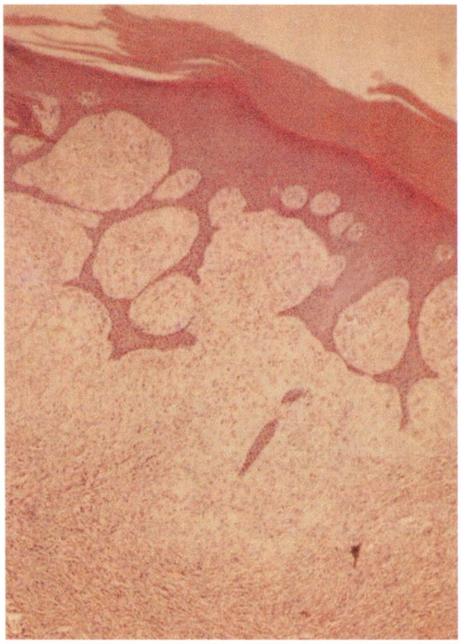

Fig. 5.14 Sarcomatoid tumor. Histology of bovine cutaneous sarcoid: it is similar to that of fibrosarcoma, but the epidermal hyperplasia is obvious with the basal layer of the epidermis growing deeper in a striated pattern, forming a "net peg," under which there are numerous tumor cells. HE ×80. (Chen Keyi)

tend to recur after excision, but do not metastasize. Histologically, they are similar to fibrosarcoma, but the skin epidermis overlying the sarcoid also grows markedly and extends into the fibrous mass like a reticulated peg.

1.4 Myxoma (Figs. 5.15 and 5.16)

Myxoma is a benign tumor derived from intrinsic connective tissue and it occurs in cattle, horses, mules, rabbits, and dogs. It is characterized by a large amount of mucus-like material in the interstitium, mainly composed of hyaluronic acid, and tumor cells derived from fibroblasts that have undergone degenerative changes.

1.5 Lipoma (Figs. 5.17, 5.18, 5.19, and 5.20)

Lipoma is benign tumor composed of mature fat cells, and most of the tumors are unencapsulated and poorly defined. Strips of connective tissue are sometimes observed in the tumor, and areas of necrosis and dystrophic calcifications are present in larger tumors, which can also progress into mucinous changes.

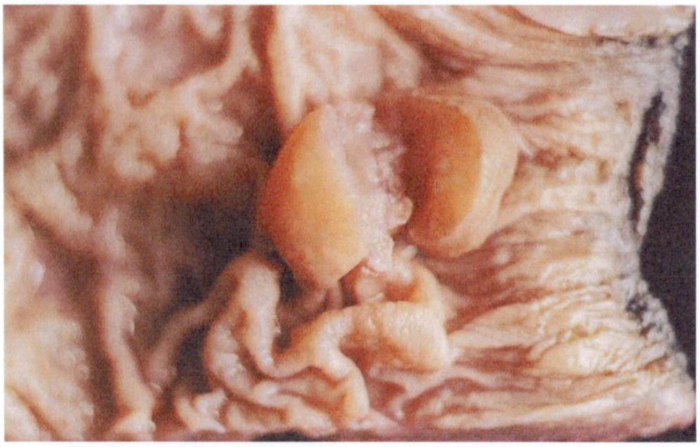

Fig. 5.15 Myxoma. Bovine rectal myxoma: the tumor is soft and well defined with yellowish, semi-translucent, and moist cutting surface. (Chen Huaitao)

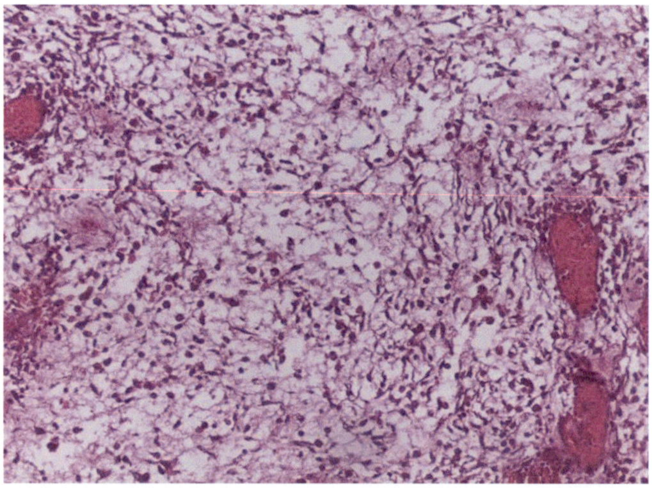

Fig. 5.16 Myxoma. Histological structure of myxoma: vascular congestion, a large amount of mucoid substance between tumor cells, sparse tumor cells, spindle or polygonal. HE ×200. (Hu Haixia)

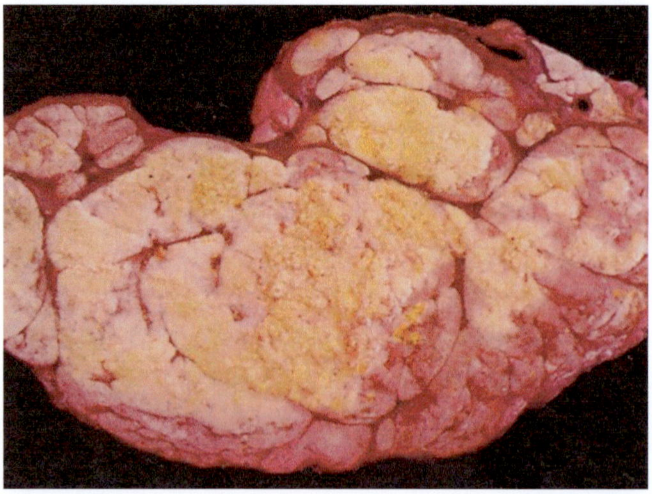

Fig. 5.17 Lipoma. Bovine lipoma: tumor section is yellowish in color and lobulated. (Chen Huaitao)

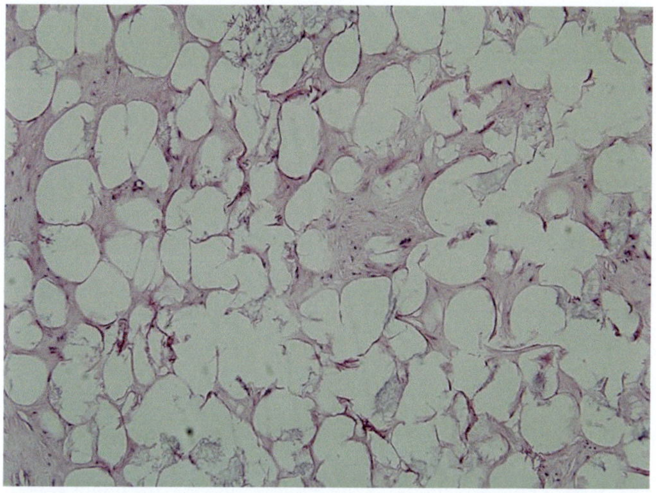

Fig. 5.18 Lipoma. Histology of bovine lipoma: it is similar to normal adipose tissue with localized connective tissue strips. HE ×100. (Chen Huaitao)

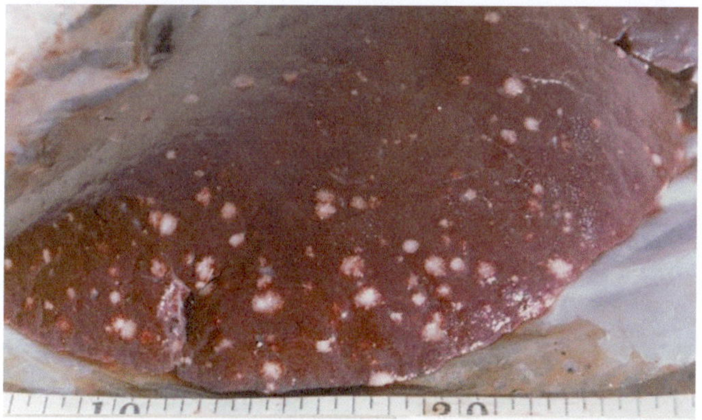

Fig. 5.19 Lipoma. Diffuse lipoma in the camel's liver: the tumor is nodular in size, hard, grayish, and well defined. (Chen Huaitao, Chen Hualan)

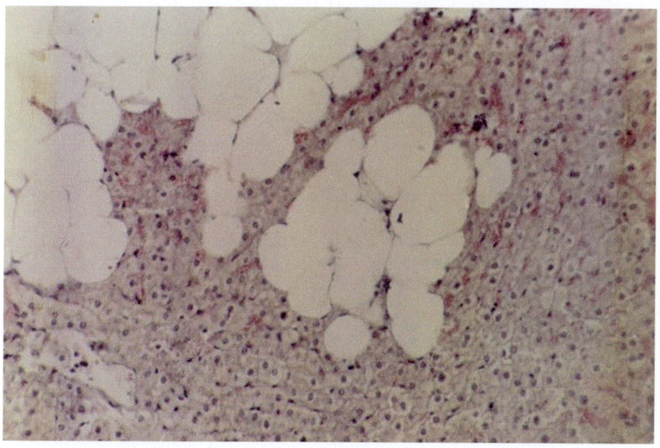

Fig. 5.20 Lipoma. Histology of camel liver lipoma: tumor cells resemble adipocytes, are arranged in clumps, and clearly delineated from surrounding liver tissue. HE ×400. (Chen Huaitao, Chen Hualan)

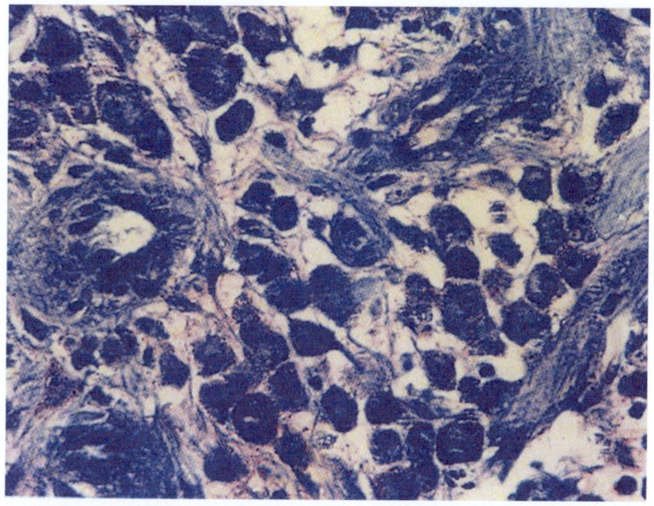

Fig. 5.21 Mastocytoma. Canine mastocytoma: tumor cells are distributed in clusters, and basophilic granules are present in cytoplasm. Mast cell staining method ×400. (Liu Baoyan et al.)

1.6 Mastocytoma (Mast Cell Tumor) (Fig. 5.21)

Mastocytoma is a malignant tumor and is the most common canine skin mesenchymal tumor; it also occurs in swine, but it is rare in other domestic animals. The tumor often occurs in the skin or viscera. Histologically, the tumor consists of differentially differentiated mast cells that are round, oval, polygonal, or narrow in shape with oval nuclei. Poorly differentiated tumors may appear as multinucleated, bizarre cells.

1.7 Leiomyoma (Figs. 5.22 and 5.23)

Leiomyoma is a benign tumor composed of mature smooth muscle cells with variable amount of collagen formation in the tumor tissue (the collagen is abundant in some cases). The tumor cells are characterized by an elongated striped shape with a rod-shaped nucleus and non-striated myogenic fibers in cytoplasm.

1.8 Leiomyosarcoma (Figs. 5.24 and 5.25)

This is a malignant tumor of smooth muscle tissue, consisting of long spindle-shaped cells. A variable amount of non-striated myogenic fibers are present in cytoplasm, and perinuclear translucent gaps are often observed. The cells are often cross-linked in bundles. The cells are more in number than in the leiomyoma, and the tumor giant cells as well as mitotic figures can be observed.

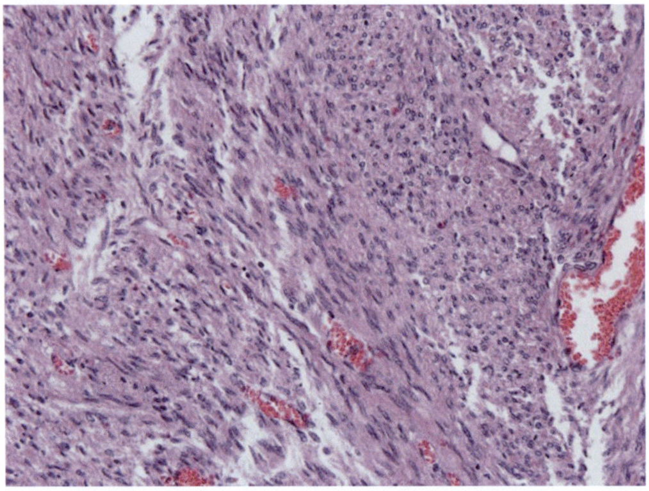

Fig. 5.22 Leiomyoma. Bovine leiomyoma: tumor cells are long and striped, with abundant cytoplasm and similar morphology to normal smooth muscle fibers, but the cells are more disarranged. HE ×400. (Chen Huaitao)

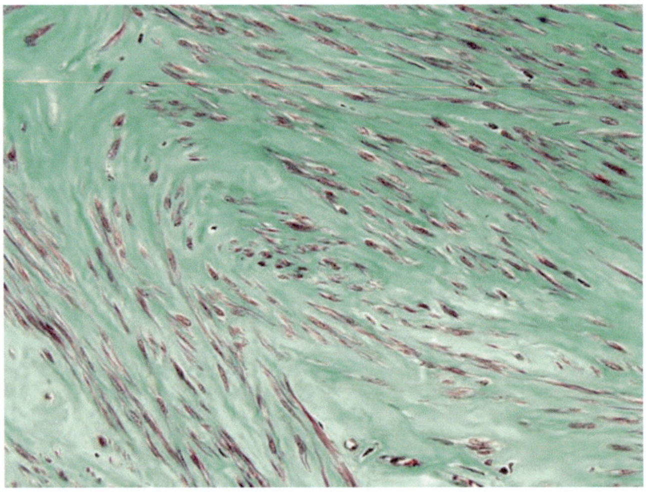

Fig. 5.23 Leiomyoma. The heterogeneity of the tumor cells is low, which is similar to the smooth muscle fibers. The tumor cells are long shuttle-shaped, located among collagen fibers; the collagen fibers are stained green, and the muscle fibers are stained red, and the nuclei are blue. Masson's modified trichrome stain ×400. (Gansu Agricultural University, Veterinary Pathology Laboratory)

1.9 Rhabdomyoma (Fig. 5.26)

This is a relatively rare benign tumor consisting of syncytial cells with pale stained and foamy nuclei. The cytoplasm is eosinophilic and often vacuolated due to the presence of glycogen. The striated cells are pretty common.

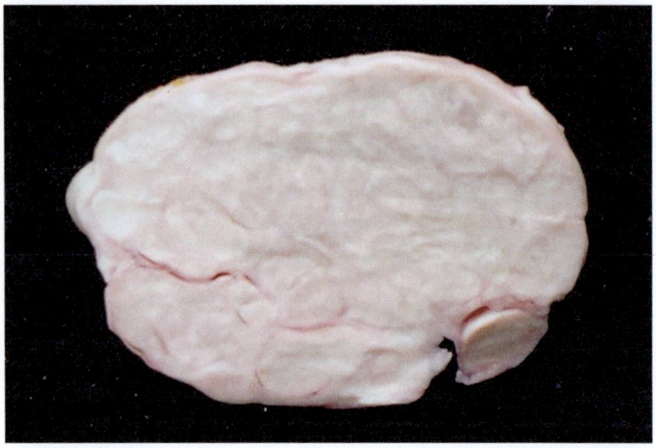

Fig. 5.24 Leiomyosarcoma. Mule leiomyosarcoma: the tumor is nodular, hard, and pale red in section, with is lobulated into several lobes by connective tissue. (Chen Huaitao)

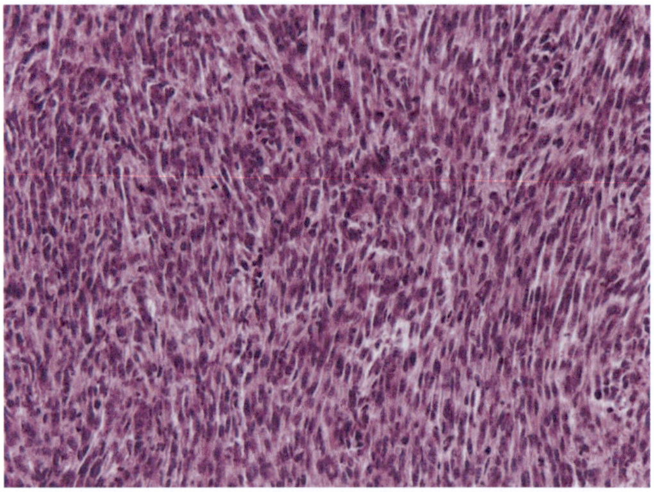

Fig. 5.25 Leiomyosarcoma. Histological structure of leiomyosarcoma: the histological structure is similar to leiomyoma, but the arrangement is more disorganized. The tumor cells are more heterogeneous with mitotic figs. HE ×400. (Chen Huaitao)

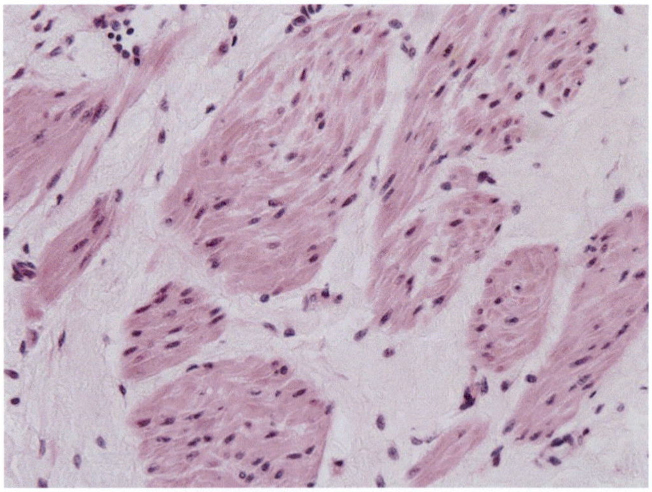

Fig. 5.26 Rhabdomyoma. Tumor cells are rich in cytoplasm, unevenly stained with visible striation, and there are plenty of collagen fibers in the tumor tissue. HE ×400. (Veterinary Pathology Unit, Gansu Agricultural University)

1.10 Hemangioma

Hemangiomata are a group of benign tumors consisting of different types of proliferating blood vessels, and the tumors are poorly boundaried.

1.10.1 Capillary Hemangioma (Fig. 5.27)

1.10.2 Cavernous Hemangioma (Figs. 5.28 and 5.29)

1.11 Hemangiosarcoma (Figs. 5.30 and 5.31)

Hemangiosarcoma originates from vascular endothelial cells; hence, it is also named hemangioendotheliosarcoma or malignant hemangioendothelioma. This tumor is highly

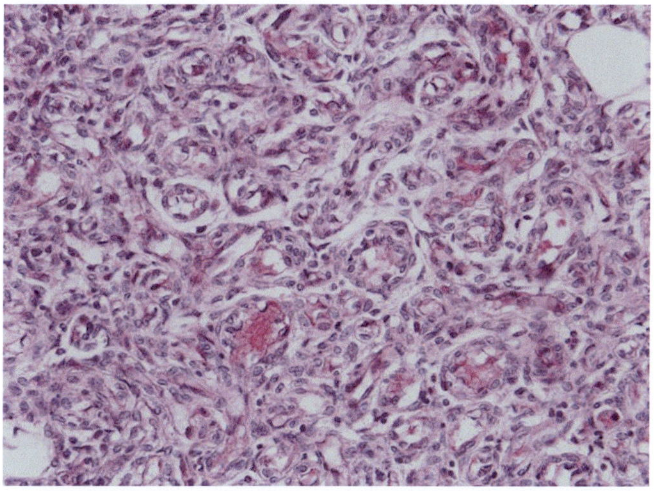

Fig. 5.27 Capillary hemangioma. The tumor tissue consists of abnormally proliferating capillaries. HE ×400. (Chen Huaitao)

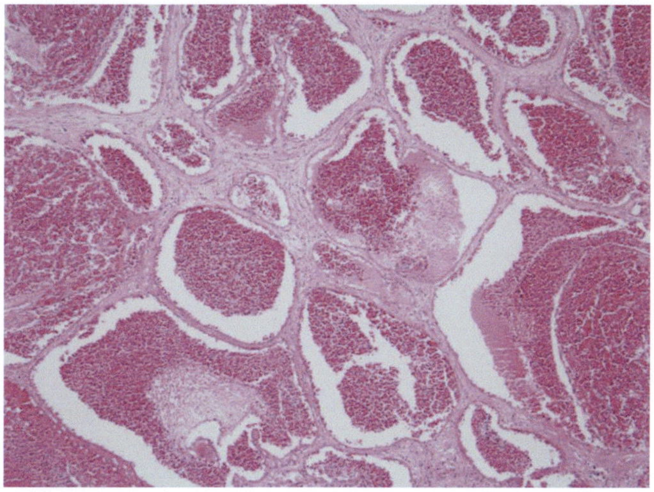

Fig. 5.28 Cavernous hemangioma. The tumor tissue consists of dilated blood sinuses of variable sizes, the walls of which are lined with flattened epithelium, the lumen is often filled with red blood cells, and there is variable amount of connective tissue among the sinuses. HE ×100. (Chen Huaitao)

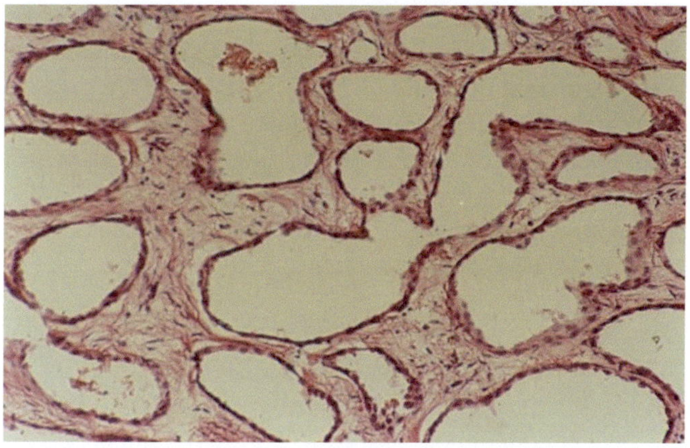

Fig. 5.29 Bovine cavernous hemangioma. The structure is similar to that of Fig. 5.28, but the sinus lumen of the vessels are mostly empty due to blood loss. HE ×200. (Chen Huaitao)

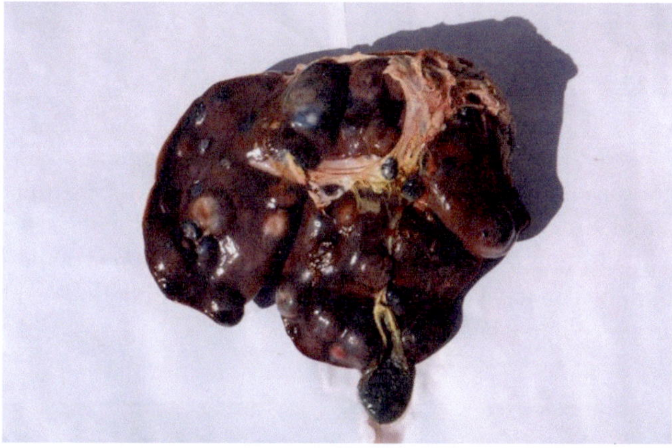

Fig. 5.30 Hemangiosarcoma. Hemangiosarcoma of the sheep liver: grayish or blackish-red tumor nodules of varying sizes are present on the surface of the liver, usually with depressions at the center of larger nodules. (Chen Huaitao, Haas)

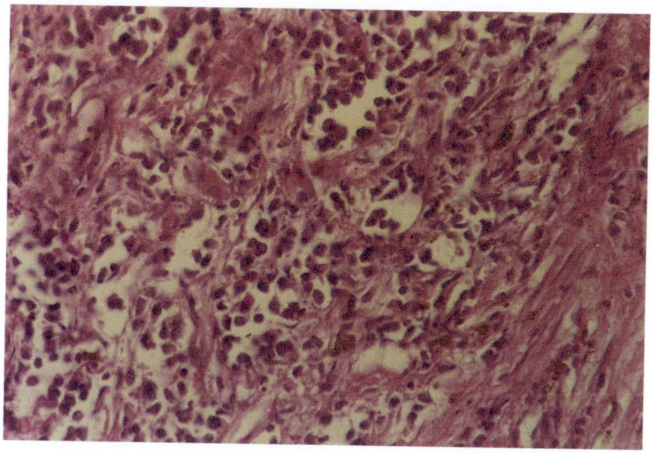

Fig. 5.31 Hemangiosarcoma. Hemangiosarcoma of the sheep liver: the hepatic sinusoid endothelial cells show malignant proliferation, with high atypia of tumor cells, some of which grow toward the lumen of the vessels or even into the lumen. The vessels are in different sizes with irregular lumen and small amount of connective tissue among the vessels. HE ×400. (Chen Huaitao)

malignant and is histologically characterized by irregular anastomosis of vessels with each other. The vessels are lined with single or multiple layers of atypical pleomorphic endothelial cells. There are gaps made up of the malignant endothelial cells in some areas in the tumor tissue, in which erythrocytes are present, based on which the diagnosis can be made. There are many mitotic figures. Angiosarcomas often metastasize to various organs.

1.12 Lymphangioma (Fig. 5.32)

This is a benign tumor consisting entirely of lymphatic vessels of variable sizes lined with a single layer of endothelial cells, which may be classified as capillary, spongy, or cystic types. Congenital lymphangiomas (malformations) occur in both domestic animals and humans.

1.13 Mesothelioma (Figs. 5.33 and 5.34)

Mesothelioma is a benign tumor originating from pleural or peritoneal mesothelial cells. It appears as solitary or multiple nodular or wrinkled tumor without infiltration or metastasis, and the tumor cells are often spindle-shaped, resembling fibrous connective tissue, and some are epithelioid and arranged into islands.

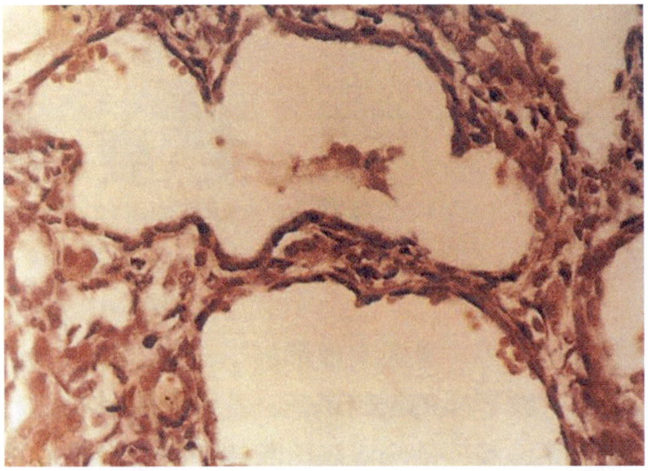

Fig. 5.32 Lymphangioleioma. Hepatic lymphadenoma in sheep: the tumor tissue consists of many cystic cavities of similar size and irregular morphology to lymphatic vessels, with interstitial connective tissue containing blood vessels. HE ×400. (Liu Baoyan et al.)

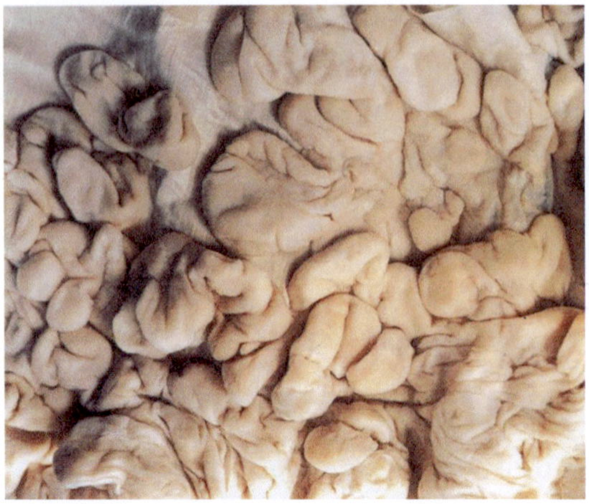

Fig. 5.33 Mesothelioma. Bovine pleural mesothelioma: tumors grow in wrinkled patterns with soft texture and irregular shape. (Xue Dengmin)

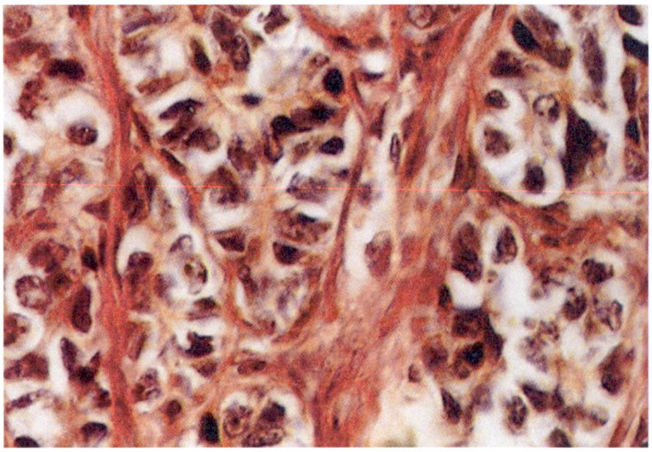

Fig. 5.34 Mesothelioma. Mesothelioma of chicken intestine: tumor cells are rectangular or polygonal, with large and deeply stained nuclei, divided by mesenchyme into glandular vesicle-like or island-like structures. van Gieson ×400. (Li Baoyan et al.)

2 Tumors of Systems

2.1 Tumors of the Nervous System

2.1.1 Glioma

2.1.1.1 Astrocytoma (Fig. 5.35)

The tumor originates from astrocytes and is more common in dogs, cats, and cattle, and although they can occur in any part of the central nervous system, they are more commonly observed in the cerebral hemisphere of dogs.

2.1.1.2 Oligodendroglioma (Fig. 5.36)

This tumor originates from oligodendrocytes and commonly occurs in dogs. This tumor is mostly located in the frontal and pyriform lobes of the cerebral hemispheres and originates in the white matter.

2.1.2 Neurofibroma (Fig. 5.37)

Neurofibromata are benign tumors that occur from connective tissue cells of the perineurium and therefore all contain a connective tissue component. In the tumor tissue, the tumor cells are arranged outwardly with the nerve fibers or nerve bundles in the center, so there will be areas that are primarily neurilemmomata, or sections that are primarily like fibromata. Tumors can occur in cerebral nerves, spinal nerve roots, spinal ganglia, and peripheral as well as sympathetic nerves. It commonly occurs in cattle and cats.

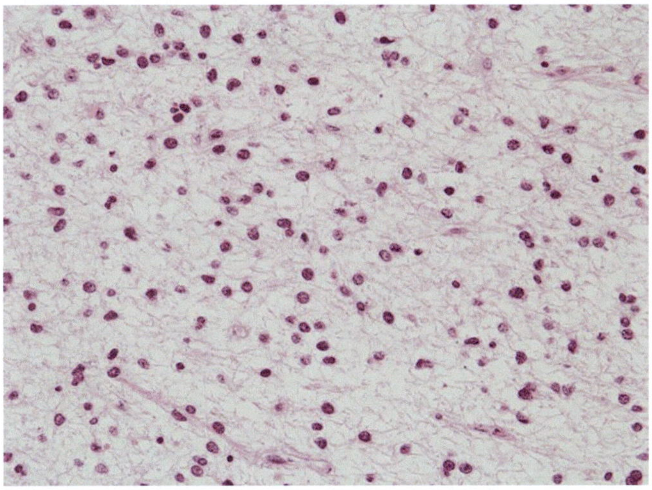

Fig. 5.35 Astrocytoma. Canine brain astrocytoma: tumor cells are relatively well differentiated, loosely arranged with small size, large nuclei, mostly round or oval, darkly stained. Glial fibers are rich. HE ×400. (Veterinary Pathology Unit, Gansu Agricultural University)

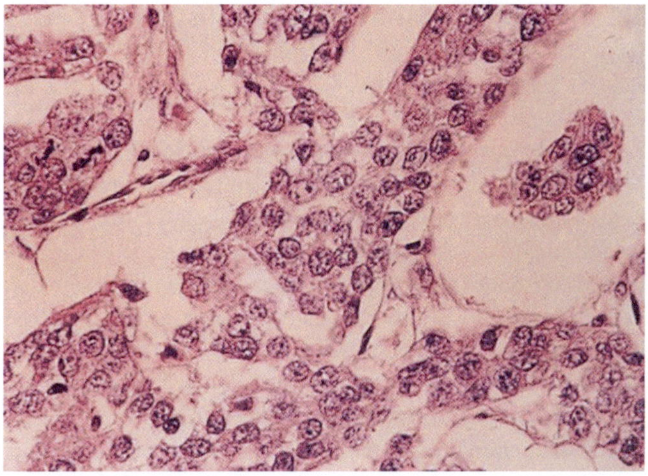

Fig. 5.36 Oligodendroglioma. Canine cerebral oligodendroglioma: tumor cells aggregated into nests, with basically similar cell size in round or polygonal shape, densely arranged. The nuclei are round, deeply stained, with a perinuclear bright ring for each cell, resembling a honeycomb structure. HE ×400. (Liu Baoyan et al.)

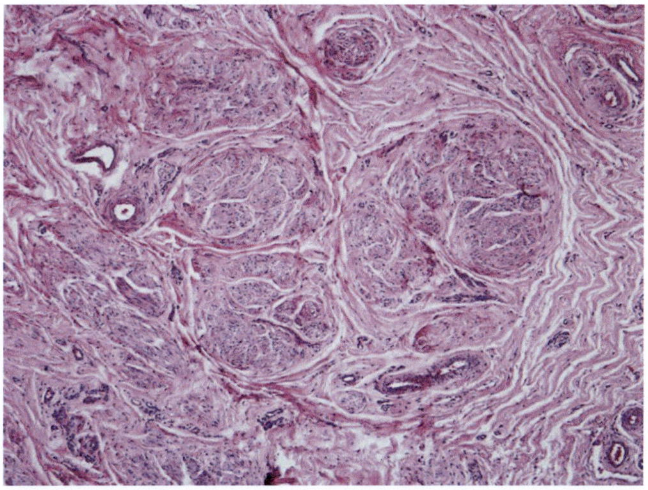

Fig. 5.37 Neurofibroma. This image shows that the tumor cells originated from the nerve bundle membrane cells. The tumor cells are heavily proliferated and interspersed with each other, in which the nerve bundle is visible across. HE ×100. (Chen Huaitao)

2.2 Tumors of the Endocrine System

2.2.1 Adrenal Tumors

2.2.1.1 Adrenal Cortical Adenoma (Fig. 5.38)

This is a benign tumor that occurs mainly in cattle and older dogs. The tumor varies in size from small ones buried only in the adrenal gland to large ones that may protrude to the surface. The tumor tissue is yellowish in color and calcium salt deposits often occur; necrosis and hemorrhage are observed in larger cases.

2.2.1.2 Adrenal Cortical Carcinoma (Fig. 5.39)

This is a malignant tumor that occurs in the adrenal cortex occasionally in cattle and older dogs. The adrenal gland with cancer is markedly enlarged and brittle, often with cyst, hemorrhage, necrosis, and calcium-salt deposition in the tumor. The tumor cells are prone to invade surrounding tissues and the posterior vena cava as well as metastasize to other organs.

2.2.2 Thyroid Tumors

2.2.2.1 Thyroid Adenoma (Figs. 5.40 and 5.41)

Thyroid adenomata are benign tumors originating from the epithelial cells of the thyroid follicles in dogs, cats, cattle, and horses. The tumors are generally small, nodular, white, or yellowish in color, with a distinct capsule, well-defined, and solid texture. Histologically, they can be classified into follicular adenomata and papillary adenomata.

2.2.2.2 Thyroid Carcinoma (Figs. 5.42 and 5.43)

It is a malignant tumor originating from the follicular epithelium of the thyroid gland and can occur in dogs, cats, and

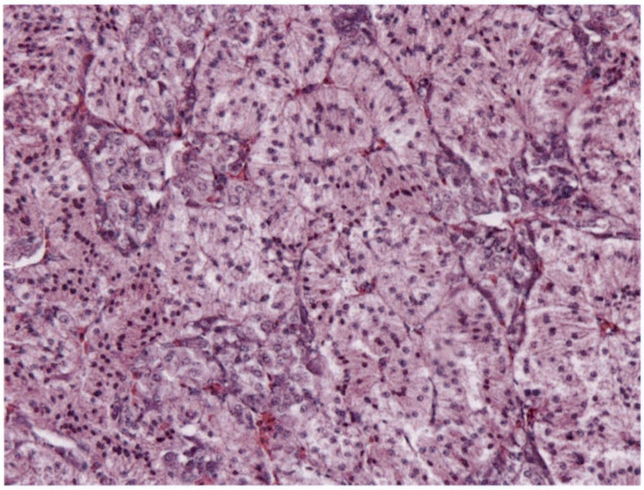

Fig. 5.38 Adrenal cortical adenoma. Tumor cells are similar to the adrenal cortex cells, in cords or high column, with abundant cytoplasm, light eosin staining. Tumor cells are often arranged in adenoid or clusters, interspersed with blood vessels and fibers. HE ×200. (Veterinary Pathology Unit, Gansu Agricultural University)

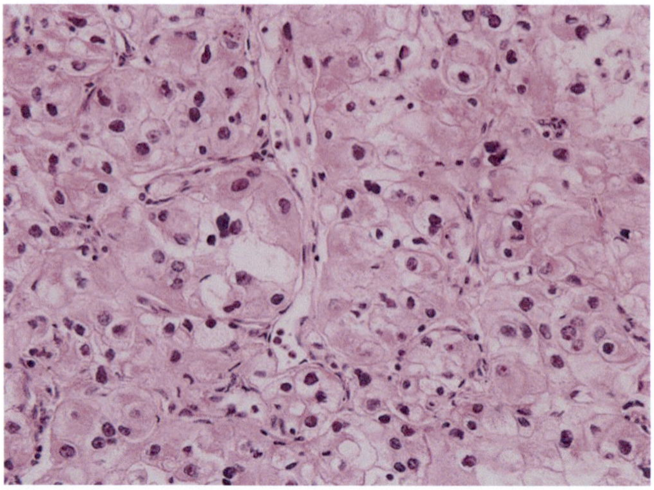

Fig. 5.39 Adrenal cortical carcinoma. The tumor cells are large in size, polygonal in shape, with cytoplasm lightly stained and even vacuolated. The cellular atypism is high and the nuclei are vesicular, with obvious mitotic fig. HE ×400. (Veterinary Pathology Department, Gansu Agricultural University)

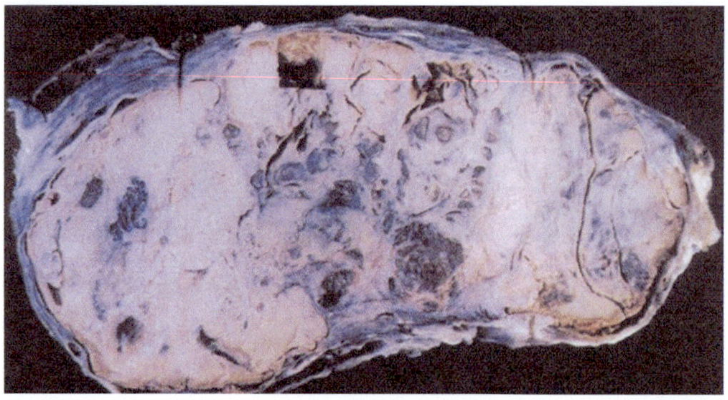

Fig. 5.40 Thyroid adenoma. Bovine thyroid adenoma: well-defined tumor with capsule, on the cut surface of which the areas of hemorrhage and necrosis are present. (Xue Dengmin)

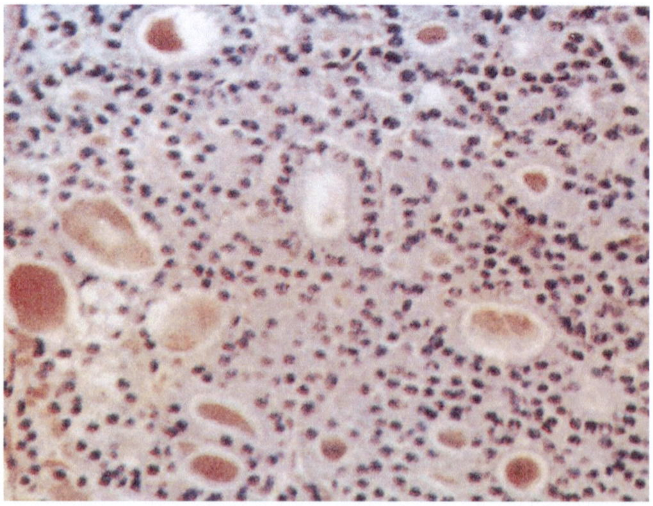

Fig. 5.41 Thyroid adenoma. The tumor tissue is mainly composed of acinus of varying sizes, the epithelium of the vesicles is mostly cuboidal, with a relatively uniform morphology, often without mitotic figures. Many vesicle lumens are filled with secretions. But solid structures can also be observed. HE ×200. (Xue Dengmin)

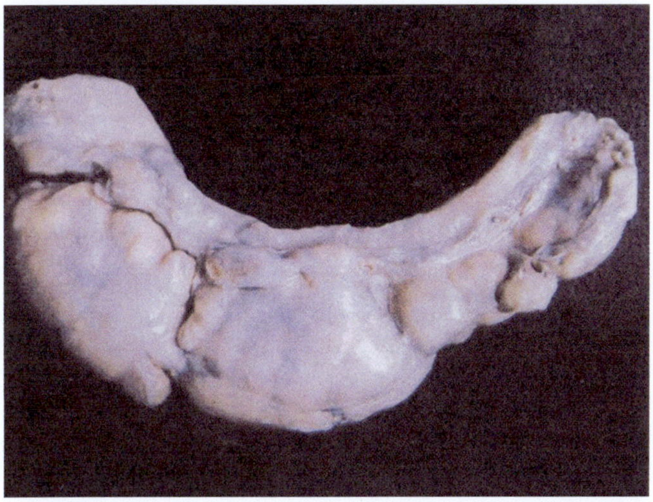

Fig. 5.42 Thyroid carcinoma. Enlarged bovine thyroid gland with yellowish-brown nodules of variable sizes present on the surface, not well circumscribed with a hard texture. (Xue Dengmin)

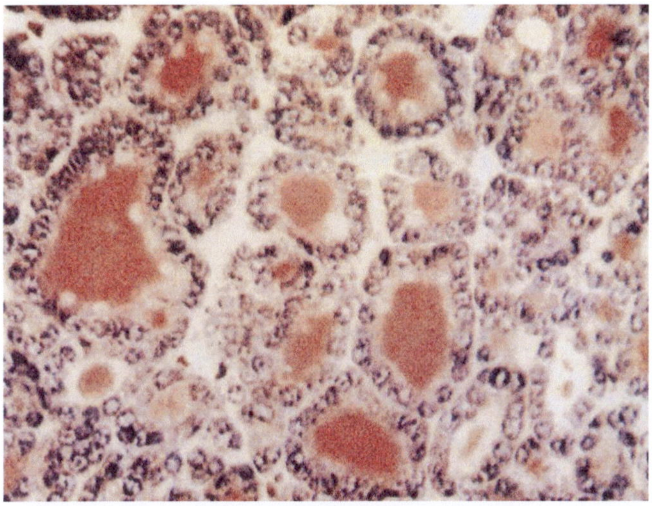

Fig. 5.43 Thyroid carcinoma. The carcinomatous tissue is mainly composed of acini of different sizes, and they were somewhat similar to those of the normal thyroid gland, but the epithelial cells of the acinus are actively mitotic, with vesicular nuclei and obvious mitotic figures; the lumen of the vesicles is filled with variable amount of colloid. HE ×200. (Xue Dengmin)

other animals. Metastasis to the lungs via the bloodstream is common in early stages, while lymph node metastasis is rare. The appearance of the tumor is similar to that of thyroid adenoma, but the capsule is often incomplete and tumor cells often infiltrate to the surrounding tissue with hemorrhage, necrosis, calcification, and cystic changes. According to the growth characteristics and degree of differentiation of cancer tissue, it can be classified into follicular carcinoma (malignant adenoma), solid carcinoma and solid-follicular carcinoma, papillary carcinoma, squamous cell carcinoma, and anaplastic (undifferentiated) tumor. Among these tumors, the solid and solid-follicular carcinomas are most often observed in dogs, while papillary adenocarcinomas occur most often in cats and humans, but they are rare in dogs.

2.2.3 Tumors of the Pancreas (Figs. 5.44, 5.45, and 5.46)

The pancreas histologically includes the pancreatic gland (exocrine division) and islets (endocrine division), both of which can develop adenomas and adenocarcinomas, more commonly in dogs and cats, but rarely in cattle, horses, sheep, and pigs. Pancreatic adenomas are nodular, encapsulated, and the ductal type is predominant, but the acinar type is rear in histology. Pancreatic adenomas are histologically classified into small ductal, large ductal, and glandular cell types with incomplete encapsules and metastases to the liver, local lymph nodes, as well as peripancreatic tissues before the onset of symptoms. Islet cell adenomas are usually small nodular in shape and can be histologically classified as giant islet, ribbon or trabecular, and rosette node types. Islet cell carcinoma shows a similar morphology to adenoma, but the cancer cells are denser with high atypism, and they invade nearby pancreatic parenchyma and metastasize.

A common tumor of the pancreas is adenocarcinoma of the pancreas.

2.3 Tumors of the Skin and Its Derivatives

2.3.1 Papilloma (Figs. 5.47, 5.48, 5.49, 5.50, and 5.51)

Cutaneous papillomas, also known as squamous cell tumors, are benign tumors that occur from squamous epithelium and can be caused by infectious agents (viruses) or non-infectious factors. Infectious ones occur in a variety of animals, including horses, cattle, sheep, rabbits, and dogs with multiple tumors, while non-infectious ones occur in dogs, laboratory animals, and other animals often with solitary tumor. Papillomas can occur on the skin all over the body, especially on the head, neck, chest, abdomen, breasts, vulva, lips, and limbs. The tumors are papillary, nodular, or cauliflower-headed and may be with pedicles and are well circumscribed. Histologically, the epidermis of the skin shows protruding growths, each protrusion being axially centered on connective tissue and covered with a thicker layer of less regularly arranged epidermis. Papillomas occurring on basal cells are called basal cell papilloma and are more common in dogs and cats, mostly solitary. The tumor cells are small, with little cytoplasm, and lack of intercellular bridges between tumor cells.

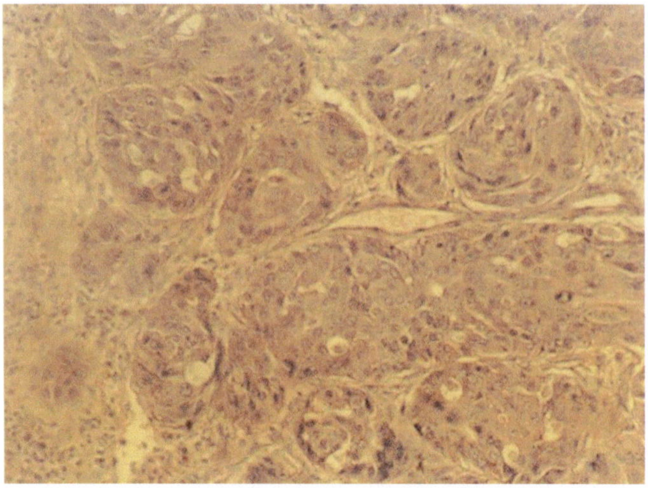

Fig. 5.44 Adenocarcinoma of the pancreas. Adenocarcinoma of the pancreas in yellow cattle: the cancer nests are in clusters of cells of varying sizes, without tubular structures, and the cancer nests are separated by a small amount of connective tissue. HE ×200. (Guangxi Nanning Meat Combined Processing Plant)

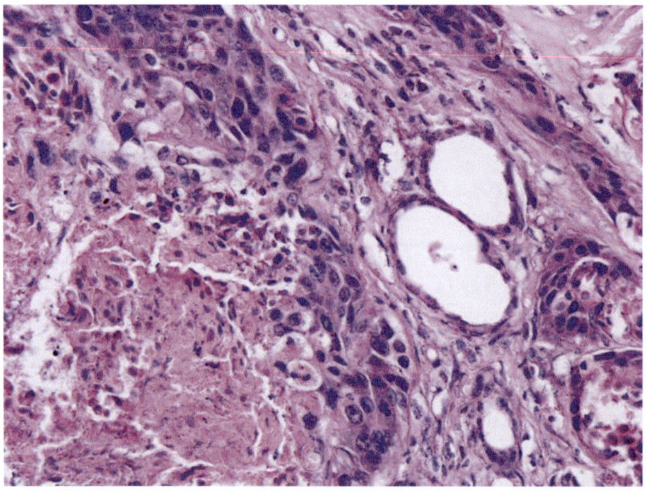

Fig. 5.45 Adenocarcinoma of the pancreas. Adenocarcinoma of pancreas in the yellow cattle: In addition to the mass nests, the glandular duct-like structures are present in the cancerous tissue. The carcinomatous cells are with high atypism, and the mitotic figures can be observed. Some cancer cells underwent necrosis. HE ×400. (Guangxi Nanning Meat Joint Processing Plant)

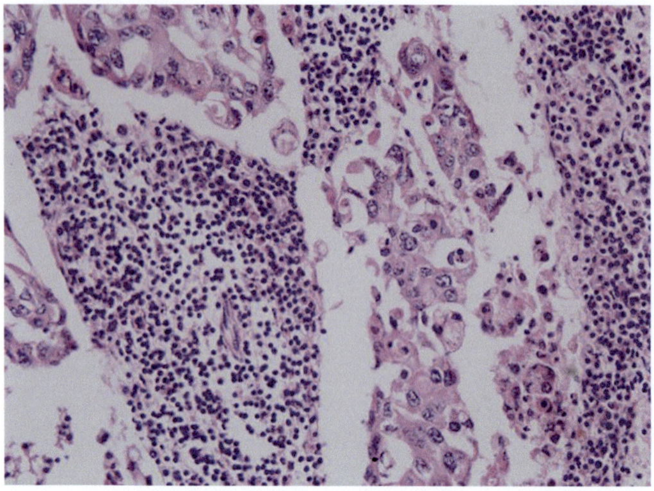

Fig. 5.46 Adenocarcinoma of the pancreas. Bovine mesenteric lymph nodes: A relatively large amount of metastatic pancreatic adenocarcinomatous cells are present in both the cortical and medullary lymph sinuses of the lymph nodes. HE ×400. (Guangxi Nanning Meat Combined Processing Plant)

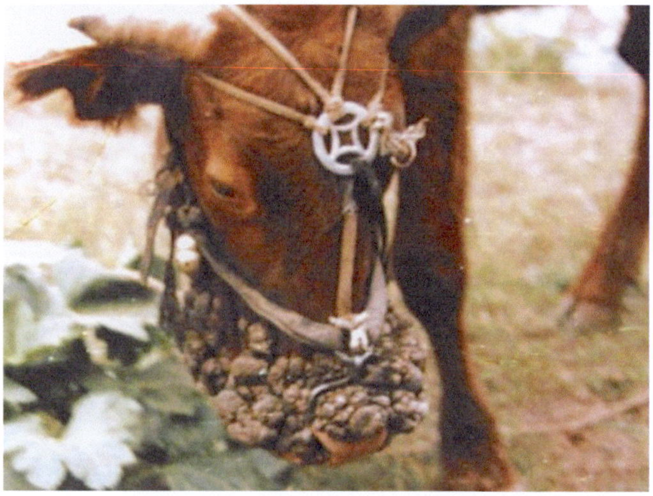

Fig. 5.47 Papilloma. Infectious papilloma on the cattle skin of the mouth and lips: a large number of cauliflower-like tumor nodules with a hard texture are present on the mouth and lips of the affected cattle. (Wang Xinhua)

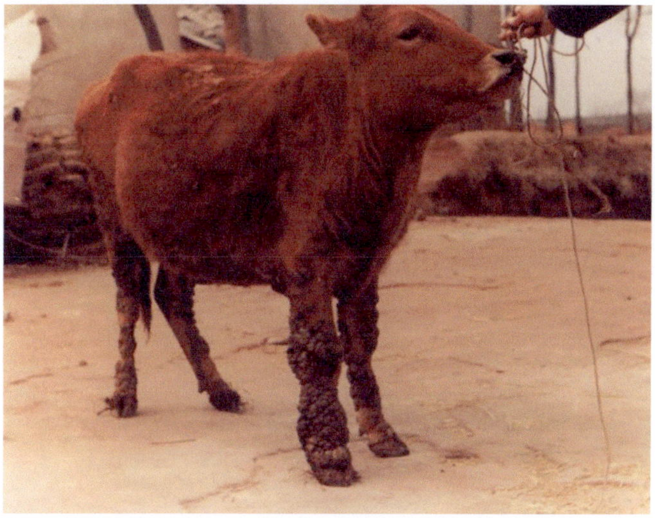

Fig. 5.48 Papilloma. Infectious papilloma on the skin of the extremities of the cattle: the skin of the extremities is almost covered with cauliflower-shaped or nodular papillomas. (Zhou Shiqi)

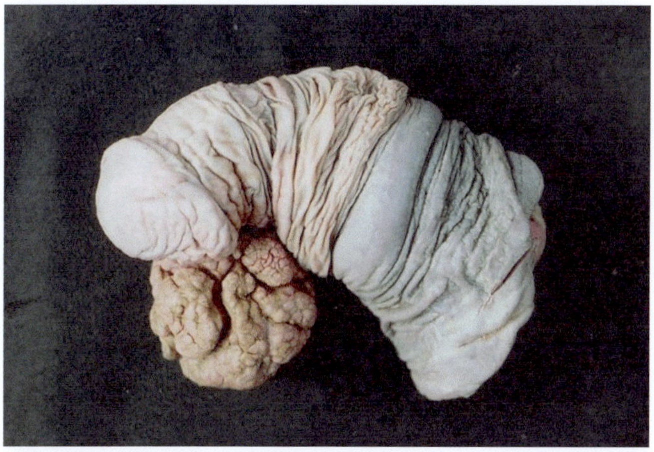

Fig. 5.49 Papilloma. Mule genital papilloma: a nodular tumor with hard texture is present on the glans foreskin, and its surface is uneven. (Veterinary Pathology Unit, Gansu Agricultural University)

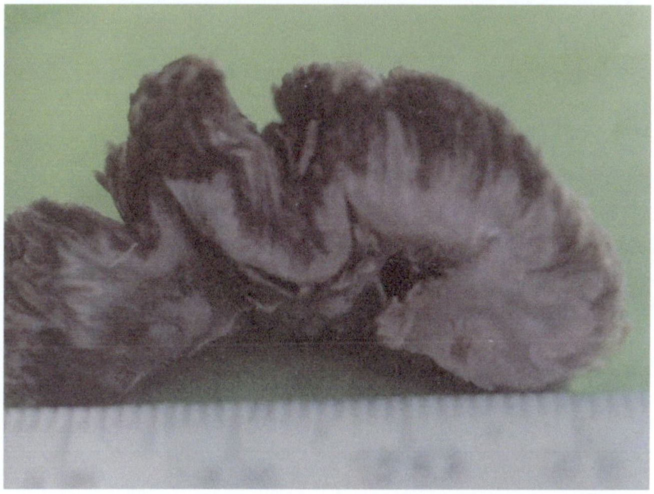

Fig. 5.50 Papilloma. The section of cutaneous papilloma in sheep: the skin grows outward and many protrusions are formed with obvious surface keratinization. (Veterinary Patholo gy Unit, Gansu Agricultural University)

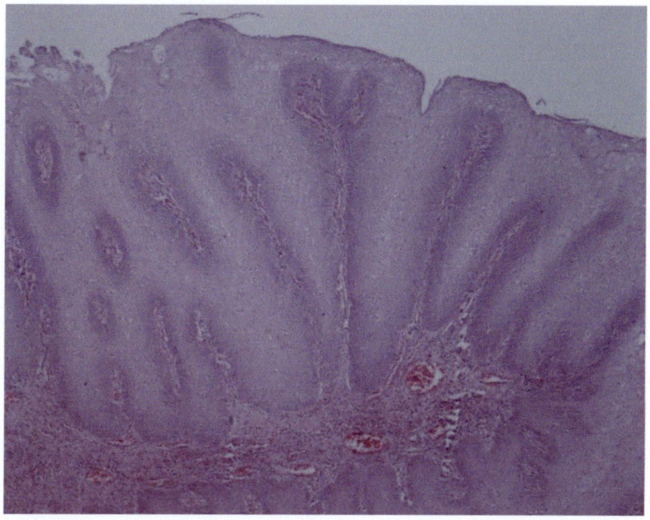

Fig. 5.51 Papilloma. Cutaneous papilloma: The tumor grows exophytically, forming finger-like protrusions of varying sizes, with connective tissue as its axis, and the peripheral tumor cells resemble the squamous epithelium of normal skin, but with marked proliferation and irregular arrangement. HE ×40. (Wang Wenhui)

2.3.2 Squamous Cell Carcinoma (Figs. 5.52, 5.53, 5.54, 5.55, 5.56, 5.57, 5.58, 5.59, 5.60, 5.61, 5.62, and 5.63)

Squamous cell carcinoma, also known as squamous epithelial carcinoma or epidermoid carcinoma, or simply squamous carcinoma, is a malignant tumor that occurs from squamous epithelial cells of the skin or skin-type mucosa. It can also occur on non-squamous epithelium (e.g., nasal, bronchial, uterine mucosa) after squamous epithelial metaplasia. It is common in older or adult horses, cattle, sheep, dogs, and cats, with the exception of pigs. Histologically, malignant transformation of epidermal cells not only thickens the local superficial layer (carcinoma in situ) but can also continue to grow and break through the basement membrane to infiltrate deeper tissues, forming differently shaped clusters of cancer cells known as cancer nests (cancer nest).

The cancer cells in the nests are differently differentiated, with the highly differentiated ones having a keratinized center. In poorly differentiated ones, cells are keratinized only in single, and intercellular bridges are uncommon. Karyorrhexis can still be observed in carcinoma cells, rather than pyknosis as in well-differentiated ones, and mitotic figures are common in all kinds of squamous carcinomas, and more common in poorly differentiated ones. Inflammatory cells often infiltrate the superficial layer of squamous carcinoma. Basal cell carcinoma is a malignant tumor originating from the basal cells of the skin. The nests of carcinoma are often irregular, in the form of masses or islands, without carcinoma pearls and intercellular bridges.

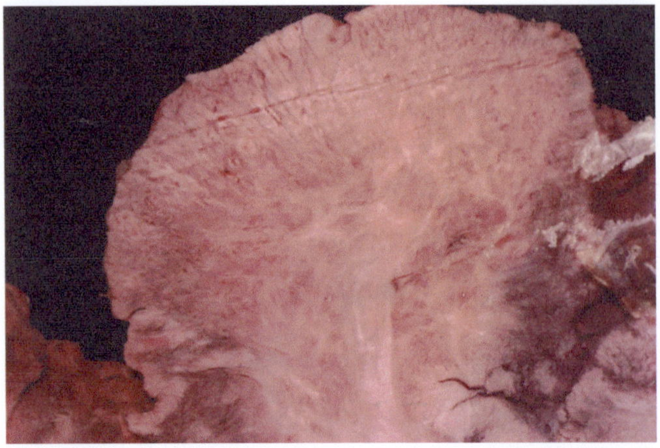

Fig. 5.52 Squamous cell carcinoma. Section of equine pubic sheath squamous cell carcinoma: the tumor tissue shows infiltrative growth resulting in swelling of the pubic sheath, and when taking a closer look, the small gray-white stripes and speckled nests of carcinoma can be observed in the section, and the skin in the tumor lesion is usually necrotic and hemorrhagic. (Veterinary Pathology Unit, Gansu Agricultural University)

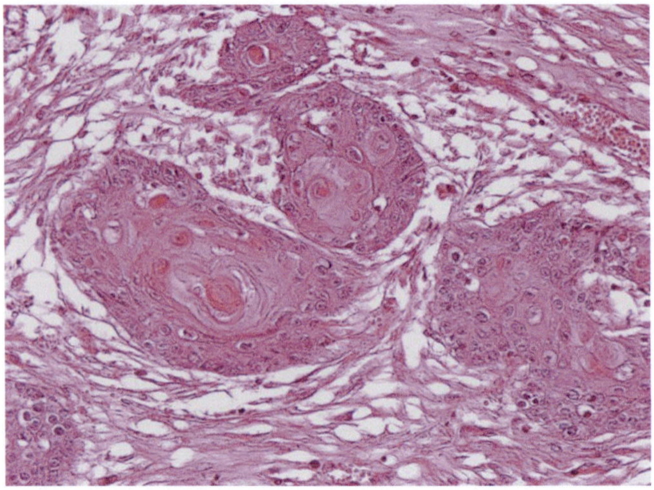

Fig. 5.54 Squamous cell carcinoma. Squamous cell carcinoma of bovine skin: the carcinoma cells in the nest show severe atypia with mitotic figure; partial keratinization in the central part of the nest is present. HE ×400. (Chen Huaitao)

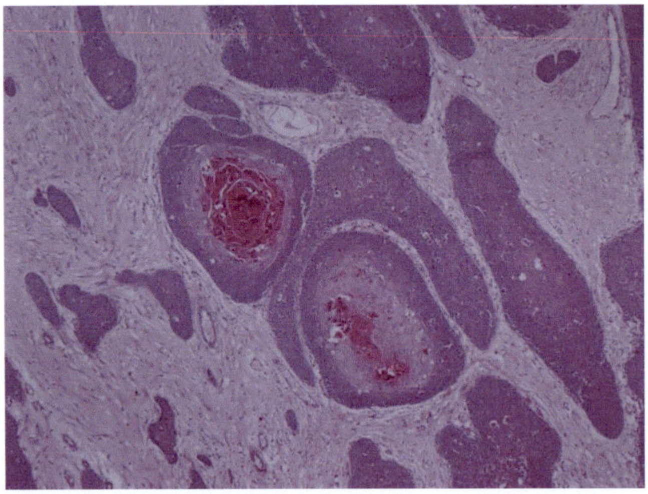

Fig. 5.53 Squamous cell carcinoma. Squamous carcinoma of the skin: the cancerous tissue breaks through the basement membrane and grows infiltratively like a tree root into deeper tissues, forming clusters of cancer cells in different sizes and shapes, i.e., cancer nests, with keratinization in the center of larger nests (called cancer beads) and dense connective tissue between the nests. HE ×100. (Wang Wenhui)

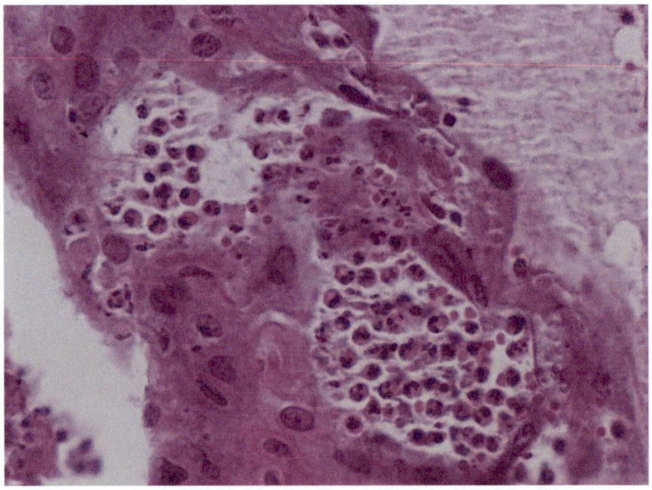

Fig. 5.55 Squamous cell carcinoma. Skin squamous cell carcinoma: superficial cancerous tissue is often infected, so severe neutrophil infiltration is present. HE ×400. (Wang Wenhui)

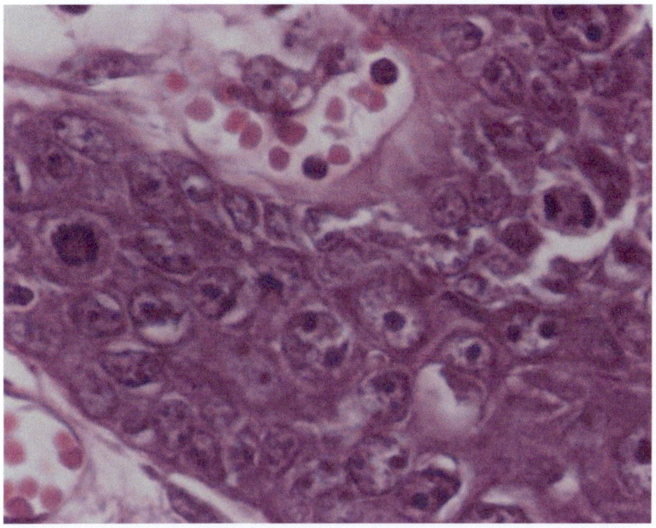

Fig. 5.56 Squamous cell carcinoma. Skin squamous cell carcinoma: cancer cells show severe atypia, obvious mitotic figure (▽), large and clear nuclei. HE ×400. (Wang Wenhui)

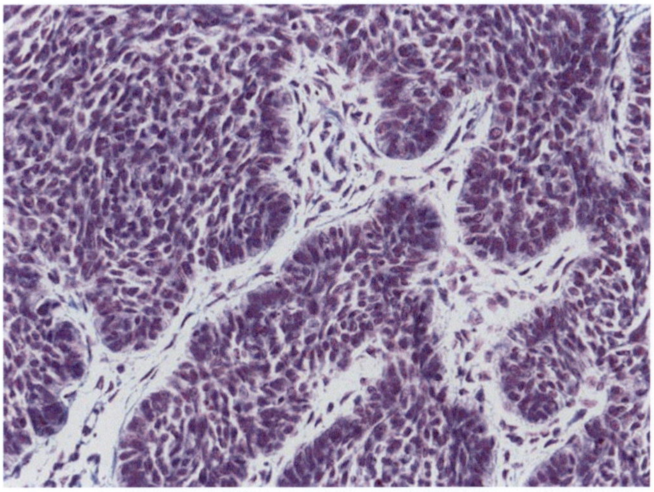

Fig. 5.57 Squamous cell carcinoma. Basal cell carcinoma of the skin: tumor cells are densely arranged and form irregular strips or island-like nests without cancer pearls and intercellular bridges. HEA ×400. (Chen Huaitao)

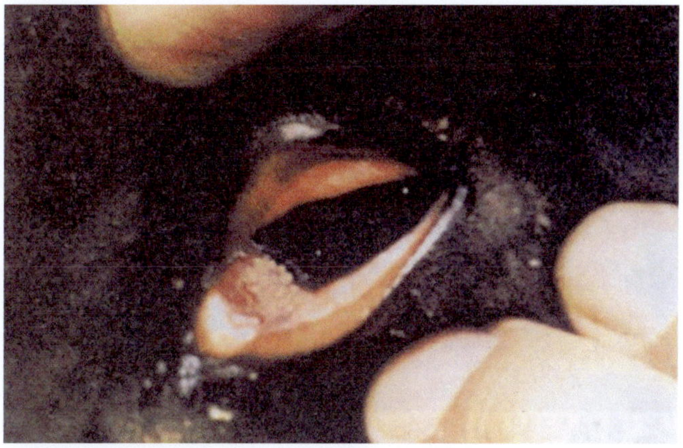

Fig. 5.58 Squamous cell carcinoma. Bovine transient membrane carcinoma (third eyelid carcinoma): This is a relatively common type of squamous carcinoma of the bovine eye. Initially, there is a yellowish, fine-grain-sized tumor lesion growing on the transient membrane, and in severe cases, it forms a distinct nodular mass and protrudes from the inner corner of the eye. (Chen Huaitao)

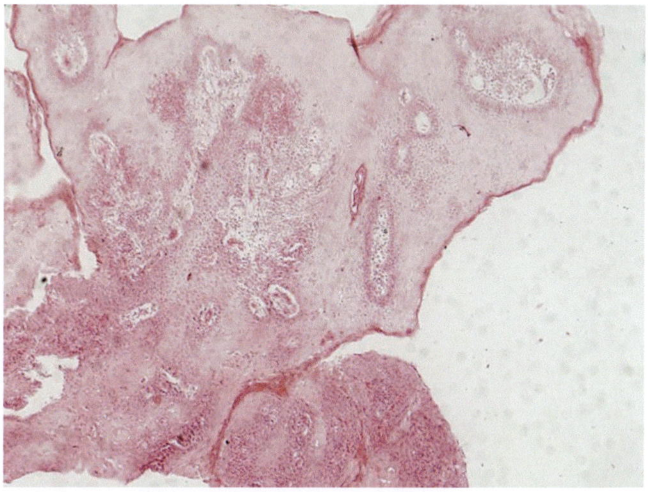

Fig. 5.59 Squamous cell carcinoma. Third eyelid carcinoma in bovine: irregular outgrowth of cancerous tissue toward the third eyelid surface, with scattered connective tissue axes seen in the protrusions. HE ×100. (Chen Huaitao)

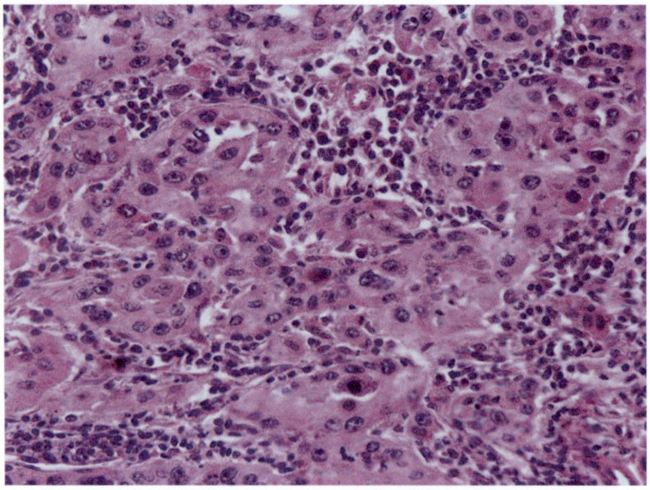

Fig. 5.60 Squamous cell carcinoma. Third eyelid carcinoma in bovine: Clusters of carcinoma cells of varying sizes are present in the lamina propria of third eyelid with infiltration of plasma cells and other inflammatory cells among them. HE ×400. (Chen Huaitao)

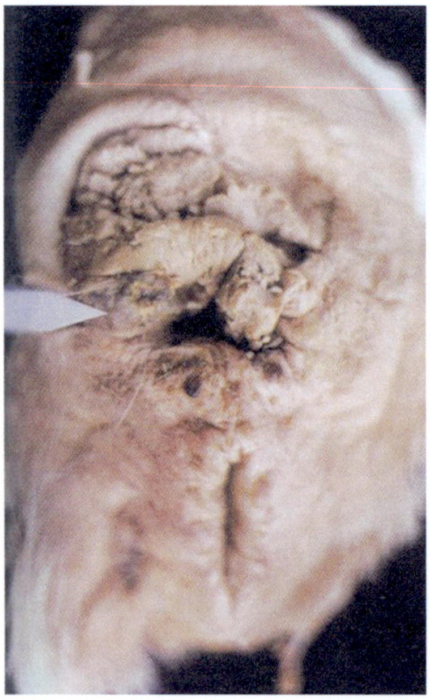

Fig. 5.61 Squamous cell carcinoma. Anal carcinoma in goat: the skin near the anus is uneven (↑), with local tissue necrosis and bleeding. (Veterinary Pathology Unit, Gansu Agricultural University)

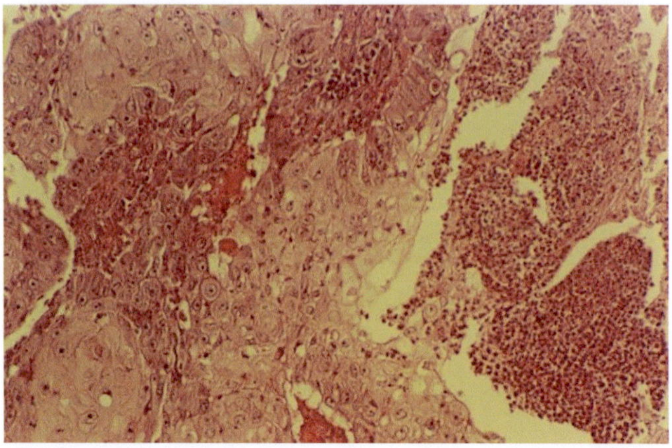

Fig. 5.62 Squamous cell carcinoma. Goat anal carcinoma: cancer cells are in a continuous nest, no keratin pearl formation is observed, nucleoli are obvious, double nucleoli are common; there is a large infiltration of neutrophils on the surface of the carcinoma and between the nests, bleeding was also observed. HE ×200. (Veterinary Pathology Laboratory, Gansu Agricultural University)

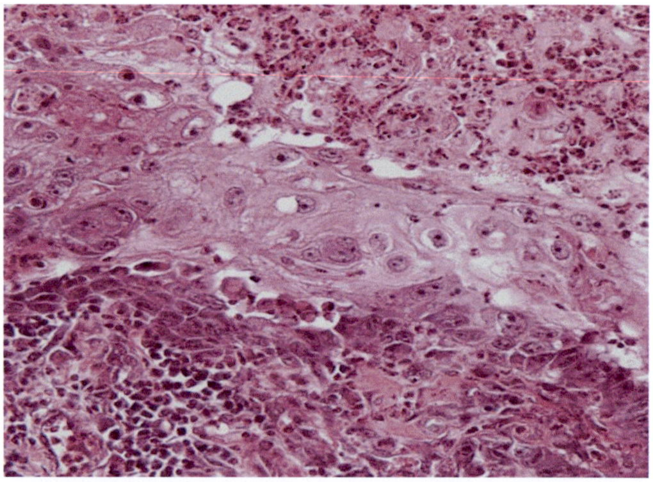

Fig. 5.63 Squamous cell carcinoma. Goat anal cancer: the atypia of cancer cells is obvious, and there are often more inflammatory cells infiltrating near the cancer nest. HE ×400. (Veterinary Pathology Unit, Gansu Agricultural University)

2.3.3 Malignant Melanocytoma (Figs. 5.64, 5.65, 5.66, 5.67, 5.68, and 5.69)

Malignant melanocytomas are malignant tumors that originate from the transformation of raw melanocytes occur in a wide variety of livestock and fish, with canines and equines being the most susceptible animals. In dogs, they often occur in the mouth or skin, and in equines, the primary site of the tumor is often at the tail root, near the anus, or in the perineum. The tumor may start growing relatively slowly in the skin, but once metastasized, it can spread to many parts of the body. The tumors vary in size with black or smoky gray color in cut surface. The tissue is composed of melanin-containing tumor cells, which vary greatly in size and shape

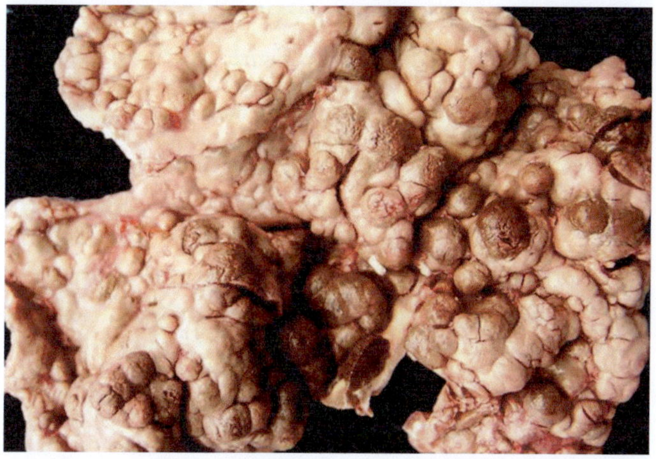

Fig. 5.64 Malignant melanoma. Equine pleural metastatic melanoma: There are variable-sized, dense tumor nodules present on the pleural surface, and the tumors are smoky gray or black because of the melanin contained in the tumor cells. (Veterinary Pathology Unit, Gansu Agricultural University)

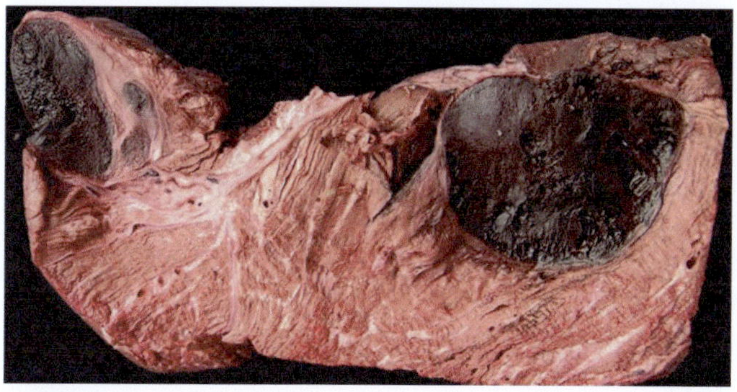

Fig. 5.65 Malignant melanoma. Equine metastatic melanoma of the muscle: A well-circumscribed black tumor nodule is present in muscle section. (Veterinary Pathology Unit, Gansu Agricultural University)

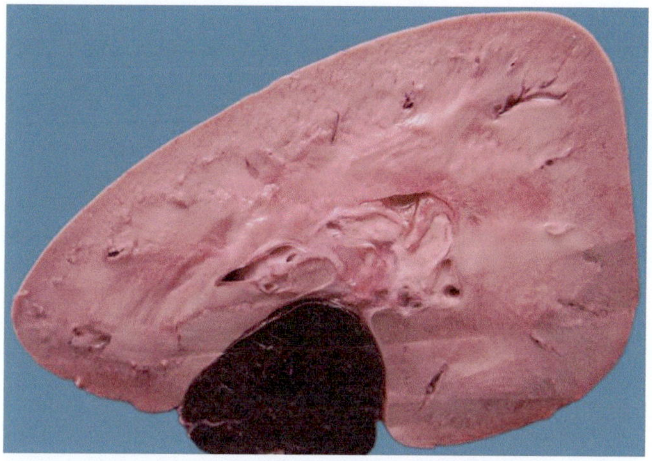

Fig. 5.66 Malignant melanoma. Metastatic melanoma of the equine renal hilum: The metastatic tumor is formed in the renal hilum in the form of black mass. (Veterinary Pathology Unit, Gansu Agricultural University)

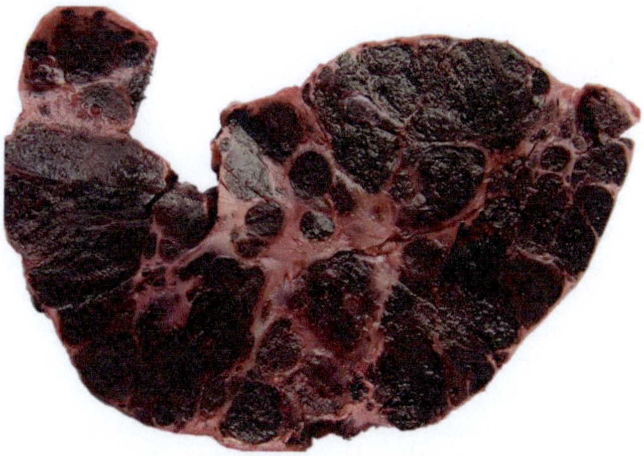

Fig. 5.67 Malignant melanoma. Metastatic melanoma of equine lymph nodes: The lymph node is enlarged and deformed, with the entire lymph node almost occupied by metastatic growth of melanoma tissue. (Veterinary Pathology Unit, Gansu Agricultural University)

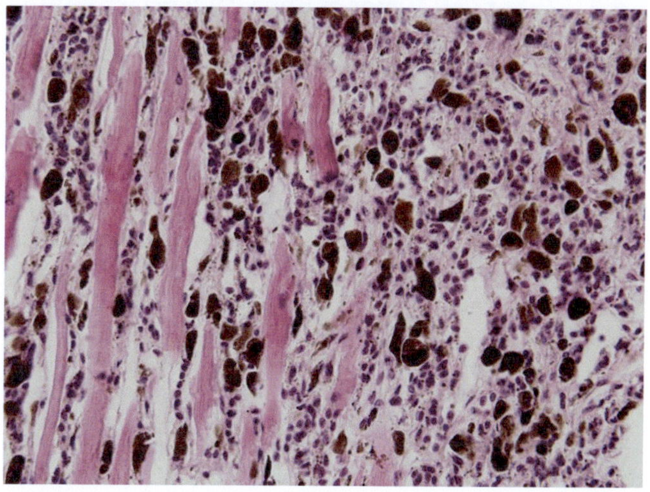

Fig. 5.68 Malignant melanoma. Muscle metastatic melanoma: a large number of tumor cells containing melanin particles are seen between the striated muscle, with homogenization and breakage of the striated muscle fibers, or atrophy and disappearance. HE ×400. (Chen Huaitao)

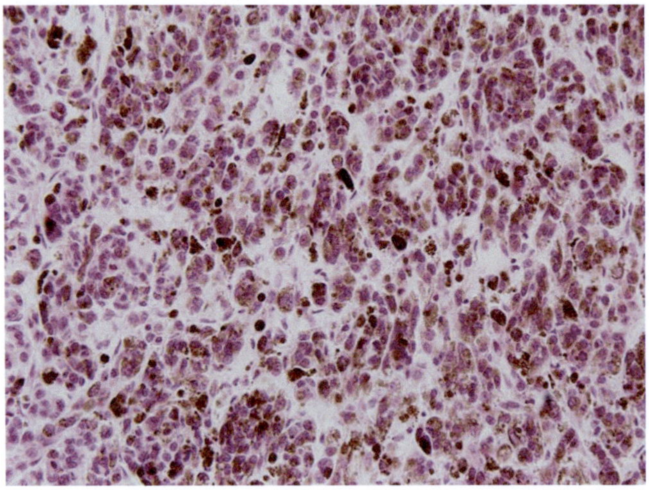

Fig. 5.69 Malignant melanoma. Hepatic metastatic melanoma: a number of melanoma cells scattered in the liver tissue. HE ×400. (Chen Huaitao)

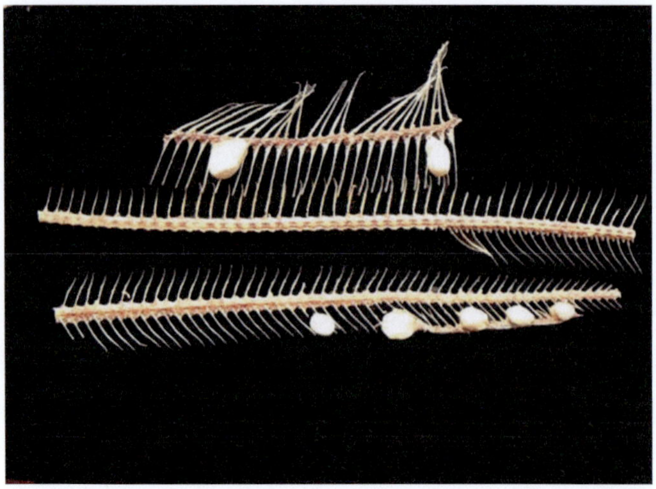

Fig. 5.70 Osteoma. Osteoma of the hairtail: this image shows the common sites of the osteoma occurring (muscle has been removed).The tumor is round or oval nodular in shape and often located on the dorsal or ventral side of the spine. The upper part is the anterior half of the hairtail bone and the lower part is the posterior half of the bone. (Chen Huaitao)

2.4 Tumors of Bone

2.4.1 Osteoma (Fig. 5.70)

Osteomata are benign tumors of bone in which the tumor cells originate from osteoblasts in the outer or inner lining of the bone. They occur less frequently in domestic animals including horses, cattle, and dogs, mainly in the skull and mandible but also in the bones of the extremities. The tumors are round or flat, protrude from the bone surface, and consist of dense or cancellous bone in section. Osteomata are common in hairtail, with round and solitary or multiple tumors. Histologically, the osteoma is mostly surrounded by periosteum and irregular bone plates, and internally consists of bone trabeculae of varying thickness and length, interconnected in a network, with connective tissue among the trabeculae.

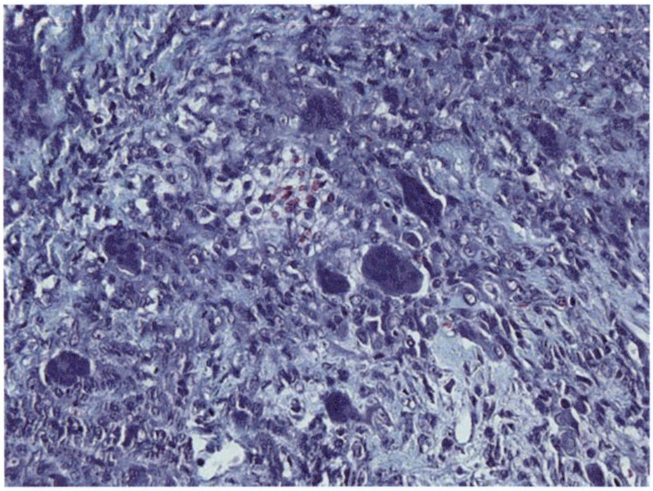

Fig. 5.71 Giant cell tumor of bone. Giant cell sarcoma: The tumor tissue consists of spindle-shaped or ovoid mononuclear tumor cells and osteoblast-type multinucleated tumor giant cells; the former are numerous and dense, with obvious atypia and mitotic figures, and the latter are less frequent and scattered among the tumor tissue. The nuclei also show atypia with high vascularity in the tumor tissue. HEA ×400. (Chen Huaitao)

2.4.2 Giant Cell Tumor of Bone (Osteoclastoma) (Fig. 5.71)

Giant cell tumor of bone, also known as osteoblastoma, arises from undifferentiated mesenchymal tissue in the bone marrow. It occurs in dogs and cats at the end of long bones, the vertebrae, and ribs. It is classified into two types: benign giant cell tumor and giant cell sarcoma, and the latter is malignant. The tumor often occurs at one end of the tubular backbone, with a flesh-like texture in solitary or multiple tumors. The tumor is poorly circumscribed, often with hemorrhage, necrosis, and formation of fluid-containing cysts.

2.4.3 Chondroma (Fig. 5.72)

Chondromata are benign tumors of cartilaginous tissue, the main component of which is mature hyaline cartilage. The tumor cells originate primarily from cartilaginous tissue within the bone marrow cavity but may also originate from connective tissue in the epiphysis or subepiphysis. The tumors occur in adult sheep, dogs, horses, and cats, and they are hard and solid, resembling hyaline cartilage, and may undergo mucinous degeneration or calcification.

2.4.4 Chondrosarcoma (Fig. 5.73)

Chondrosarcomata are malignant tumors of cartilaginous tissue that originate in the marrow cavity or in the outer lining of the bone and are most often observed in dogs, sheep, and occasionally in cats and horses. The tumors are commonly found in flat bones and are similar in appearance and texture to chondroma, but are prone to mucinous degeneration and hemorrhage with necrosis.

2.4.5 Myeloma (Fig. 5.74)

Myeloma, also known as plasma cell myeloma, is a malignant tumor that occurs from plasma cells in the bone marrow. The tumor begins in the bone marrow, progresses outward, and may metastasize further to internal organs. The blood and urine of affected animals have increased levels of abnormal globulin. The tumor occurs mostly in the vertebrae, pelvis, ribs, and long bones of dogs, while it is rare in other animals.

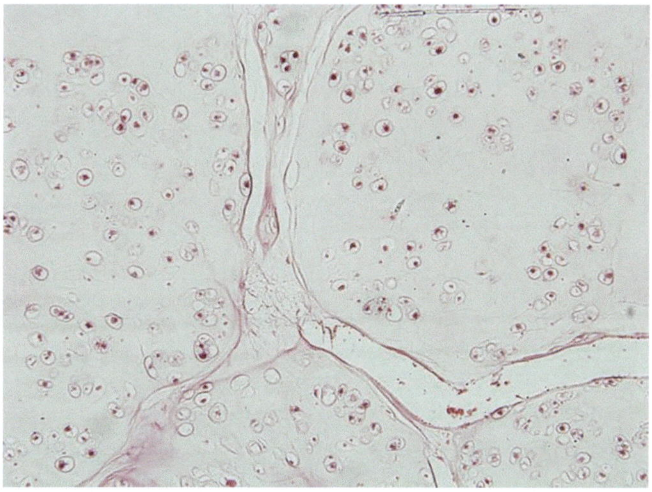

Fig. 5.72 Chondroma. The tumor tissue is mainly composed of chondrocytes and cartilage stroma, and the tumor tissue is separated into lobules of different sizes by connective tissue. Tumor cells at the edges of the lobules are generally small and numerous, with less stroma and often calcium salt deposits, while tumor cells in the center of the lobules are large, more mature, and more similar to mature chondrocytes. HE ×100. (Chen Huaitao)

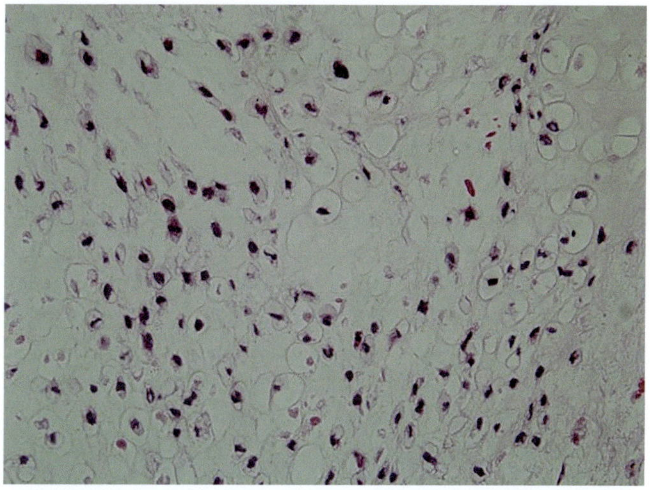

Fig. 5.73 Chondrosarcoma. The tumor tissue is somewhat similar to cartilage tissue, but the tumor cells are abundant with severe atypia. Some tumor cells are obese and contain meganuclei or binuclei, and the splitting image is obvious. HE ×400. (Chen Huaitao)

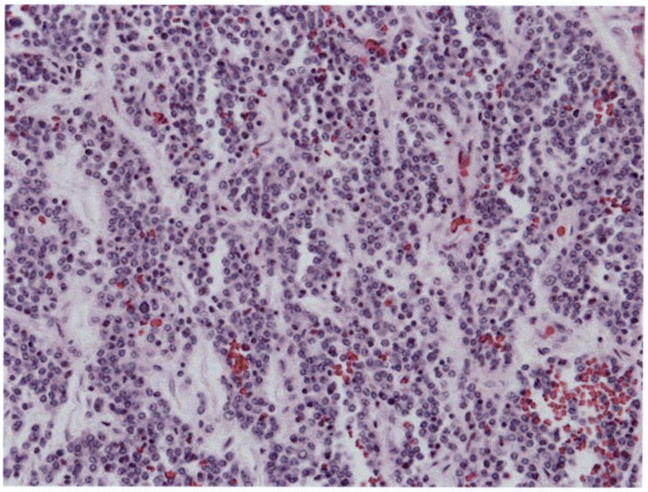

Fig. 5.74 Myeloma. The tumor tissue consists of dense but separate round or oval cells, somewhat similar to plasma cells, but with a different degree of differentiation, little interstitium, and few intertumor cell reticular fibers. HE ×400. (Veterinary Pathology Unit, Gansu Agricultural University)

2.5 Tumors of Lympho-Hematopoietic Tissue

2.5.1 Lymphosarcoma (Figs. 5.75, 5.76, 5.77, 5.78, 5.79, 5.80, and 5.81)

Lymphosarcoma, or lymphoma, also known as malignant lymphosarcoma, is a malignant tumor of lymphoid tissue. Its anatomical types include multicentric (lymph nodes and organs such as the spleen and liver), digestive tract, thymus with other organs. Histologically, they are classified into five types according to the degree of differentiation: stem cell, which is poorly differentiated, histocytic or reticulate cell, lympho-blastic, prolymphocytic, and lymphocytic types.

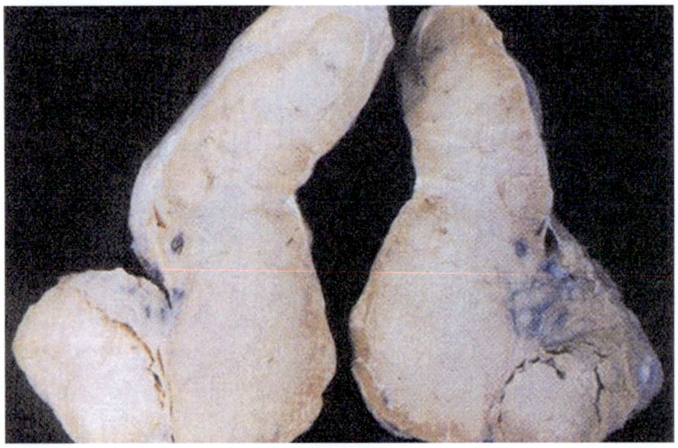

Fig. 5.75 Lymphosarcoma. Superficial cervical lymph node in goat: the lymph node is highly enlarged, deformed, about ten times larger than normal ones, firm in texture, grayish-red on cut surface, with encapsulated nodules. (Xue Dengmin)

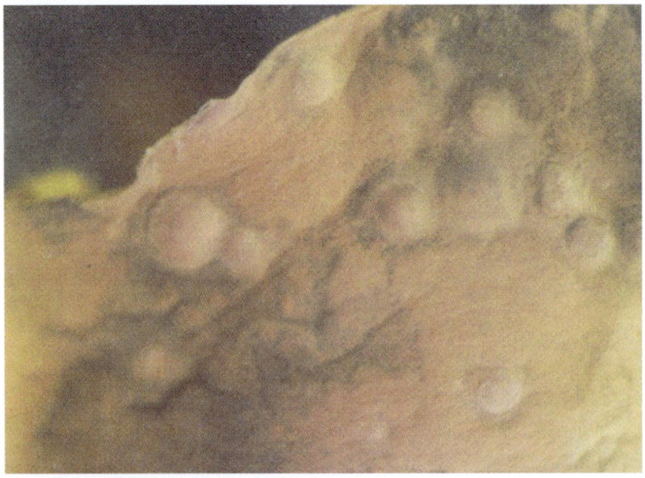

Fig. 5.76 Lymphosarcoma. Sheep's liver: some round, slightly elevated tumor nodules of variable sizes are present on the surface of the liver. They are grayish in color and well circumscribed. (Xue Dengmin)

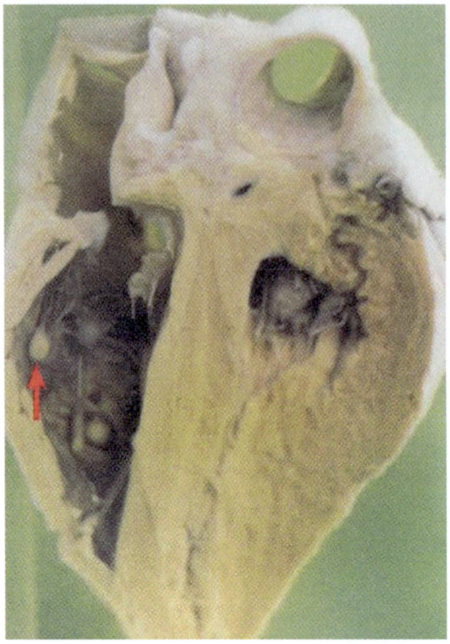

Fig. 5.77 Lymphosarcoma. Sheep's heart: several round tumor grayish-white nodules are present on the right endocardium. (Xue Dengmin)

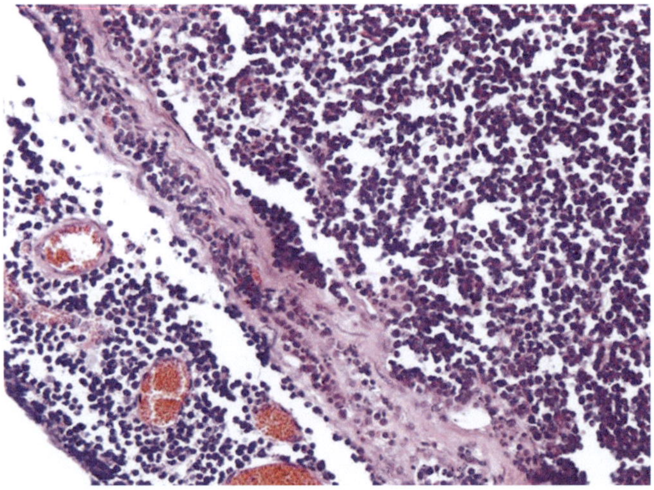

Fig. 5.78 Lymphosarcoma. Goat lymph nodes: massive proliferation of tumor cells both inside and outside of the lymph nodes; the strip of connective tissue in the middle of the figure is the lymph node perithelium. HE ×400. (Xue Dengmin)

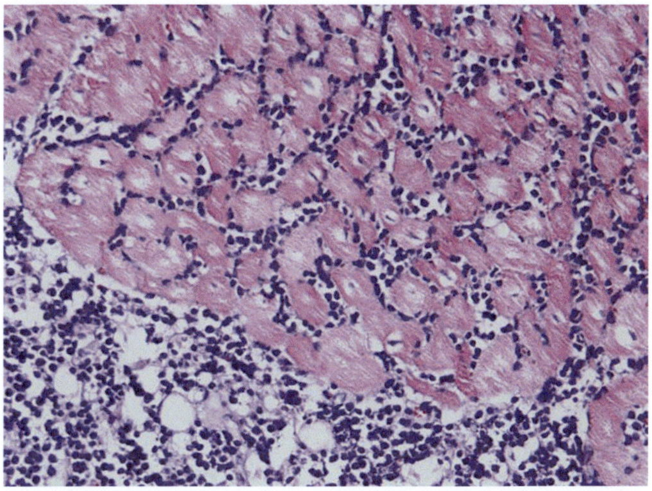

Fig. 5.79 Lymphosarcoma. Sheep heart: a large number of lymphosarcoma cells in variable sizes and morphology are scattered and accumulated between myocardial fibers and under the epicardium. HE ×400. (Xue Dengmin)

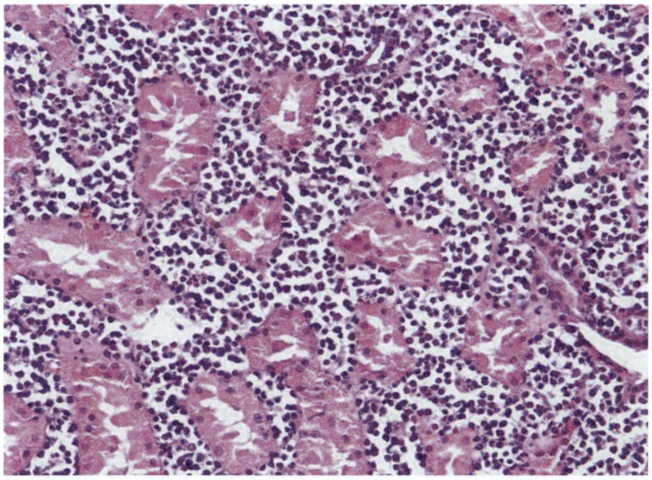

Fig. 5.80 Lymphosarcoma. Sheep kidney: there is a large proliferation of tumor cells in the interstitium of the kidney, so the interstitium is widened and the tubules are atrophied or degenerated with necrosis. HE ×400. (Xue Dengmin)

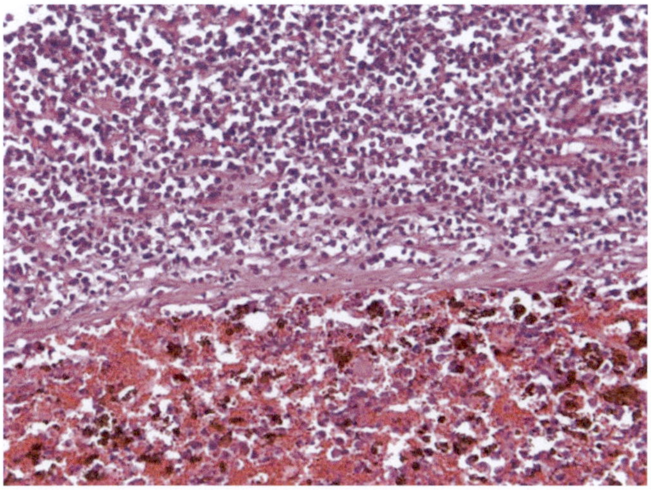

Fig. 5.81 Lymphosarcoma. Sheep spleen: massive infiltration of tumor cells in the spleen peritoneum. HE ×400. (Xue Dengmin)

2.5.2 Myelogenic Leukemia (Figs. 5.82, 5.83, and 5.84)

Myeloid leukemia, also known as granulocytic leukemia, is less common in various domestic animals and is characterized by diffuse infiltration of tumor cells in the bone marrow, liver, and lymph nodes, with severe tissue damage and a tumor lesion where the tumor cells are clustered, which can show a green appearance due to the peroxidase-containing tumor cells; the green color can disappear quickly when the tumor cells are exposed to air, but the green color can reappear with hydrogen peroxide on it. The tumor cells are from different developmental stages of the granulocyte lineage, some of which are dominated by poorly differentiated medulloblast (myeloid) cells with mitotic figures, while others are dominated by well-differentiated granulocytes with lobulated nuclei.

2.6 Tumors of the Respiratory System (Figs. 5.85 and 5.86)

The common tumor of the respiratory system is pulmonary carcinoma, which occurs mainly in older dogs, cats, and cattle. It is mostly adenocarcinoma histologically, with a few squamous cell carcinomas, and interstitial carcinomas (small cell interstitial carcinomas and large cell interstitial carcinomas).

2.7 Tumors of the Digestive System

2.7.1 Papilloma (Figs. 5.87 and 5.88)

Papillomas can occur in several parts of the gastrointestinal tract, with the oral cavity, esophagus, and gastrointestinal mucosa being the sites with tumor occurring more frequently. Oral papillomas in dogs, cattle, horses, wolves, cats, and rabbits are mostly caused by papillomavirus and occur more frequently in young animals with multiple, but benign, tumors.

2.7.2 Gastric Adenocarcinoma (Fig. 5.89)

Gastric adenocarcinoma is a malignant tumor of the stomach that can occur in a variety of animals, more commonly in dogs, more in males than in females, and mostly in the pylorus. Ocularly, gastric adenocarcinoma is papillary, ulcerated, or diffusely thickened locally. Histologically, they can be classified as papillary, tubular, mucinous, and signet cell carcinomas. It can also be classified into intestinal, diffuse, and intermediate types according to the classification of human gastric cancer.

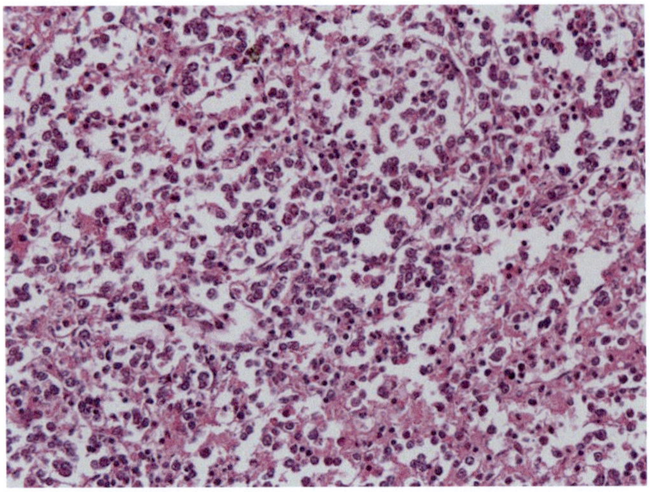

Fig. 5.82 Myeloid leukemia. Spleen: splenic tissue had been destroyed, lymphocytes are reduced, many larger medulloblasts with little cytoplasm, basophilic, and vesicular nuclei with 1 ~ 2 nucleoli are present in the splenic sinus. HE ×400. (Veterinary Pathology Unit, Gansu Agricultural University)

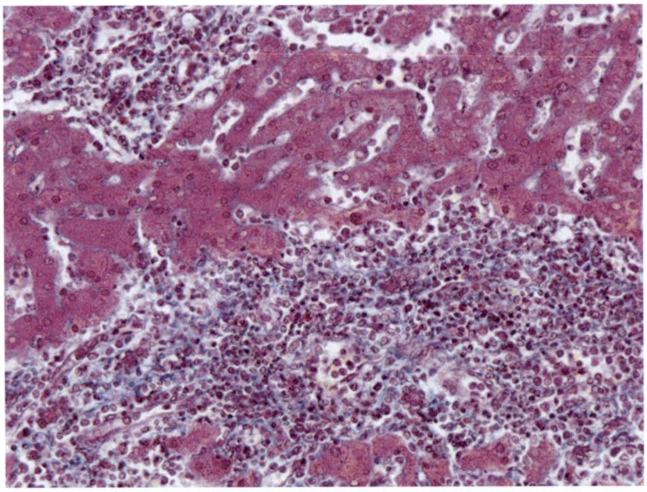

Fig. 5.83 Myeloid leukemia. Liver: foci of neoplastic cells. Tumor cells are clustered in the hepatic sinusoids and portal space. Mallory stain ×400. (Veterinary Pathology Unit, Gansu Agricultural University)

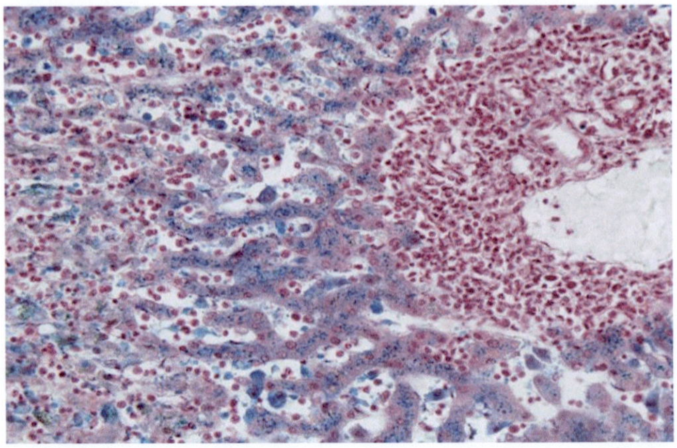

Fig. 5.84 Myeloid leukemia. Liver: there is a large collection of tumor cells in the hepatic sinusoids and in the central zone of the lobules. Prussian blue stain ×400. (Veterinary Pathology Unit, Gansu Agricultural University)

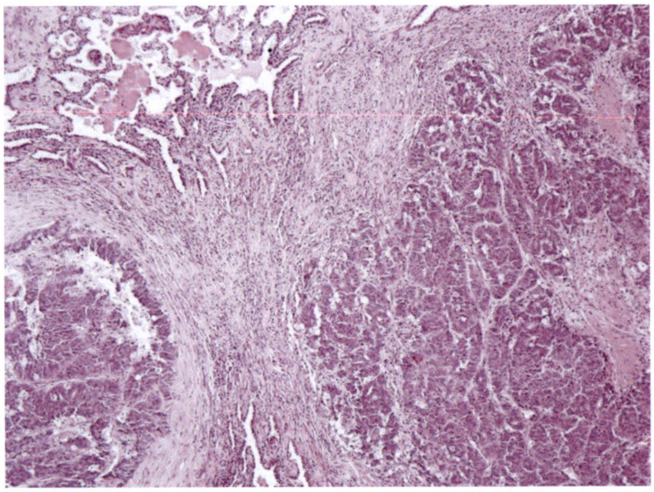

Fig. 5.85 Lung cancer. Lung cancer of bronchial epithelial-derived (adenocarcinoma): abnormal proliferation of bronchial epithelium, protruding into the lumen, forming adenocarcinoma structures with more connective tissue visible around it. HE ×100. (Veterinary Pathology Unit, Gansu Agricultural University)

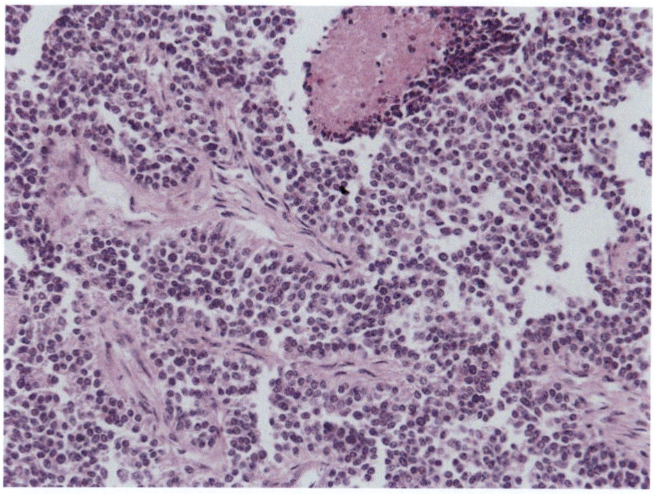

Fig. 5.86 Lung cancer. Bovine small cell interstitial carcinoma: the cancer cells are small and round, resemble lymphocytes, form small islands, and are epithelial in nature as seen from their margins; some tumor cells undergo necrosis. HE ×200. (Veterinary Pathology Unit, Gansu Agricultural University)

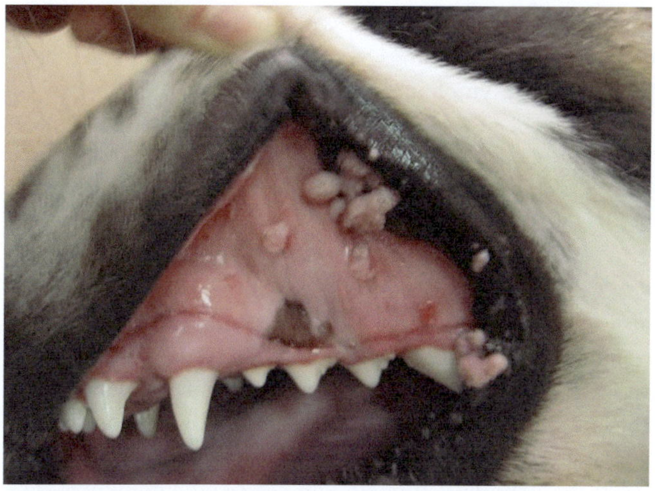

Fig. 5.87 Papilloma. Canine oral papillomas: nodular tumors, variable in size, multiple, grayish-yellow in color, and rough on surface. (Zhou Qingguo)

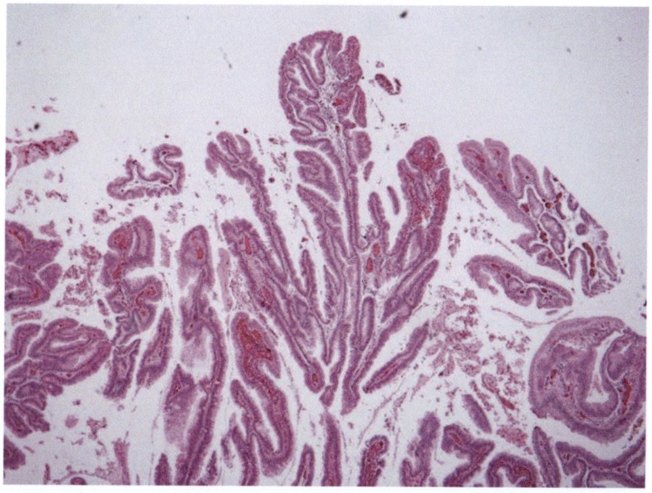

Fig. 5.88 Papilloma. Rectal mucosal epithelial papilloma: Due to abnormal proliferation of rectal mucosal epithelium, the mucosal layer forms many finger-like protrusions extending into the intestinal lumen, and the center of the protrusions contains a small amount of connective tissue. HE ×40. (Veterinary Pathology Unit, Gansu Agricultural University)

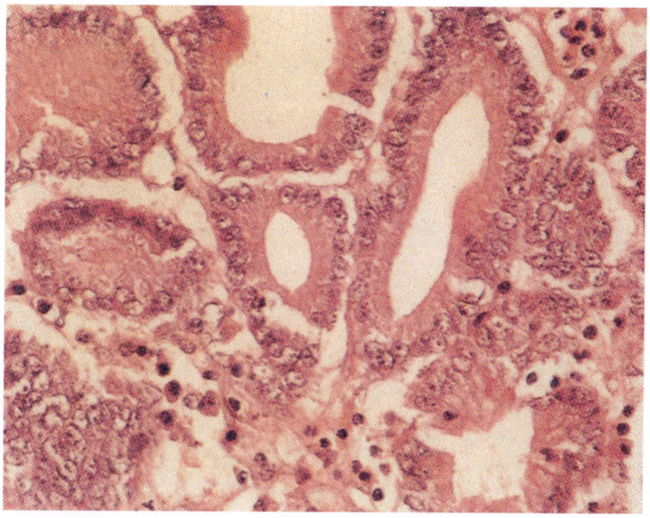

Fig. 5.89 Gastric adenocarcinoma. Adenocarcinoma of porcine gastric cardia (tubular adenocarcinoma): the cancerous tissue consists of adenoid ducts in variable sizes and a small amount of mesenchyme; the cancer cells are columnar epithelium and the mucus-like material is present in cytoplasm. HE ×400. (Liu Baoyan)

2.7.3 Intestinal Adenocarcinoma (Figs. 5.90 and 5.91)

Intestinal adenocarcinoma is a malignant tumor of the intestine that has been reported in dogs, sheep, goats, cattle, and cats. It can occur in the small and large intestine, and intestinal adenocarcinoma in dogs is commonly found in the colon and rectum of 8- to 9-year-old dogs. The tissue types of intestinal adenocarcinoma are similar to those of gastric adenocarcinoma, and there are four types, which can overlap with each other. The malignant manifestation of intestinal

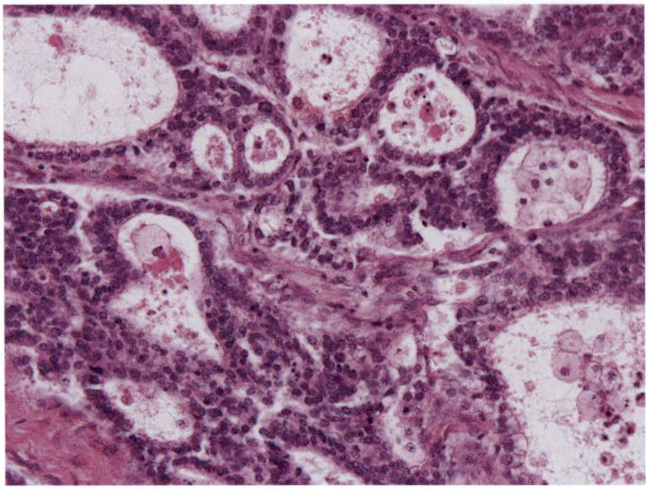

Fig. 5.90 Intestinal adenocarcinoma. Tubular-mucinous adenocarcinoma: The cancerous tissue consists of adenoid structures of variable sizes and irregular shape and a small amount of connective tissue; the epithelium of the glandular lumen is in a single or multiple layers; and the lumen contains mucus, exfoliated epithelium, and inflammatory cells. HE ×400. (Chen Huaitao)

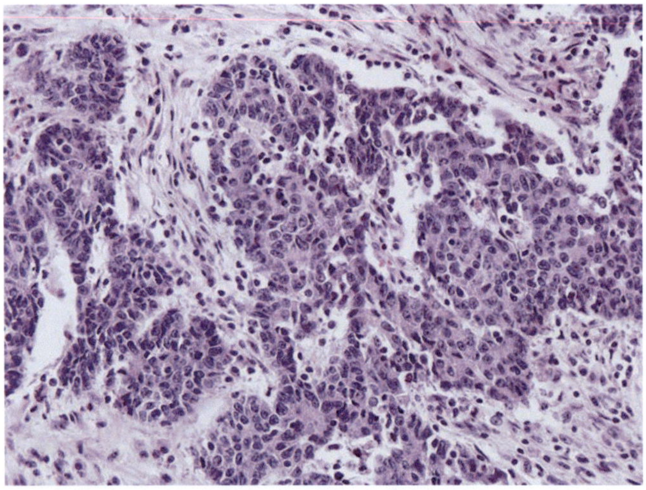

Fig. 5.91 Intestinal adenocarcinoma. Poorly differentiated adenocarcinoma: Most of the cancer cells form an irregular mass of cells without a glandular lumen, with a small amount of connective tissue and severe atypia. HE ×400. (Chen Huaitao)

adenocarcinoma is that most of the cancers can metastasize extensively and often metastasize to mesenteric lymph nodes, abdominal lymph nodes, abdominal organs, and the liver.

2.7.4 Hepatocellular Adenoma (Fig. 5.92)

Hepatocellular adenomas are well-differentiated tumors with cells that resemble normal hepatocytes but are generally larger, with morphologic changes, and often vacuoles, some glycogen and fat the cytoplasma, so the cytoplasm is clear. The tumor cells are mostly arranged in a trabecular or glandular vesicle pattern. The tumor tissue is well circumscribed. It looks like nodules, is soft, and is yellowish in color.

2.7.5 Hepatocellular Carcinoma (Figs. 5.93, 5.94, and 5.95)

It is a malignant tumor of the hepatocytes, which varies greatly in malignancy. The cancer cells either resemble hepatocytes or are extremely dissimilar, with severe atypia and many mitotic figures. Hepatocellular carcinoma can occur with hemorrhage, necrosis, steatosis, and bile pigment infiltration; hence, it shows mottled appearance. Small intrahepatic metastases may occur around the primary hepatocellular carcinoma foci, followed by metastasis to the hilar lymph nodes, with hematogenous metastases occurring first in the lungs.

2.7.6 Cholangiocellular Carcinoma (Figs. 5.96 and 5.97)

Cholangiocarcinoma, also known as intrahepatic bile duct carcinoma, is composed of components of bile duct-like epithelium with extremely irregular lumen size and shape, cuboidal, columnar, or flattened epithelial cells that may form papillary projections, or solid cell cords or small foci that appear as adenosquamous carcinomas. Cholangiocarcinoma is often with plenty of interstitium. The carcinoma occurs in dogs, cats, and cattle, and it can metastasize to local lymph nodes and peritoneum.

2.8 Tumors of the Urinary System

2.8.1 Nephradenocarcinoma (Fig. 5.98)

Renal adenocarcinoma, also known as renal cell carcinoma, occurs more frequently in older dogs and cattle and can also occur in horses, sheep, and pigs. These tumors are solitary, nodular, often located in the anterior part of the kidney, variable in size, and grayish or grayish-yellow in appearance, with hemorrhage and necrosis. Histologically, it can be classified into papillary, tubular, and clear cell carcinomas. The tumor may metastasize to renal lymph nodes, distant lymph nodes, lungs, and other organs.

2.8.2 Nephroblastoma (Figs. 5.99 and 5.100)

Nephroblastoma, a relatively common renal tumor in young animals, occurs most commonly in pigs, chickens, and rabbits, and also in cattle, dogs, horses, sheep, goats, cats, even some fish. Nephroblastoma shows some of the characteristics of incomplete differentiation of the embryonic kidney at the primitive stage. Histologically, poorly differentiated epithelial structures and different mesenchymal components such as fibers, mucus, fat, muscle, cartilage, and bone-like tissue can be observed. Epithelial cells, tumorigenic tubules, embryonic glomerular structures, and a small amount of fibroid-like tissue can be present in the tumor.

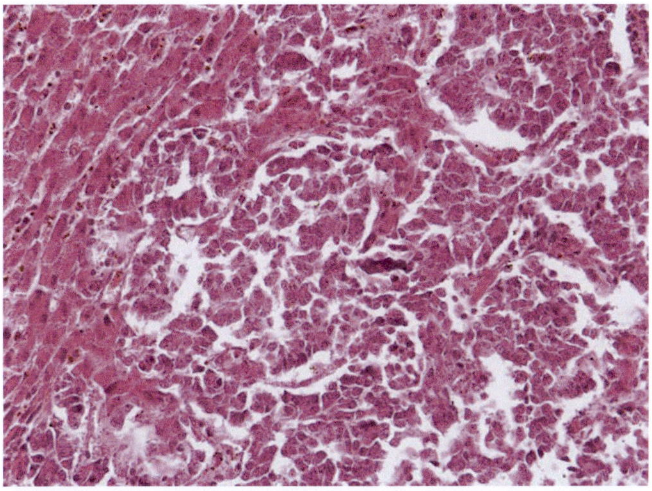

Fig. 5.92 Hepatocellular adenoma. Hepatocellular adenoma in pigs: tumor cells are arranged in strips or small clusters, whose shape is similar to normal hepatocytes, and the surrounding hepatocytes are compressed and atrophied. HE ×400. (Chen Huaitao)

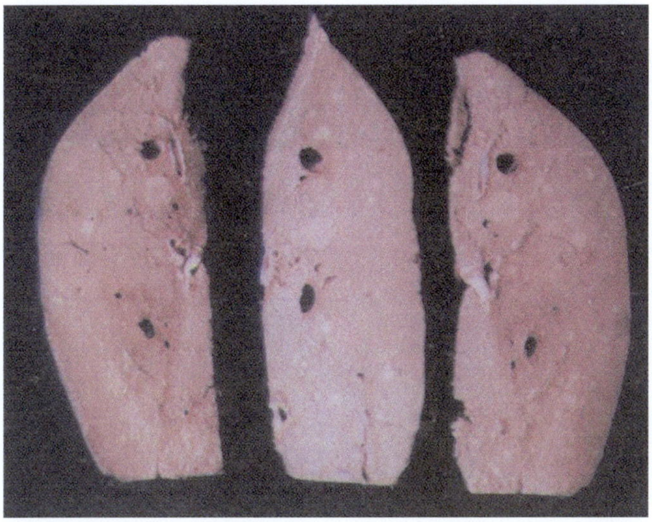

Fig. 5.93 Hepatocellular carcinoma. Sheep liver cancer: many round yellowish-white tumor nodules of various sizes are present on the surface and section of the liver, which are clearly defined but without capsule. (Xue Dengmin)

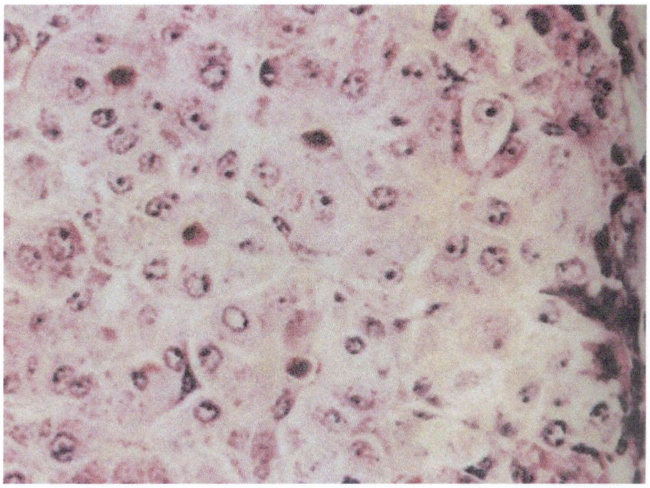

Fig. 5.94 Hepatocellular carcinoma. Sheep liver cancer: cancer cells resemble hepatocytes, large and lightly stained, surrounding hepatocytes are compressed and atrophied. HE ×400. (Xue Dengmin)

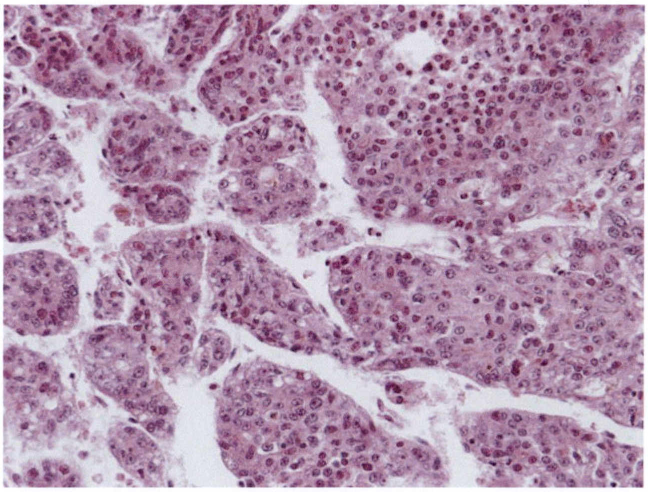

Fig. 5.95 Hepatocellular carcinoma. Porcine hepatocellular carcinoma: The carcinoma cells are arranged in cell clusters or strips, with eosinophilic granules and vacuoles in cytoplasm, and the nuclei are obvious, with mitotic figures. ×400. (Chen Huaitao)

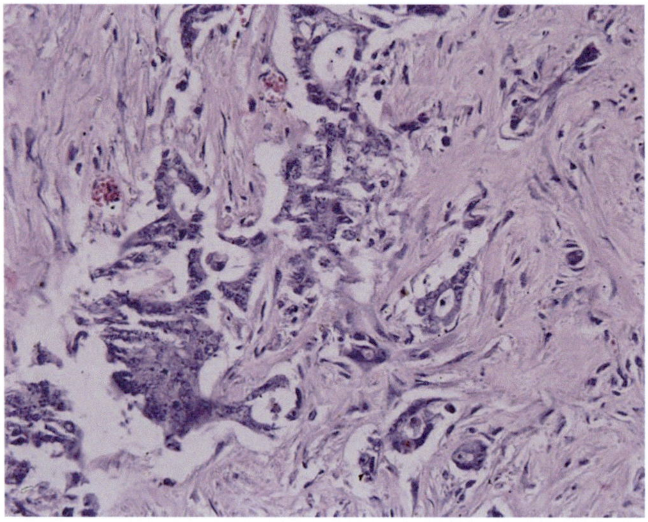

Fig. 5.96 Cholangiocarcinoma. Bovine cholangiocarcinoma: Cancer cells are arranged in extremely irregular glandular ducts, strips, or small clusters, with obvious atypia, abundant collagen fibers in the interstitium. HE ×400. (Chen Huaitao)

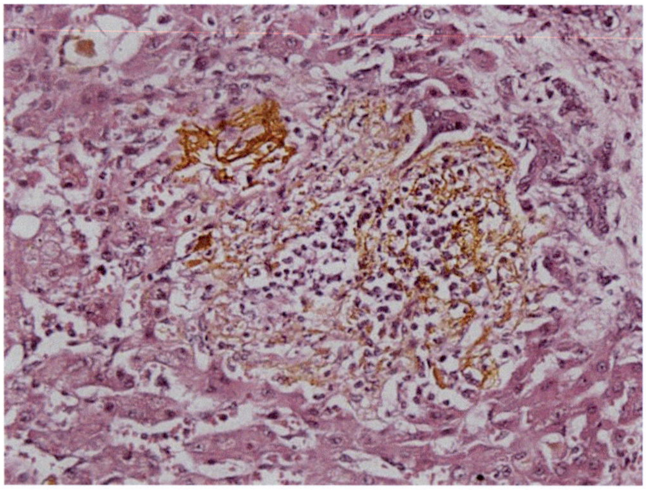

Fig. 5.97 Cholangiocarcinoma. Cholangiocarcinoma consists of irregular bile duct-like structures. Cholangiocarcinoma leads to the formation of "bile lakes," hence it is named cholangiocarcinoma bile lakes, and the yellow color is the bile pigment of the bile lakes. HE ×400. (Chen Huaitao)

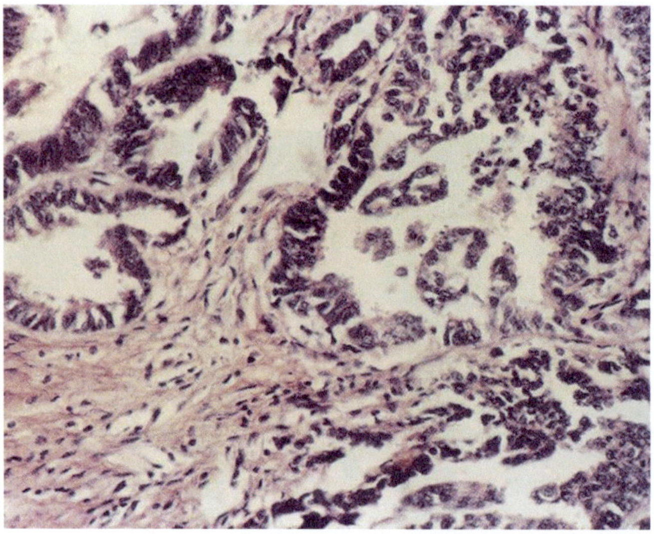

Fig. 5.98 Nephradenocarcinoma. The tumor cells are cuboidal or columnar in shape, with abundant cytoplasm, slightly basophilic, deeply stained, well circumscribed, and visible mitotic figs. HE ×140. (Zhang Xujing)

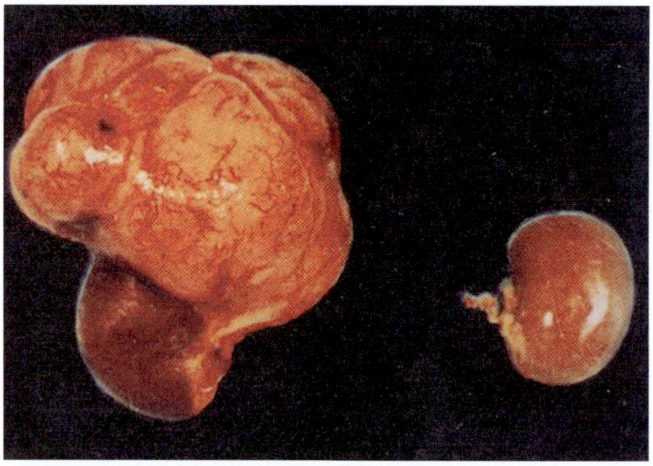

Fig. 5.99 Nephroblastoma. A large tumor formed in the anterior part of the rabbit kidney, with a normal-sized control kidney on the right. (Ding Liangqi)

2.8.3 Papilloma of the Bladder (Fig. 5.101)

Papilloma of the bladder is a benign tumor that originates from the bladder epithelium, but it often shows the potential of malignant transformation and recurrence. It occurs most often in adult or older animals. Papillomas account for approximately 17% of the bovine bladder primary tumors and 14% of dogs. Histologically, papillomas are composed of papillary structures with a fibrous, vascular center and a mesenchyme surrounded by no more than six layers of transitional epithelium outside. The tumor cells resemble normal transitional epithelium without significant atypia, and the few normal mitotic figures can be observed in the basal layer.

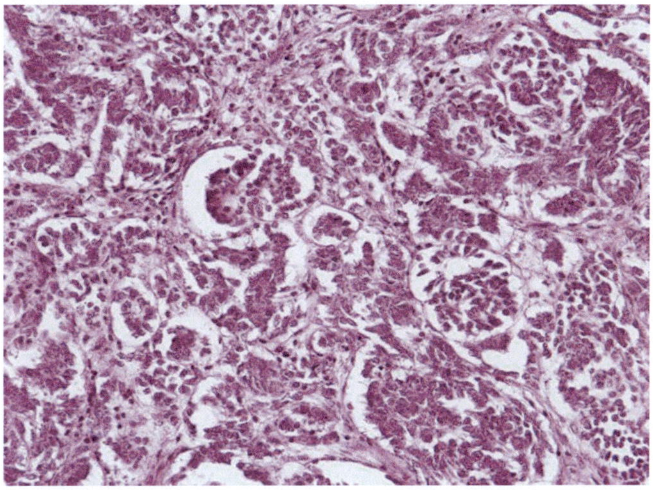

Fig. 5.100 Nephroblastoma. The tumor tissue consisted mainly of poorly differentiated tumor cells with glomerular and tubular-like structures, among which is few fibrous tumor-like tissue. HE ×400. (Chen Huaitao)

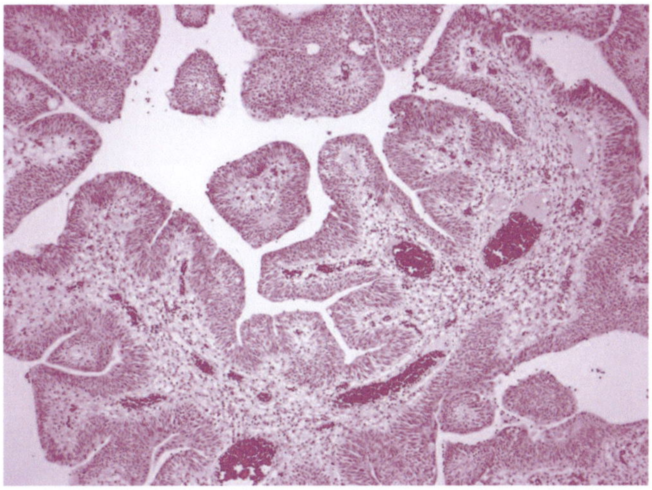

Fig. 5.101 Papilloma. Bovine bladder choroidal papilloma: continuous papillary growth of bladder mucosal epithelium protruding into the bladder with a small amount of connective tissue in the protrusion. HE ×100. (Xu Loren)

2.9 Tumors of the Reproductive System

2.9.1 Tumors of the Male Genital Organs

2.9.1.1 Seminoma (Figs. 5.102, 5.103, and 5.104)

Seminoma, also known as germinocarcinoma or spermatogenic carcinoma, is a less malignant tumor that evolves from the primitive germ cells of the testis. The tumor is a common testicular tumor and commonly occurs in dogs and also in equine animals, cattle, sheep, and chickens. The tumors occur unilaterally or bilaterally with the testes enlarged. The tumor is mostly nodular and often is lobulated by connective tissue, with capsule, solid texture, and gray or grayish-red

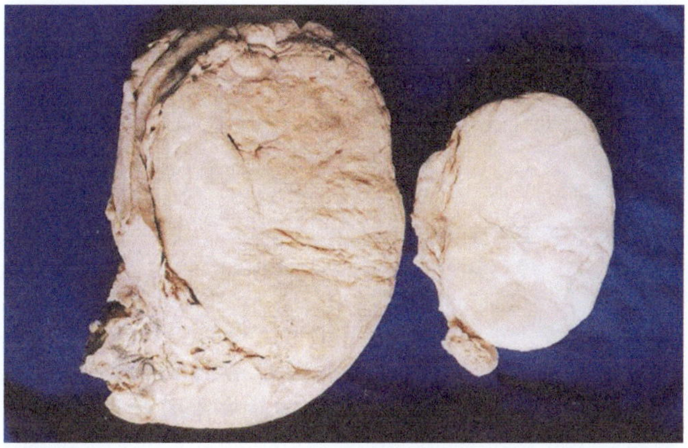

Fig. 5.102 SeminomaLeft: Bovine seminoma. The testicle is highly enlarged and firm, with yellowish-white section and hemorrhagic as well as necrotic foci; right: normal-sized testis. (Xue Dengmin)

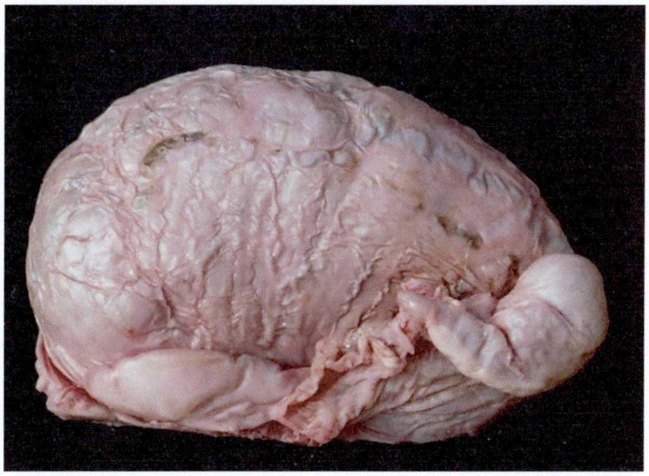

Fig. 5.103 Seminoma. Seminoma in a donkey: The affected testis is significantly enlarged and firm due to massive proliferation of tumor tissue. (Chen Huaitao)

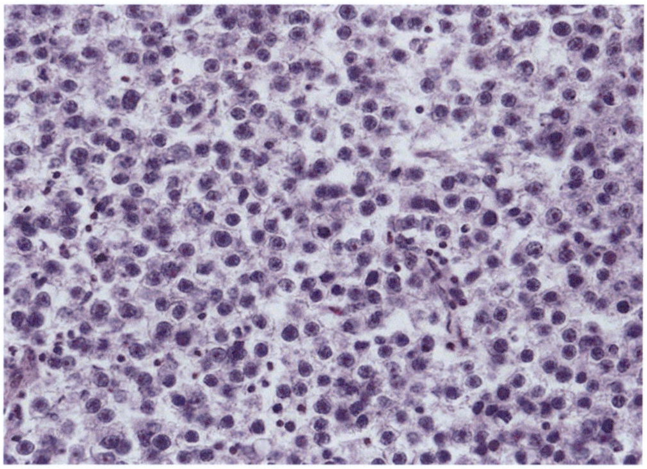

Fig. 5.104 Seminoma. Bovine seminoma: The tumor cells are polygonal, with lightly stained cytoplasm, large and round nuclei, thick nuclear membrane, obvious mitotic figures, obvious nucleoli, eosinophilic, more lymphocytic infiltration in the interstitium, and loss of original testicular structures. HE ×400. (Chen Huaitao)

cut surface, occasional hemorrhage, and necrosis. Histologically, the tumor cells differentiate to varying degrees, and most tumors are well-differentiated typical seminomatous tumors with little atypia and lymphocytic infiltration.

2.9.1.2 Teratoma (Fig. 5.105)

Teratomata are tumors of embryonic tissue origin, consisting of polyembryonic tissue that mostly exhibit maturation and occasionally contain a single embryonic component. Teratomata occur in the testes, ovaries, and occasionally other parts of the body in humans and animals. In animals, it occurs most commonly in the cryptorchid testes of horses aged 1 to 5 years; it is less common in dogs, cats, cattle, pigs, and birds, mainly in adults or olders. A wide variety of different mature and embryonic tissues can be observed in the tissues. Mature teratomata are common in animals, and they are benign, often cystic, and in which almost all the same or similar tissues as in adult animals can be seen, such as epithelium, cartilage, muscle, hair, teeth, nerve tissue, and glands; immature teratomas are most often seen in humans, are generally malignant, and are often solid.

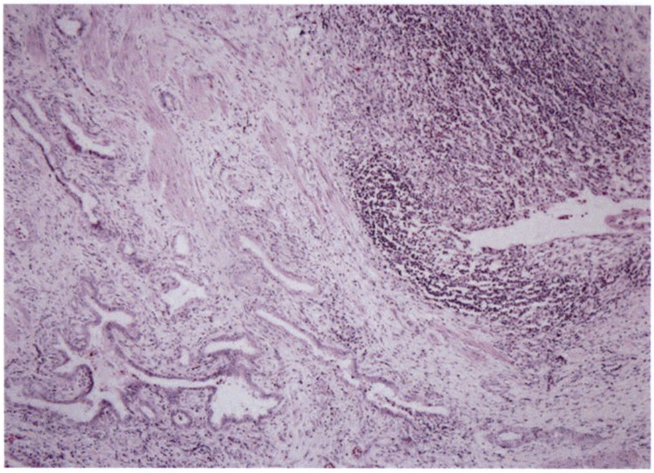

Fig. 5.105 Teratoma. Testicular teratoma: The tumor is composed of acini, ducts, lymphoid tissue, smooth muscle, and connective tissue, etc. The acini and ducts are lined with columnar epithelium. HE ×100. (Veterinary Pathology Unit, Gansu Agricultural University)

2.9.2 Tumors of the Female Genital Organs

2.9.2.1 Ovarian Cystadenoma (Fig. 5.106)

Ovarian cystadenomas originate from the epithelium (mesothelium) of the ovarian surface and the ovarian mesenchyme beneath it and can be classified into serous cystadenoma and mucinous cystadenomas. Serous cystadenoma are predominant in domestic animals, which can occur in dogs and cats, whereas mucinous cystadenomas are extremely rare. Cystadenomas consist of numerous thin-walled sacs containing clear, bright plasma, with protrusions on the wall, which is covered by a single layer of well-differentiated cuboidal, low, or ciliated columnar epithelium, without mitotic figures. The axis of the papillary protrusions is composed of fibrous connective tissue.

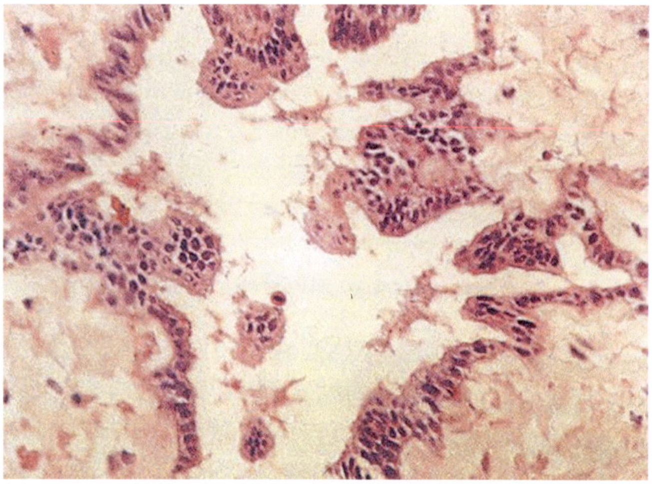

Fig. 5.106 Ovarian cystadenoma. Bovine ovarian cystadenoma (serous cystadenoma): The cyst cavity wall is lined with a single layer of columnar epithelium with papillary formation. HE ×400. (Liu Baoyan et al.)

2.9.2.2 Granulose Cell Tumor (Fig. 5.107)

Granulose cell tumor originates from the sex cord and is one of the common tumors in various domestic animals. The tumor often occurs on one side in a lobulated mass with a yellowish-white cut surface, and cysts, hemorrhage, as well as necrosis are often present in the tumors. Histologically, the tumor cells resemble normal granulose cells, with similar cell size, lightly stained cytoplasm, indistinct cell borders, and round, ovoid, or irregular nuclei. The nuclei are vacuolated, with generally few mitotic figure and obvious nuclear grooves. The tumor cells are arranged in follicular, clustered or diffuse pattern. Stromal cell areas or luteinized areas (large tumor cells with lipid-like cytoplasm) are often observed in granulose cell tumor tissue.

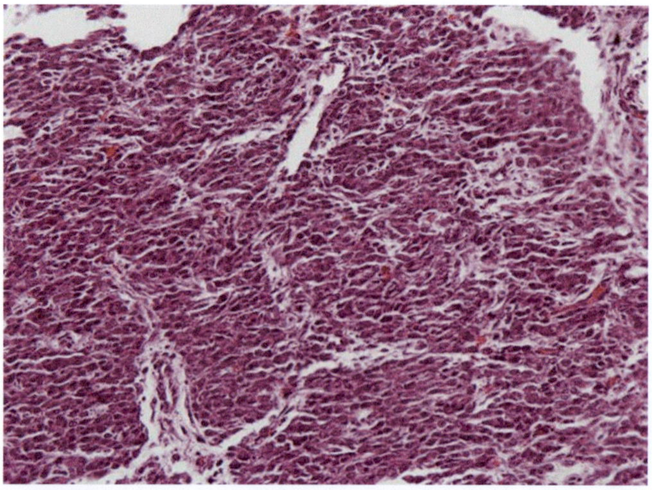

Fig. 5.107 Granulose cell tumor. Ovarian granulose cell tumor: tumor cells resemble normal granulose cells in a diffuse arrangement. HE ×400. (Veterinary Pathology Unit, Gansu Agricultural University)

2.9.2.3 Luteoma (Fig. 5.108)

Luteomata are rare and have been reported in cows, dogs, and sows. Luteomata are tumors originating from the ovarian corpus luteum cells, which are located in the ovarian cortex or medulla with nodular shape, variable sizes, and brownish or grayish-yellow color.

2.9.2.4 Teratoma (Fig. 5.109)

2.9.2.5 Mammary Adenoma (Fig. 5.110)

Mammary adenoma is a simple, small tubular benign tumor consisting of the secretory epithelium of the mammary gland. This tumor occurs in female dogs and cats as well as other animals.

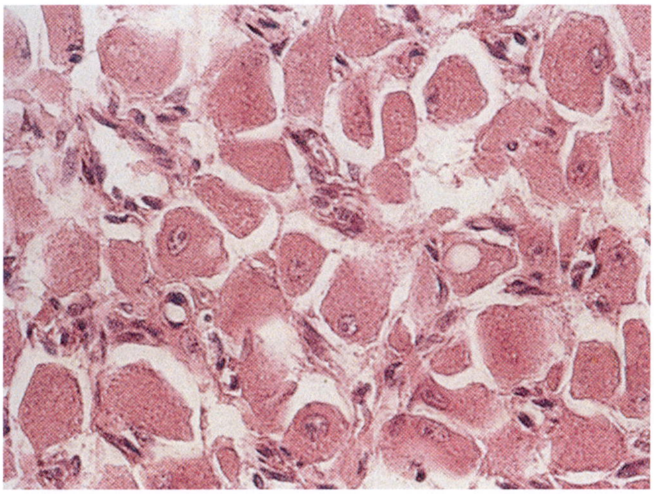

Fig. 5.108 Luteoma. The tumor cells are similar to luteal cells. They are polygonal in shape, with abundant cytoplasm, filled with fine lipid droplets and distinct nuclei. (Liu Baoyan et al.)

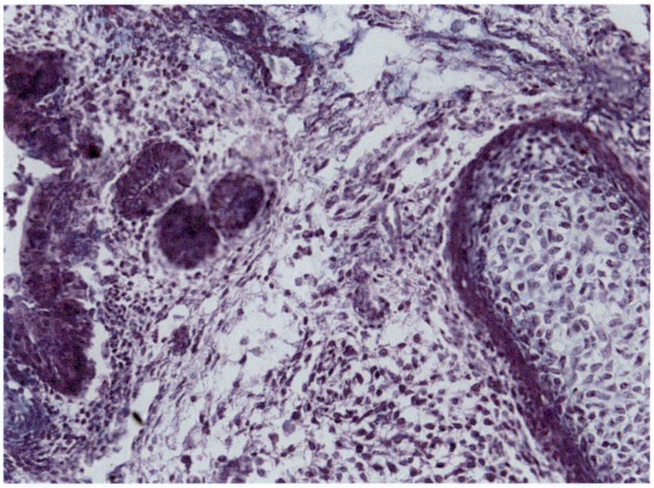

Fig. 5.109 Teratoma. Ovarian teratoma contains polyembryonic tissue, and the glandular bursa as well as follicle-like structures are present with connective tissue and cartilage-like tissue too. HEA ×400. (Chen Huaitao)

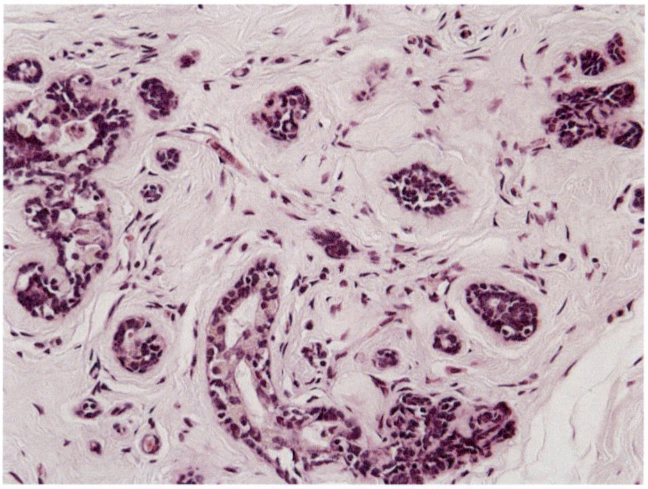

Fig. 5.110 Mammary adenoma. The tumor consists mostly of a single layer of epithelial tubules and vesicles surrounded by fibrous connective tissue. HE ×400. (Chen Huaitao)

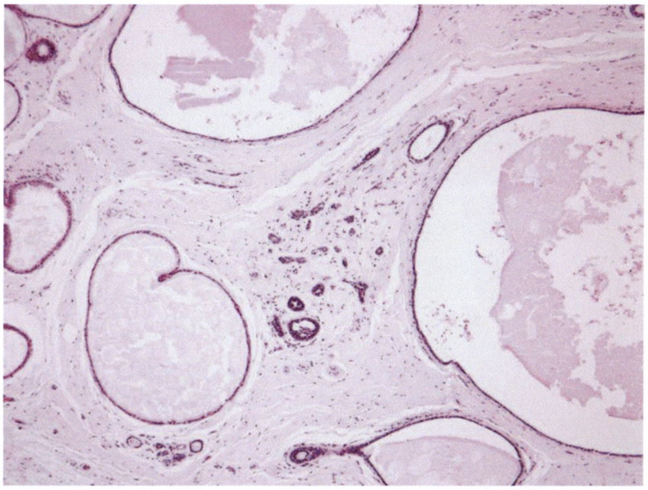

Fig. 5.111 Adenofibroma. Peritubular adenofibroma: Abnormal hyperplasia of connective tissue is present at the periphery of the glandular ducts. Some ducts are dilated into cysts with plenty of secretions. HE ×40. (Chen Huaitao)

2.9.2.6 Adenofibroma (Figs. 5.111, 5.112, and 5.113)

Adenofibroma is a benign tumor consisting of both abnormal proliferating fibrous and glandular tissues, which commonly occurs. The tumor is round, hard, encapsulated, grayish, or grayish-red in color, usually with small cysts present. Histologically, it can be classified into intraductal and periductal types, and mixed types can also be observed.

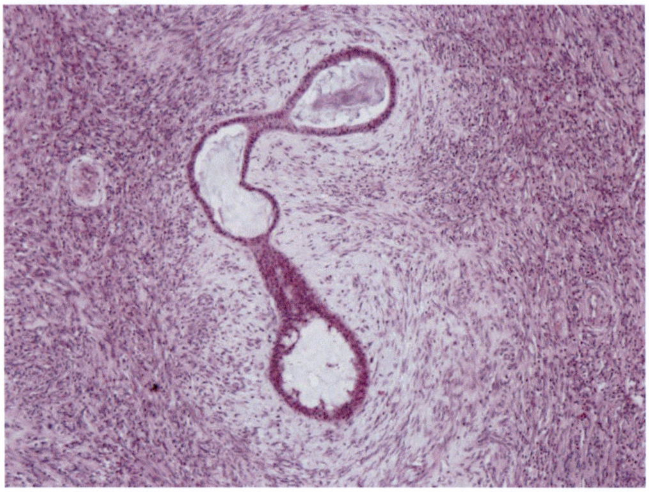

Fig. 5.112 Adenofibroma. Peritubular adenofibroma: Massive hyperplasia of connective tissue is present at the periphery of the ducts. The walls of the ducts are lined with a single layer of columnar epithelium with some secretion in the lumen. HE ×100. (Chen Huaitao)

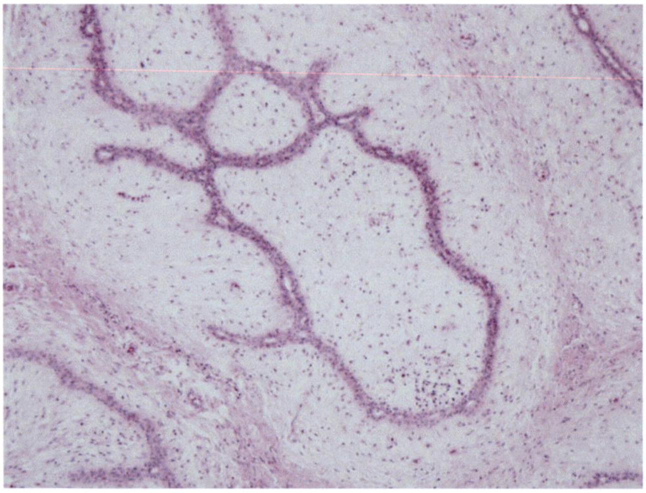

Fig. 5.113 Adenofibroma. Intraductal adenofibroma: massive proliferation of connective tissue is present at the periphery of the glandular duct, which protrudes into the lumen of the duct. The duct wall is composed of double layer of cells. HE ×100. (Chen Huaitao)

2.9.2.7 Breast Carcinoma (Breast Cancer, Mammary Cancer) (Fig. 5.114)

Breast carcinomas are malignant tumors originating from the mammary gland acini and ductal epithelium. This tumor occurs commonly in dogs, cats, and cattle, but it is rare in other animals. The tumors vary in shapes, most of which are unencapsulated and poorly circumscribed. Some of them are soft with cystic cavity, but some are hard with grayish-yellow color. Sometimes hemorrhage and necrosis are present in the lesion. Breast cancer develops fast and metastasizes easily to lymph nodes and lungs. The tissue type of this carcinoma is complex and can be classified as adenocarcinoma (tubular, papillary, papillary cystic), solid carcinoma, spindle cell carcinoma, interstitial carcinoma, squamous cell carcinoma, and mucinous carcinoma.

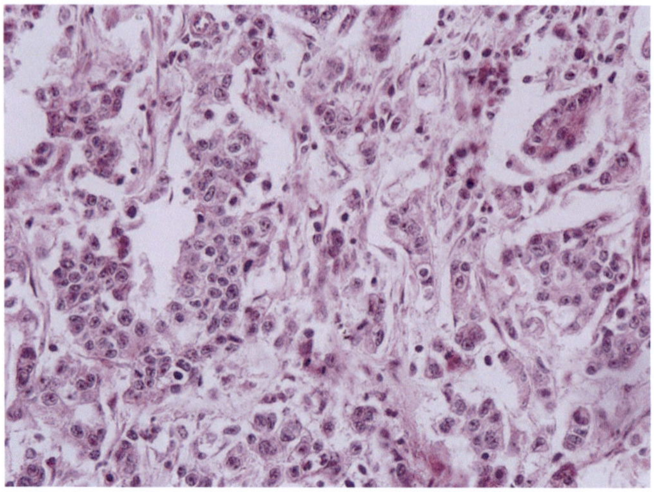

Fig. 5.114 Breast carcinoma. Bovine breast carcinoma: the cancer cells are scattered, forming irregular adenoid structures or cell clusters and strips, with severe cellular atypia and mitotic fig. HE ×400. (Chen Huaitao)

Bibliography

1. World Health Organization International Histological Classification of Tumours of Domestic Animals Expert Group (Zhu Xuanren, Chen Huaitao). International Histological Classification of Tumours of Livestock. Chongqing: Science and Technology Literature Press, Chongqing Branch; 1976.
2. WHO Expert Group on International Histological Classification of Tumours in Domestic Animals (Zhu Xuanren, Chen Wanfang et al.). International Histological Classification of Tumors of Livestock. Chongqing: Science and Technology Literature Press, Chongqing Branch; 1978.
3. Xujing Z. Color atlas of animal pathology examination. Beijing: China Agricultural Press; 2003.

Pathology of the Digestive System

6

1 Gastritis

1.1 Acute Gastritis

According to the nature of the inflammatory exudate and the characteristics of the lesion, acute gastritis can be classified into five types: acute catarrhal gastritis, hemorrhagic gastritis, necrotizing gastritis, fibrinous gastritis, and septic gastritis. The following three types are common.

1.1.1 Acute Catarrhal Gastritis (Fig. 6.1)

The features of acute catarrhal gastritis are diffuse congestion of the gastric mucosa, with the surface being covered by a large amount of mucus.

1.1.2 Hemorrhagic Gastritis (Figs. 6.2 and 6.3)

The gastric mucosa shows diffuse, punctate, or patchy hemorrhage, and its surface is covered with a large amount of reddish-brown mucus. Histologically, the mucosal epithelium is degenerated, necrotic, and exfoliated, and the lamina propria as well as the submucosa are edematous, with numerous red blood cells and inflammatory cell infiltration.

1.1.3 Necrotic Gastritis (Figs. 6.4 and 6.5)

This type of gastritis is diffuse or focal and often presents as a necrotic dry crust or ulcer.

1.2 Chronic Gastritis (Fig. 6.6)

Most of the chronic gastritis is transformed from acute gastritis. It is characterized by marked hyperplasia of connective tissue in the lamina propria and submucosa, inflammatory cell infiltration, and atrophy of glands in the lamina propria due to the compression of connective tissue, while some glands show compensatory hyperplasia.

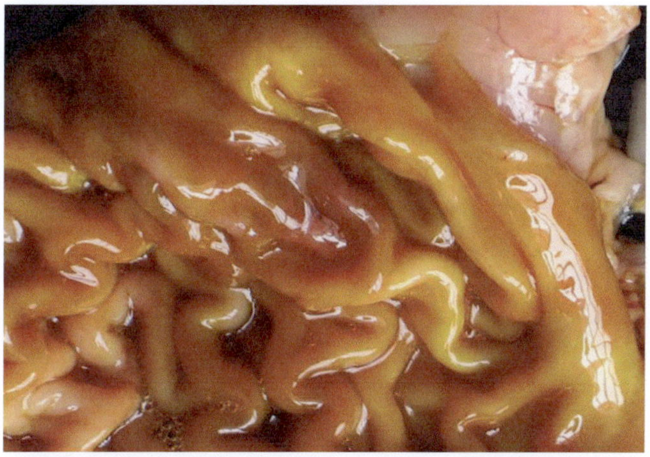

Fig. 6.1 Acute catarrhal gastritis. The gastric mucosa is congested and flushing, with a large amount of mucus adhering to the mucosal surface. (Jia Ning)

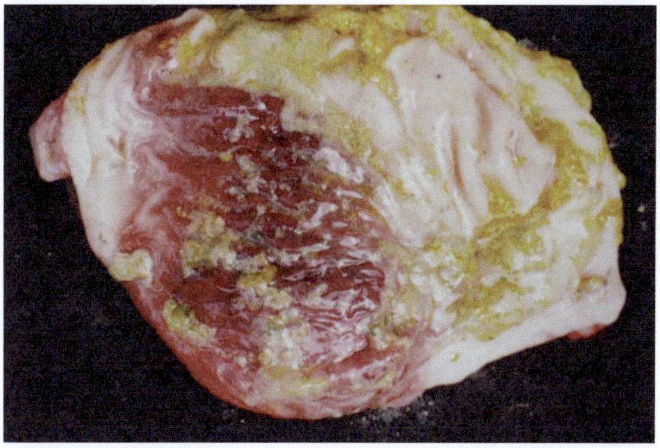

Fig. 6.2 Hemorrhagic gastritis. Swine fever. The mucosa at the fundus of stomach is flushing with diffuse hemorrhage and exfoliation of mucosa. (Li Xiaoming)

H. Chen, *Color Atlas of Veterinary Pathology*, https://doi.org/10.1007/978-981-96-7617-0_6

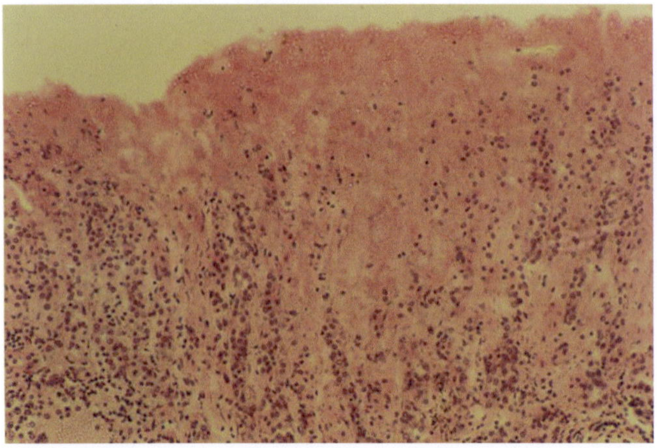

Fig. 6.3 Hemorrhagic gastritis. Sheep abomasum. The surface of the gastric mucosa is covered with a large number of red blood cells. The mucosal epithelium is exfoliated and has become indiscernible. The gastric interglandular vessels are congested with infiltration of inflammatory cells. HE ×200. (Chen Huaitao)

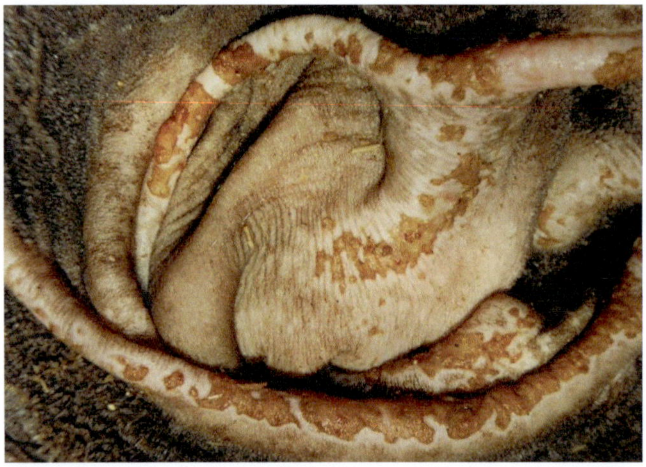

Fig. 6.4 Necrotizing gastritis. Bovine foot and mouth disease. Decaying spots of varying sizes are present on the mucosa of the rumen trabeculae carneae. (Wang Wenhui)

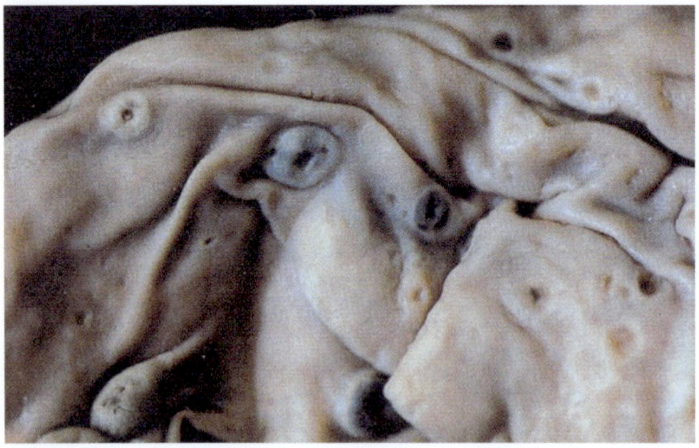

Fig. 6.5 Necrotizing gastritis. Bovine theileriosis. Many round ulcers of varying sizes are present on the abomasum mucosa, with depression in the center and elevation at the periphery. (Department of Veterinary Pathology, Gansu Agricultural University)

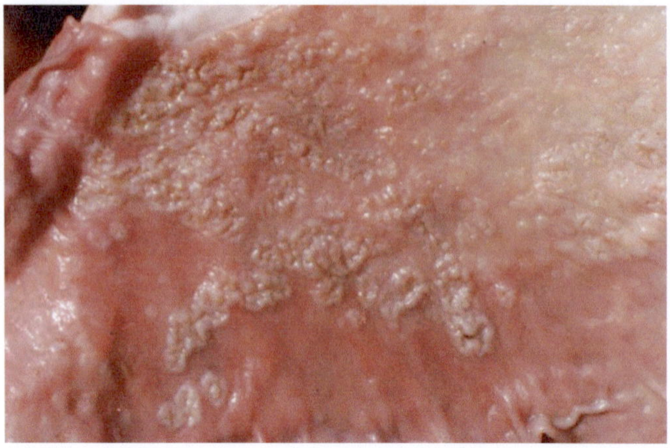

Fig. 6.6 Hyperplastic necrotizing gastritis. The abomasum mucosa of the sick bovine is thickened, and the localized mucosa is nodular, which protrudes out of the mucosal surface. (Chen Huaitao)

2 Enteritis

2.1 Acute Enteritis

Based on the nature of the inflammatory exudate and the characteristics of the lesion, acute enteritis is often classified into the following five categories.

2.1.1 Acute Catarrhal Enteritis (Figs. 6.7 and 6.8)

Acute catarrhal enteritis is characterized by flushing and swelling of the intestinal mucosa, which is covered with a large amount of serous or mucinous inflammatory exudate. Histologically, the mucosal epithelium is degenerated and exfoliated, with an increase in goblet cells and hyperproduction of mucus. The lamina propria is congested, is edematous with mild hemorrhage, and shows inflammatory cell infiltration.

2.1.2 Hemorrhagic Enteritis (Figs. 6.9 and 6.10)

The inflammation is diffuse or focal, with blood present on the mucosal surface and in the intestinal contents. The lamina propria and submucosa are markedly congested and hemorrhagic. Other changes are similar to those of acute catarrhal enteritis.

2.1.3 Suppurative Enteritis (Figs. 6.11 and 6.12)

It is characterized by a large amount of purulent exudate covering the surface of the intestinal mucosa and pus mixed with the intestinal contents, with a large infiltration of neutrophils and pus cells in the lamina propria and mucosal surface of the tissue. Other changes are the same as in acute catarrhal enteritis.

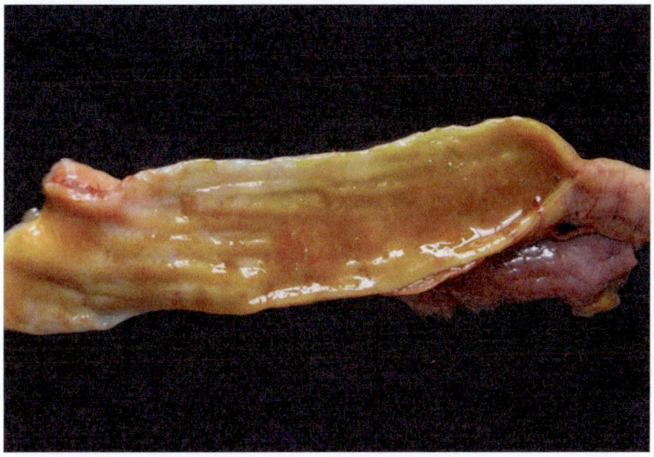

Fig. 6.7 Acute catarrhal enteritis. Canine distemper. The duodenal mucosa is congested and flushing, and the surface is covered with plenty of mucus. (Chen Huaitao)

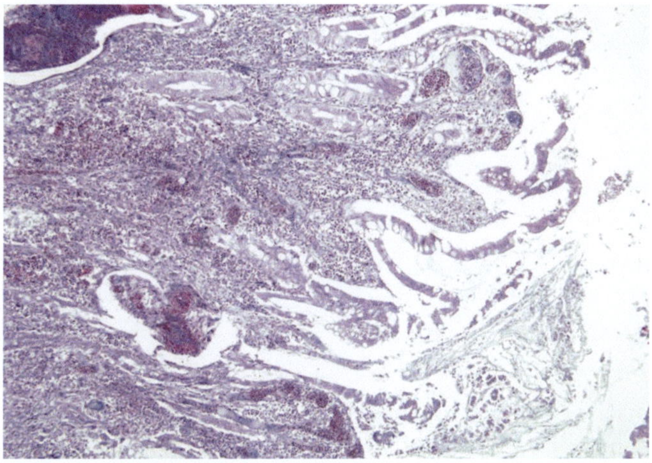

Fig. 6.8 Acute catarrhal enteritis. The lamina propria is congested with inflammatory cell infiltration, increased goblet cells in the mucosal epithelium, and enhanced secretion. Mucus and exfoliated epithelium are present on the mucosal surface. HE ×200. (Chen Huaitao)

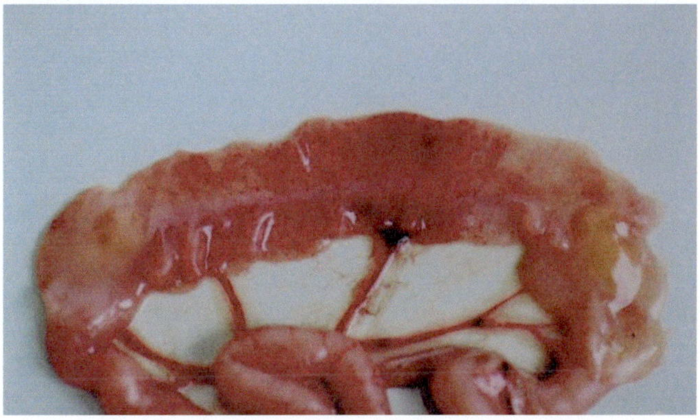

Fig. 6.9 Hemorrhagic enteritis. Acute salt poisoning in ducklings. The small intestine is congested and hemorrhagic, and the mucosa surface is covered with mucus. (Yao Jinshui)

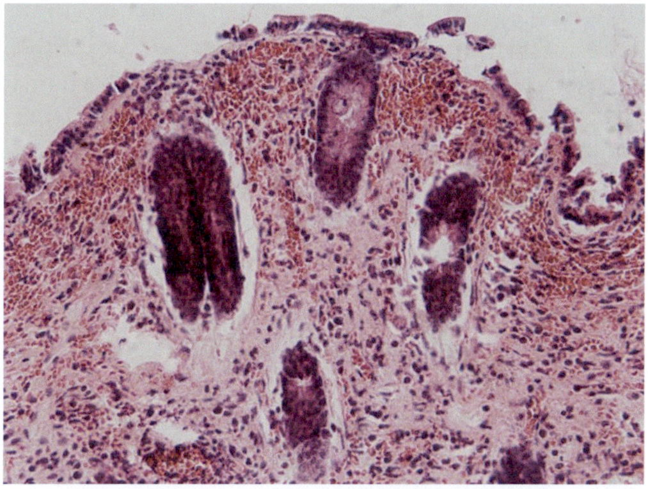

Fig. 6.10 Hemorrhagic enteritis. A large number of erythrocytes and inflammatory cells are present in the lamina propria and mucosal surface, with localized epithelial necrosis and exfoliation. The intestinal glands are degenerated and necrotized. HE ×400. (Li Xiaoming)

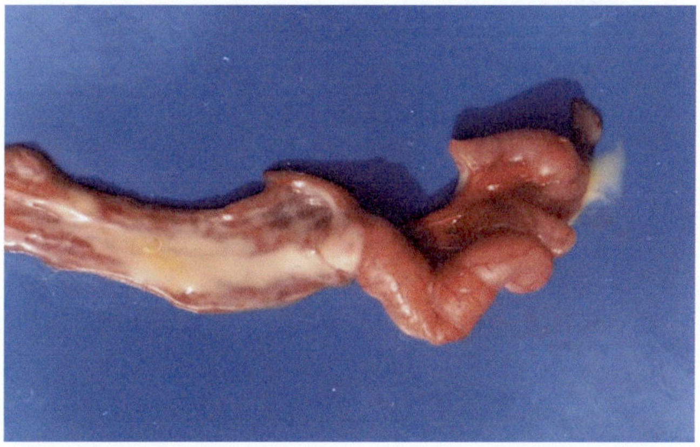

Fig. 6.11 Suppurative enteritis. The mucosa of the small intestine is congested and flushing, with a large amount of grayish-yellow paste-like contents adhering to the mucosal surface. (Wang Wenhui)

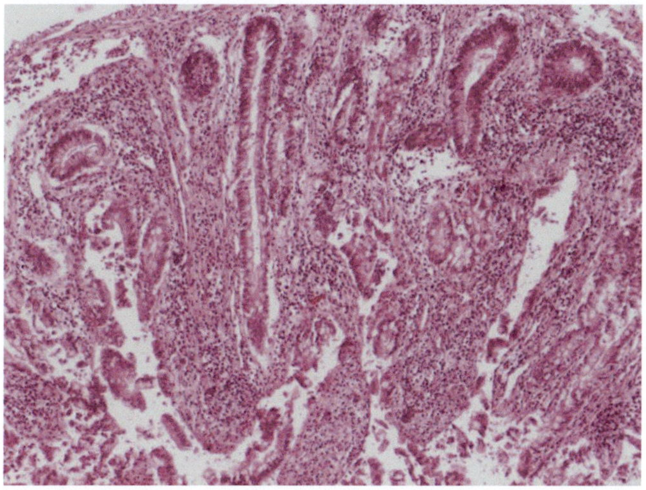

Fig. 6.12 Suppurative enteritis. A large number of neutrophils and deeply stained pus cells are present in the lamina propria; the intestinal mucosal epithelial cells are degenerated, necrotic, and detached, and some intestinal glandular epithelium is also necrotic and detached. HE ×100. (Wang Wenhui)

2.1.4 Fibrinous Enteritis (Fig. 6.13)

It is characterized by massive fibrin exudation and the formation of an easily peelable fibrinous pseudomembrane on the surface of the intestinal mucosa.

2.1.5 Fibrinonecrotic Enteritis (Figs. 6.14, 6.15, and 6.16)

It is characterized by massive fibrin exudation with severe necrosis of the intestinal tissue. The exuded fibrin and necrotic material usually coagulate together and form a solid membrane that cannot be easily peeled off.

2.2 Chronic Enteritis

There are two common types of chronic enteritis.

2.2.1 Chronic Catarrhal Enteritis (Figs. 6.17, 6.18, and 6.19)

Chronic catarrhal enteritis is mainly derived from acute catarrhal enteritis. The affected mucosa is usually covered with a large amount of mucus, and the mucosal surface is smooth or granular due to connective tissue hyperplasia. Histologically, the intestinal mucosal epithelium is degenerated, atrophied, and exfoliated. The connective tissue of the lamina propria and submucosa is markedly hyperplastic, with numerous lymphocytes, plasma cells, or eosinophils (due to parasitic parasites) infiltrating. The intestinal glands are atrophied.

2.2.2 Hypertrophy Enteritis (Fig. 6.20)

It is characterized by significant hyperplasia of the muscular layer of the small intestinal wall with changes of chronic catarrhal enteritis.

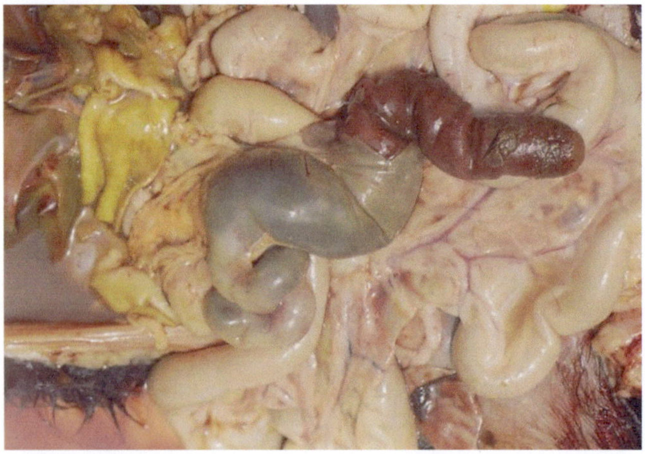

Fig. 6.13 Fibrinous enteritis. Canine intussusception: The intestinal mucosa at the affected area is congested and dark red, with fibrin membrane adhering to the surface. (Chen Huaitao)

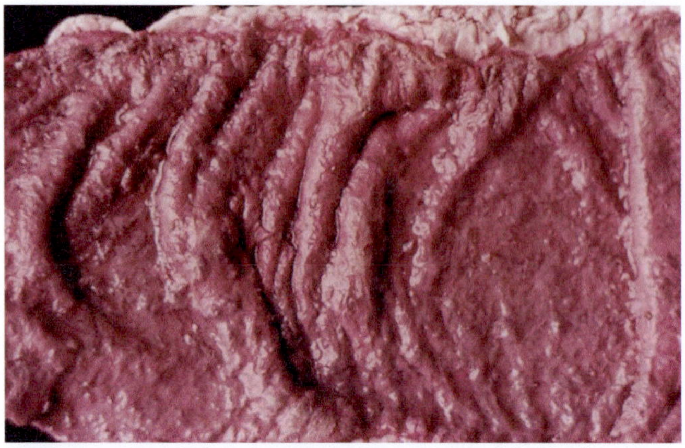

Fig. 6.14 Diffuse fibrinonecrotic enteritis. Bovine paratyphoid fever. The large intestinal mucosa is necrotized with the presence of fibrin exudation, which forms a thick layer of necrotic material. The intestinal mucosa is diffusely thickened with an uneven surface. (Veterinary Pathology Unit, Gansu Agricultural University)

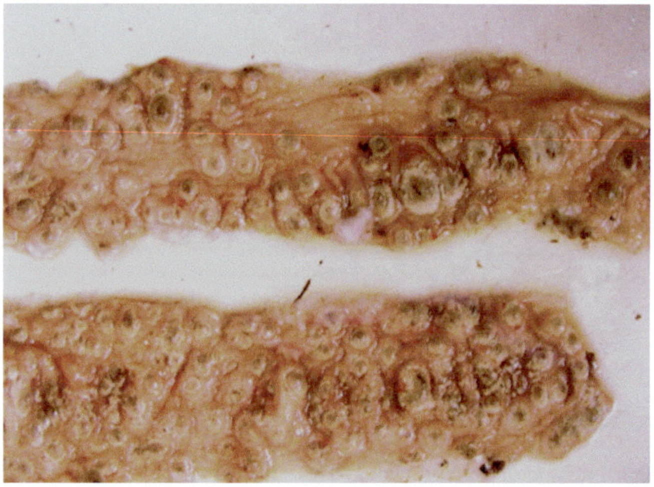

Fig. 6.15 Focal fibrinonecrotic enteritis. Chronic swine fever. Focal fibrinous necrotizing enteritis of the colonic mucosa, which is characterized by fibrin exudation with marked necrosis. The exudate and necrotic tissue coagulate together. Because the lesion protrudes from the mucosal surface in concentric circles and resembles a button, it is called button-like ulceration or button-like swelling. (Wang Xinhua)

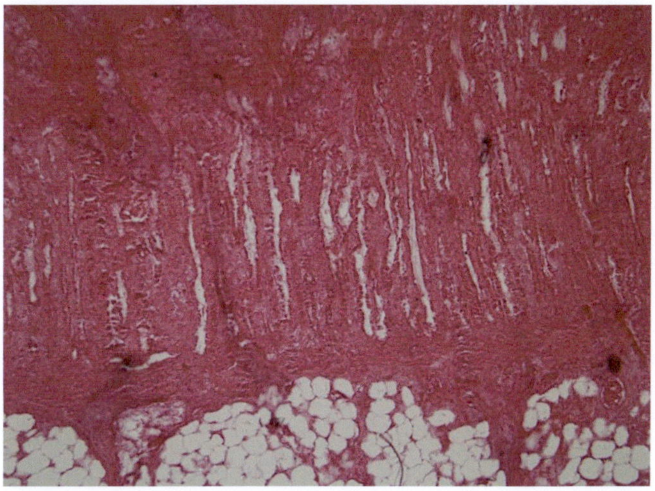

Fig. 6.16 Fibrinonecrotic enteritis. There is a large amount of fibrin exudation on the intestinal mucosal surface, which coagulates with the necrotic intestinal lamina propria. The necrotic intestinal glands are indistinctly visible. HE ×100. (Chen Huaitao)

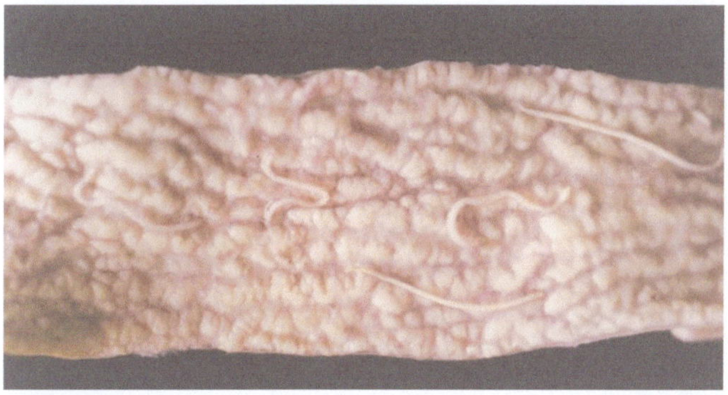

Fig. 6.17 Chronic catarrhal enteritis*Chabertia ovina*. The colonic mucosa is thickened with uneven and nodular surface. The parasites are still present on the mucosal surface. (Chen Huaitao)

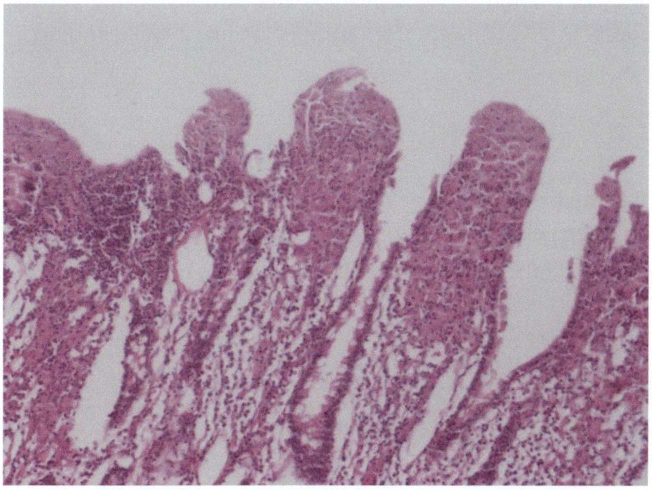

Fig. 6.18 Chronic catarrhal enteritis. Bovine paratuberculosis. Massive epithelioid cell proliferation is present in the lamina propria and submucosa of the ileum, which caused the deformation of the intestinal villi and thickening of the mucosa. HE ×100. (Wang Wenhui)

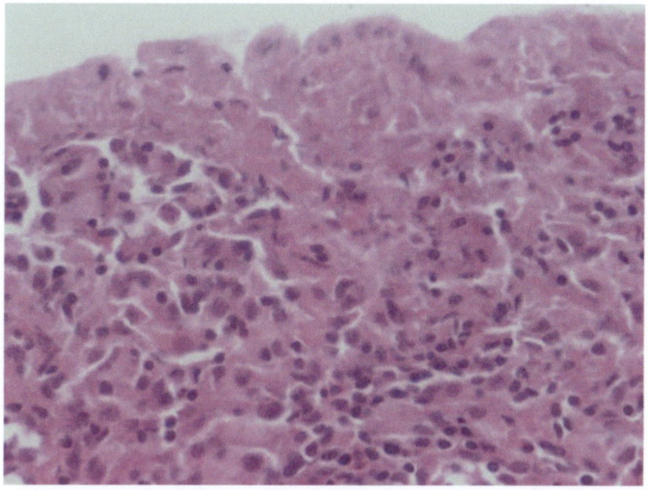

Fig. 6.19 Chronic catarrhal enteritis. Bovine paratuberculosis. A large number of epithelioid cells are present in the lamina propria of the ileal villi. Those cells are rich of cytoplasm and connect together. The epithelial cells of the intestinal mucosa are exfoliated. HE ×400. (Wang Wenhui)

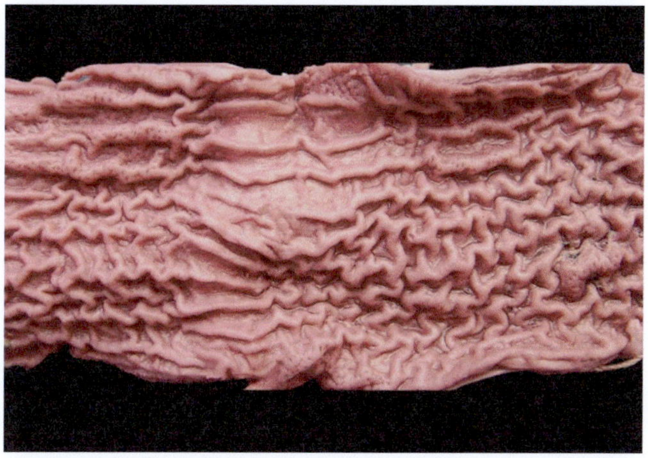

Fig. 6.20 Hypertrophic enteritis. Equine small intestine. The serosa and mucosa of the intestinal wall, especially the muscular layer, are markedly hypertrophied, with increased intestinal mucosal folds and a cerebral gyrus-like surface. (Chen Huaitao)

3 Pathological Changes of the Liver

3.1 Toxic Hepatosis and Focal Telangiectasis of Hepatic Sinusoid

3.1.1 Toxic Hepatosis (Figs. 6.21, 6.22, and 6.23)

Toxic hepatosis is a group of liver lesions characterized by severe degeneration and necrosis of hepatocytes caused by various toxic substances. It usually occurs in pigs, but also in other domestic animals. In acute cases, hepatocyte degeneration and necrosis are very severe, so it used to be called toxic

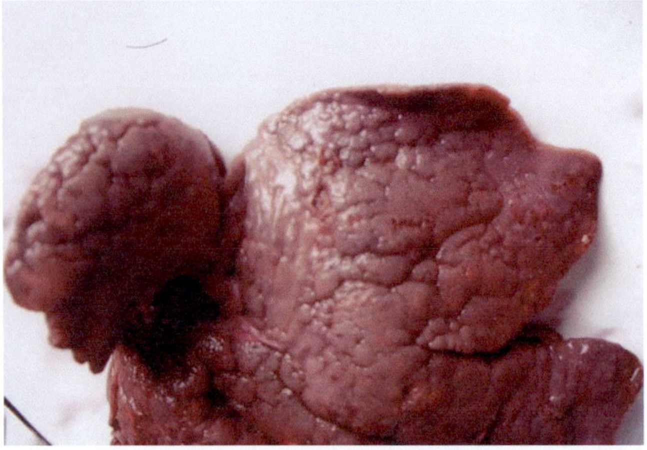

Fig. 6.21 Toxic hepatosis. Porcine toxic hepatosis (red atrophic stage): The liver is smaller, softer, unevenly colored with red patches and nodules of varying size on the surface. (Chen Huaitao)

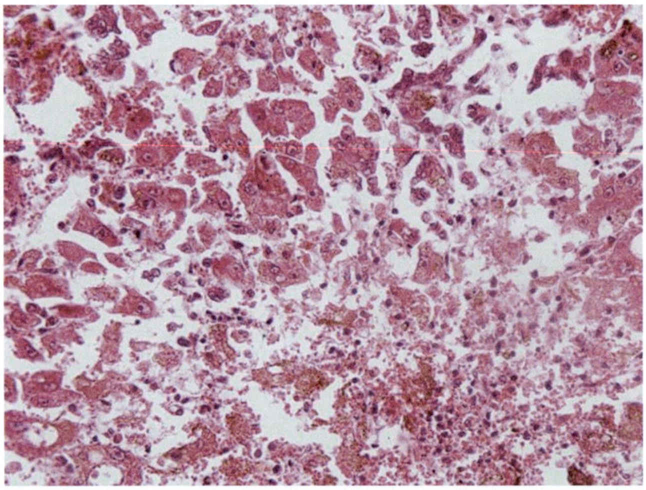

Fig. 6.22 Toxic hepatosis. Bovine moldy sweet potato poisoning. This image shows only the upper part of the hepatic lobule. The lower area is the central area of the hepatic lobule, where the hepatocytes around the central vein are completely necrotic and disintegrated, and erythrocytes as well as necrotic hepatocytes mainly remain with scattered macrophages, neutrophils, and hemosiderin-laden cells presence; the upper is the peripheral area of the hepatic lobule, where severe degeneration such as fatty change is present in the hepatocytes, and some cells are also necrotic. HE ×400. (Yang Mingqi, Chen Huaitao)

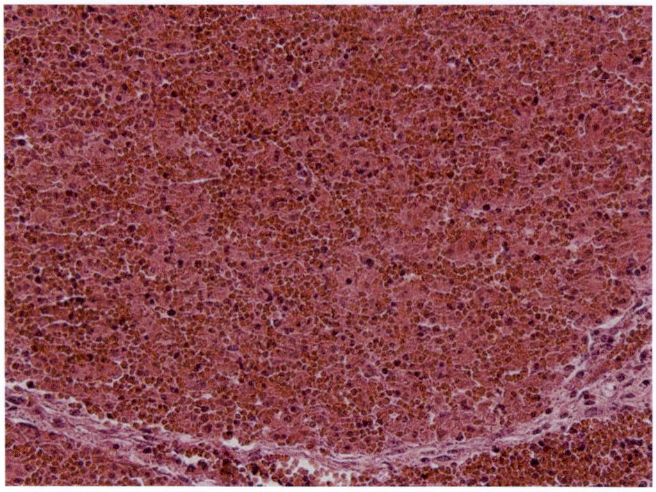

Fig. 6.23 Toxic hepatosis. Porcine toxic hepatosis: This is part of the liver lobule. The liver tissue is almost occupied by red blood cells except for a few indistinctly visible degenerated necrotic hepatocytes. The lobules are clearly defined. HE ×400. (Chen Huaitao)

liver dystrophy or acute yellow liver atrophy (yellow atrophy stage); when it lasts for a long period, the congestion and hemorrhage are present on the liver after necrosis, so it is called red liver atrophy (red atrophy stage). In chronic cases, liver fibrosis (liver stiffness) occurs. Sometimes inflammatory cell infiltration occurs, so it is also called toxic hepatitis.

3.1.2 Focal Hepatic Sinusoidal Dilatation (Figs. 6.24 and 6.25)

The cause of focal hepatic sinusoidal dilatation is not well understood and may be related to dietary deficiencies of selenium, vitamin E, and other tissue antioxidants. The sawdust-like hepatic necrotic foci may be present at the early stage of hepatic sinusoidal dilatation, which is followed by dilatation and congestion of the sinusoids and atrophy of the hepatic cords. In severe cases, the area appears like a "lake of blood."

3.2 Hepatitis

The main cause of hepatitis is biological factors; therefore, it is often classified into four categories: bacterial, viral, mycotic, and parasitic hepatitis.

3.2.1 Bacterial Hepatitis (Figs. 6.26, 6.27, and 6.28)

Bacterial hepatitis is often characterized by tissue degeneration and necrosis, formation of necrotic foci, or formation of abscesses and granulomas.

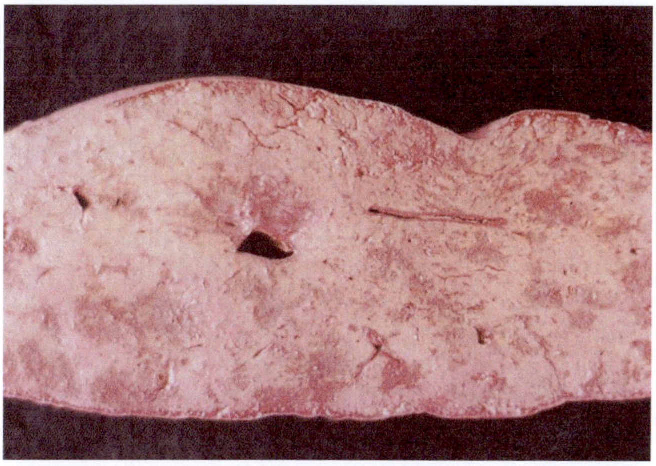

Fig. 6.24 Focal hepatic sinusoidal dilatation. Bovine liver. Dark red lesions of variable size are present in the liver section. (Chen Huaitao)

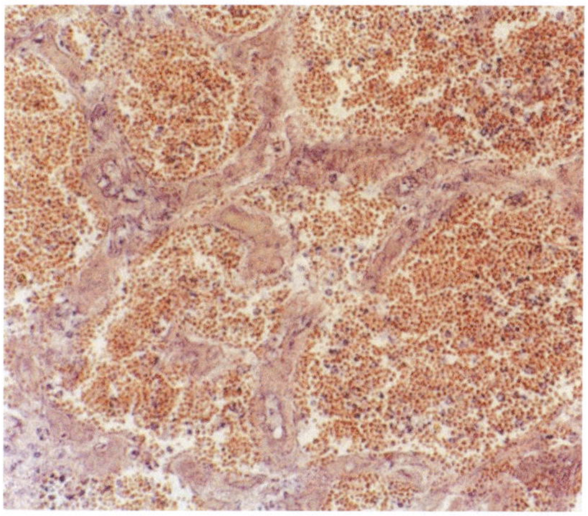

Fig. 6.25 Focal hepatic sinusoidal dilatation. Bovine liver. The hepatic sinusoids in the area of the lesion are highly dilated, filled with blood, and the hepatocytes are atrophied into long strips. HE ×200. (Chen Huaitao)

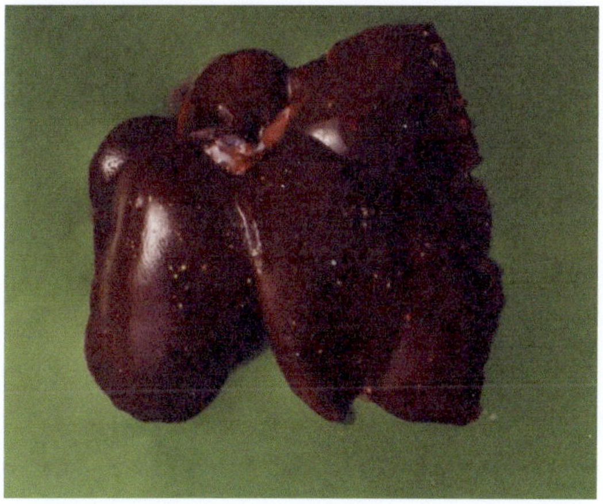

Fig. 6.26 Pasteurella hepatitis in chickens. Numerous grayish-yellow or grayish-white necrotic dots are scattered on the liver surface. (Chen Huaitao)

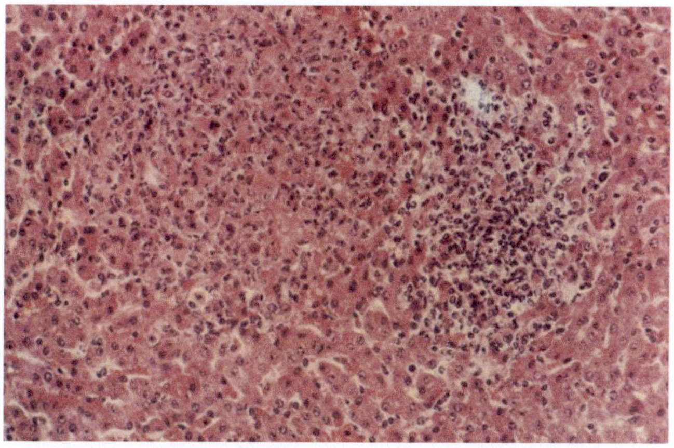

Fig. 6.27 Salmonella hepatitis in calves. Focal hepatocyte necrosis can be observed with proliferation of Kupffer cells and infiltration of inflammatory cells. HE ×200. (Liu Baoyan)

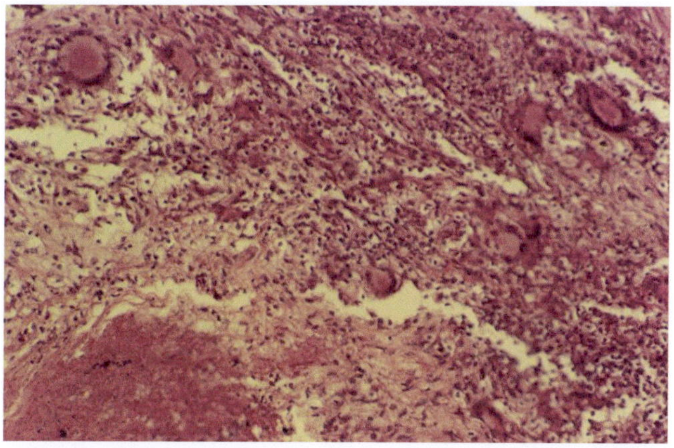

Fig. 6.28 Bovine tuberculous hepatitis. This image shows only partial of a nodule of hepatic tuberculosis. The caseous necrosis is in the center of the nodule (in the lower left), which is surrounded by epithelioid cells and multiple Langhans giant cells. HE ×200. (Wang Wenhui)

3.2.2 Viral Hepatitis (Fig. 6.29)

The viruses that cause hepatitis are mostly hepatophilic viruses that often cause degenerative changes in the liver. Some viruses causing hepatitis may also form specific inclusion bodies in the nucleus or cytoplasm of hepatocytes.

3.2.3 Mycotic Hepatitis (Fig. 6.30)

Common pathogens include *Aspergillus fumigatus*, *Aspergillus flavus*, *Aspergillus griseoides*, and *Aspergillus constructus*. Mycelium can be found in lesions caused by molds.

3.2.4 Parasitic Hepatitis (Fig. 6.31)

Parasitic hepatitis is caused by the parasitic reproduction of certain parasites in the liver parenchyma or intrahepatic bile ducts, or by the migration of larvae of certain parasites in the liver.

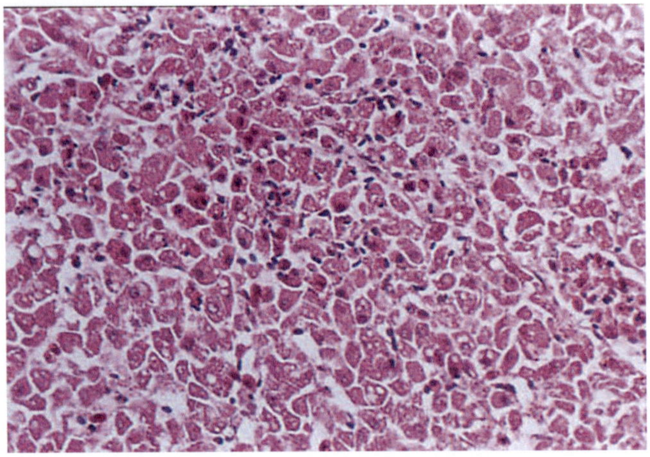

Fig. 6.29 Avian necrotic hepatitis. Chicken liver cells had fatty degeneration, coagulative necrosis, and inflammatory cell infiltration. HE ×400. (Liu Chen)

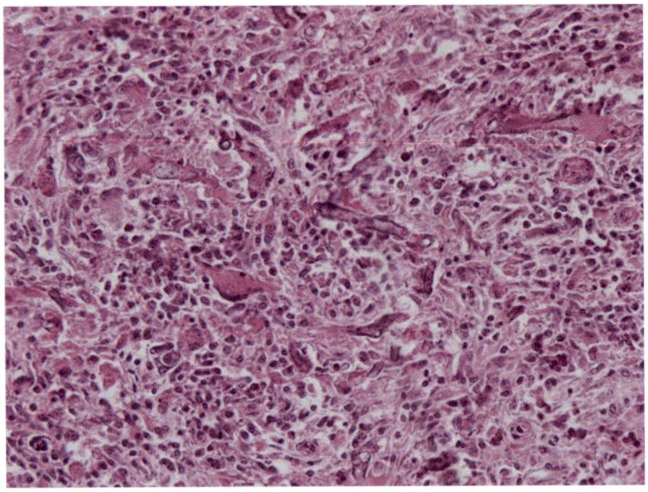

Fig. 6.30 Mycotic hepatitis in pigs. Porcine hepatic aspergillosis. Connective tissue hyperplasia and lymphocytic infiltration are present in the liver lesions with multinucleated giant cells. Note the presence of many *Aspergillus* mycelia in the hyperplastic tissue. HE ×400. (Chen Huaitao)

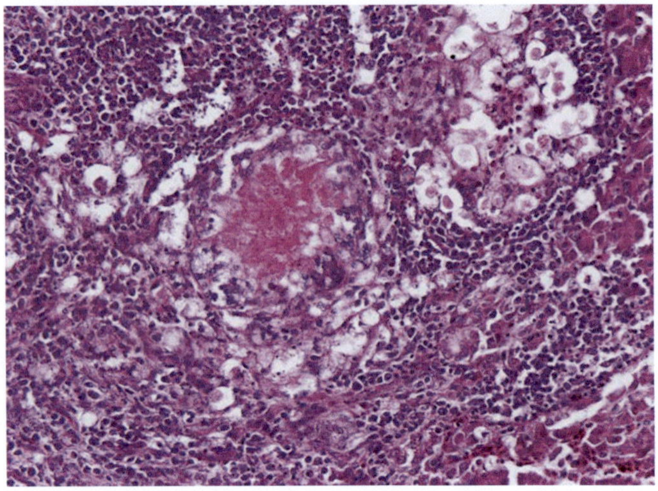

Fig. 6.31 Hepatitis in the histotrichomoniasis of chickens. A focus of necrosis is shown in the middle of this figure. The nearby connective tissue is proliferative with infiltration of lymphocytes, plasma cells, and macrophages. The giant cell formation can be observed, and a number of *Histomonas meleagridis* are present in the proliferating tissue. HE ×400. (Chen Huaitao)

3.3 Cirrhosis

Cirrhosis is caused by a variety of etiologies and is characterized by severe degeneration and necrosis of liver parenchymal cells and significant proliferation of connective tissue. As a result, the liver is often hardened and deformed. Cirrhosis can be classified into the following four types.

3.3.1 Portal Cirrhosis (Figs. 6.32, 6.33, and 6.34)

3.3.2 Postnecrotic Cirrhosis (Figs. 6.35 and 6.36)

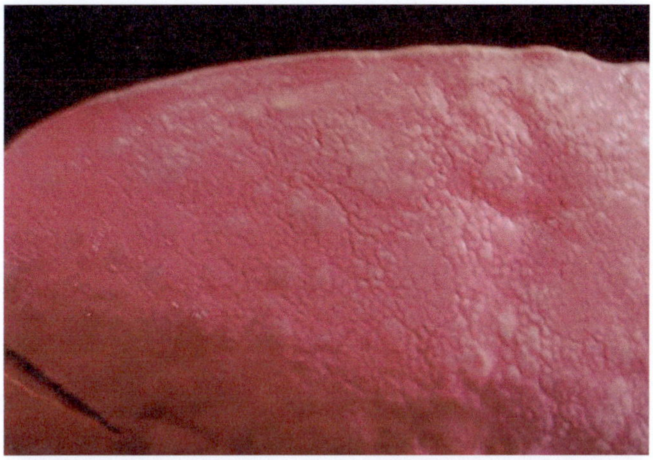

Fig. 6.32 Portal cirrhosis. Pig liver. Portal cirrhosis: The liver is enlarged with an uneven, nodular surface. (Chen Huaitao)

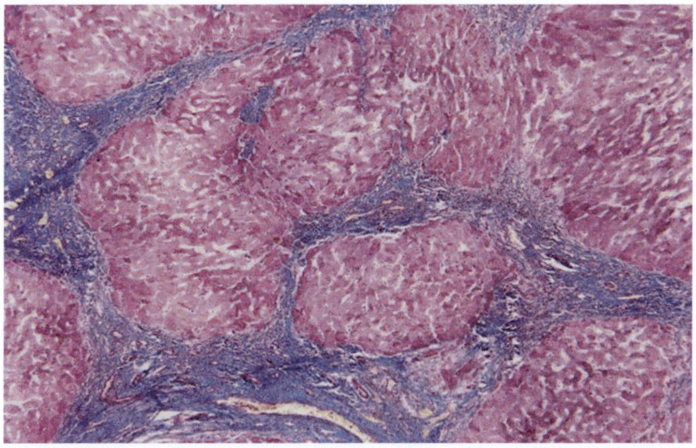

Fig. 6.33 Portal cirrhosis. The intrinsic structure of the liver is disrupted and the connective tissue proliferates, dividing the liver lobules into irregular clumps of cells called pseudolobules. Mallory connective tissue staining ×100. (Chen Huaitao)

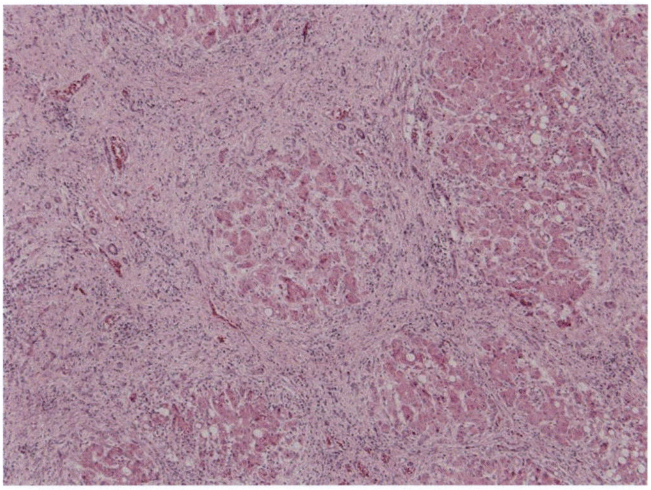

Fig. 6.34 Portal cirrhosis. The liver connective tissue is obviously hyperplastic with severe destruction of the intrinsic structure of the liver. The lobules are divided by connective tissue into cellular clumps of varying sizes (pseudolobules), which are separated by thick layers of connective tissue. A massive infiltration of inflammatory cells, mainly lymphocytes are present. In addition, new capillaries and pseudobile ducts can also be observed. HE ×100. (Chen Huaitao)

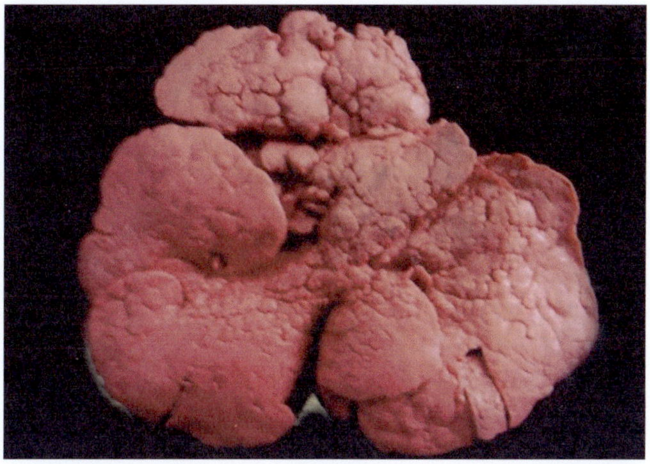

Fig. 6.35 Postnecrotic cirrhosis. Atrophic cirrhosis in pigs: The liver size is reduced and its texture is hardened with sharp edges, and nodules or grooves on the surface. (Veterinary Pathology Unit, Gansu Agricultural University)

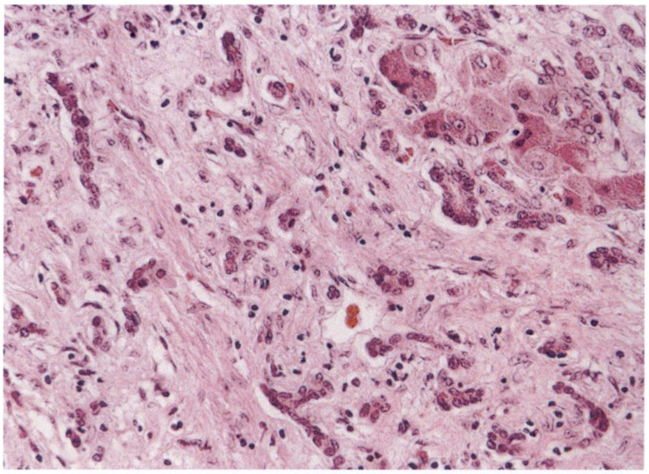

Fig. 6.36 Postnecrotic cirrhosis. Aflatoxicosis in pigs. Massive hepatocyte degeneration, necrosis, and regeneration can be observed with connective tissue hyperplasia and lymphocytic infiltration. The small bile ducts proliferate into small strips, clusters, or tubules, located in the interstitium or extending into the liver tissue. HE ×400. (Chen Huaitao)

3.3.3 Verminous Cirrhosis (Figs. 6.37, 6.38, 6.39, 6.40, and 6.41)

3.3.4 Biliary Cirrhosis (Figs. 6.42 and 6.43)

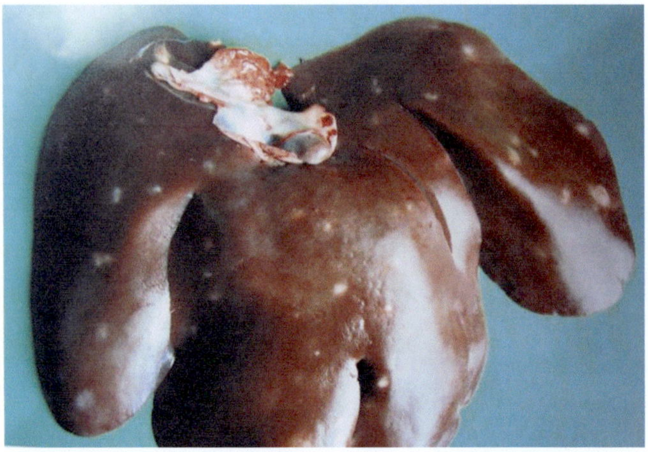

Fig. 6.37 *Ascaris lumbricoides* cirrhosis. Swine ascariasis. When *Ascaris* larvae migrate in the liver, it can cause focal interstitial hepatitis, which is called "milky spot liver." There are milky spots present on the surface of the liver, which is about 1 ~ 2 cm in diameter, and they are proliferating fibrous connective tissue. (Cheng Guofu)

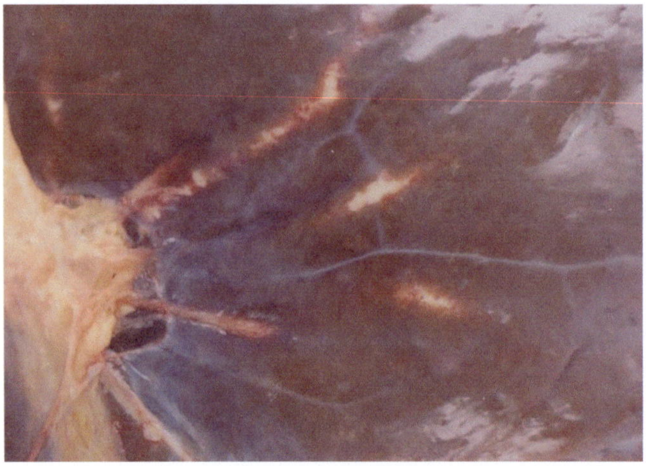

Fig. 6.38 *Fasciola hepatica* cirrhosis. Bovine fascioliasis hepatica. *Fasciola hepatica* parasitizes in the bile ducts, causing hyperplasia of the bile duct walls, so there are cord-like protrusions on liver surface. The liver becomes hard in texture. (Chen Huaitao)

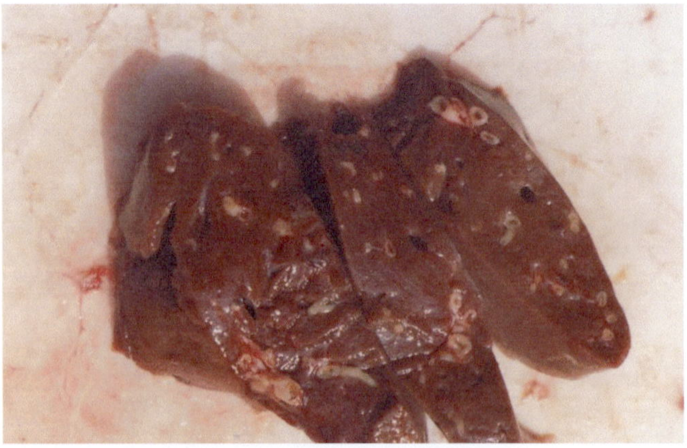

Fig. 6.39 Cirrhosis caused by dicrocoeliasis. Dicrocoeliasis in sheep. The dicrocoelium parasitizing in the small bile ducts causes hyperplasia of the bile duct walls, so the walls of the small bile ducts are markedly thickened on the liver section surface, and they are in annular form. (Chen Huaitao)

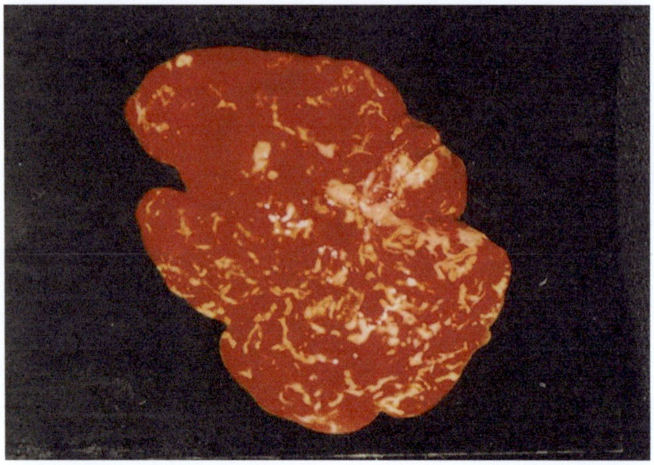

Fig. 6.40 Hepatic sclerosis caused by *Cysticercus pisiformis*. Rabbit *Cysticercus pisiformis*. Numerous curved striated hyperplastic lesions are present on the surface of the liver, which are lesions resulting from the proliferative inflammation caused by the migration of oncosphere in the liver. (Wang Yongkun)

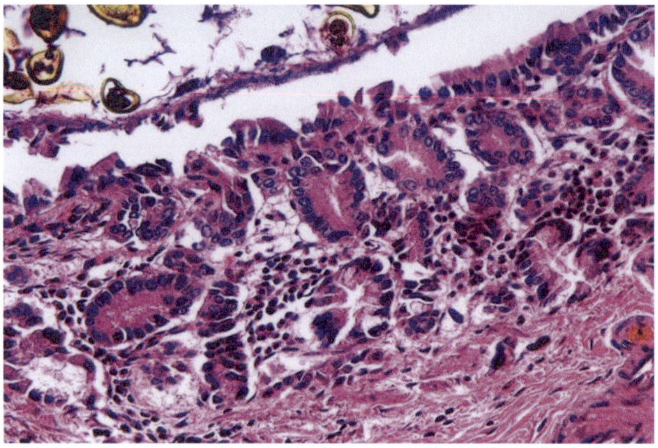

Fig. 6.41 Hepatic sclerosis caused by *Fasciola hepatica*. Sheep liver. This image shows only partial of the bile duct parasitized by *Fasciola hepatica*. The bile duct epithelium and bile duct wall glands are hyperplastic with infiltration of lymphocytes and eosinophils. The connective tissue surrounding the bile ducts is hyperplastic. A port of the *Fasciola hepatica* is shown at the upper left of the image. HE ×400. (Chen Huaitao)

4 Pancreatitis (Figs. 6.44 and 6.45)

There are acute and chronic pancreatitis. In veterinary practice, what is commonly referred to as acute pancreatitis is actually acute pancreatic necrosis, as the primary lesion is pancreatic tissue necrosis due to the direct action of pancreatic digestive enzymes. Chronic pancreatitis is often a regression of acute pancreatitis with proliferation of fibrous connective tissue and shrinking as well as wrinkling of pancreas.

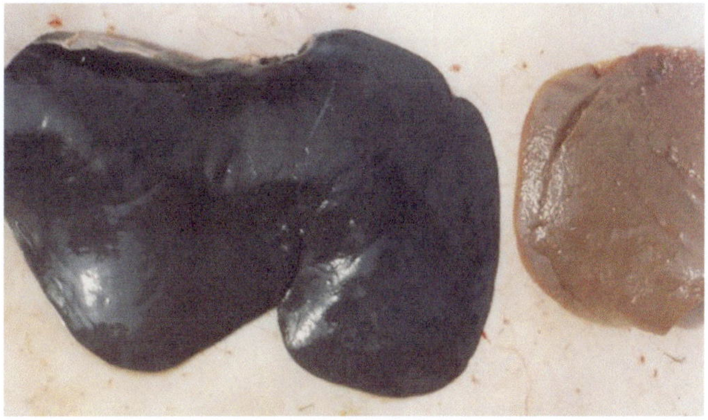

Fig. 6.42 Biliary cirrhosis. Sheep liver. Bile accumulates in the bile ducts and liver lobules after bile duct obstruction, resulting in a dark green liver with a hardened texture. The portion of a normal sheep liver is shown on the right as a control. (Chen Huaitao)

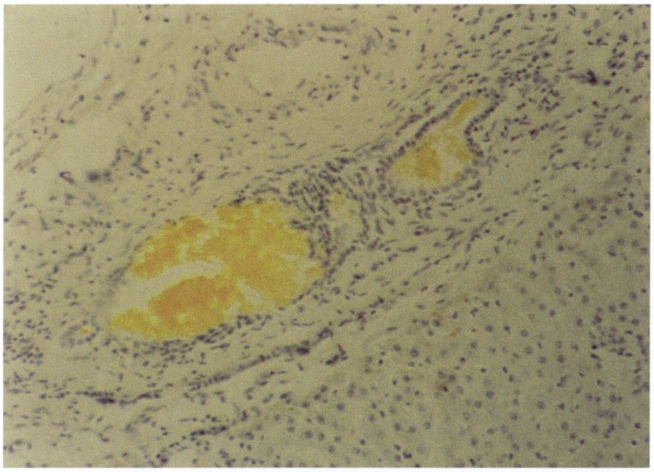

Fig. 6.43 Biliary cirrhosis. Both the large and small bile ducts are dilated and filled with yellow bile. The interstitial connective tissue is hyperplastic with lymphocyte infiltration. HE ×400. (Chen Huaitao)

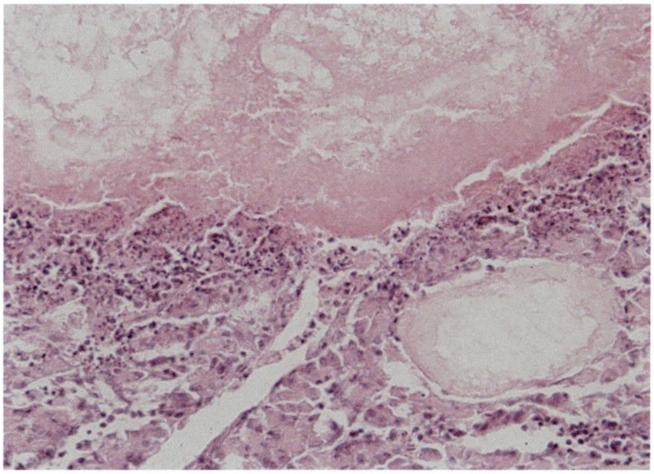

Fig. 6.44 Necrotizing pancreatitis. There are necrotic areas of varying sizes in the pancreas with distinct boundaries with adjacent tissues. The pancreatic tissue is necrotic and disintegrated in a structureless material, and the periphery of the necrotic area is infiltrated with nuclear debris and inflammatory cells. HE ×400. (Wang Wenhui)

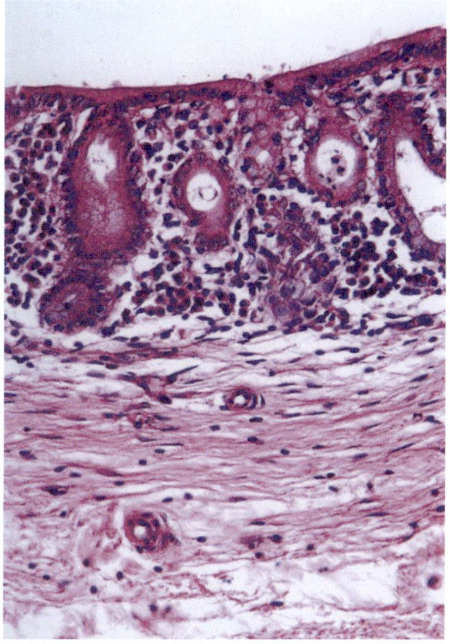

Fig. 6.45 Proliferative pancreatic ductitis. Bovine eurytrematosis. This picture shows histological changes of the pancreatic duct wall without showing the parasite *Eurytrema* in the pancreatic duct. The pancreatic duct epithelium and the glands of the pancreatic duct wall are proliferated, with massive infiltration of eosinophils and lymphocytes. The connective tissue surrounding the pancreatic duct is hyperplastic obviously. HE ×400. (Wang Wenhui)

Bibliography

1. Huaitao C, editor. Pathological anatomy of domestic animals. 3rd ed. China Agricultural Press; 2006.

Pathology of the Respiratory System

7

1 Rhinitis (Fig. 7.1)

2 Pneumonia

Pneumonia is the inflammation of the bronchioles, alveoli, and interstitial lung tissue. It is one of the most common pathological processes in the lungs.

There are various classifications of pneumonia, and based on pathological features, pneumonia can be classified into bronchopneumonia, fibrinous pneumonia, interstitial pneumonia, granulomatous pneumonia, and embolic pneumonia. Bronchopneumonia, fibrinous pneumonia, and interstitial pneumonia are common in veterinary clinical practice, but granulomatous pneumonia is also very important.

2.1 Bronchopneumonia (Figs. 7.1, 7.2, 7.3, 7.4, 7.5, 7.6, and 7.7)

Bronchopneumonia is lobular pneumonia. The histology is characterized by serum-cellular alveolar exudate, hence it is named catarrhal pneumonia.

2.2 Fibrinous Pneumonia (Figs. 7.8, 7.9, 7.10, 7.11, 7.12, 7.13, 7.14, and 7.15)

Fibrinous pneumonia, also known as lobar pneumonia, is an acute pneumonia characterized by a large amount of fibrin exuding from the alveoli.

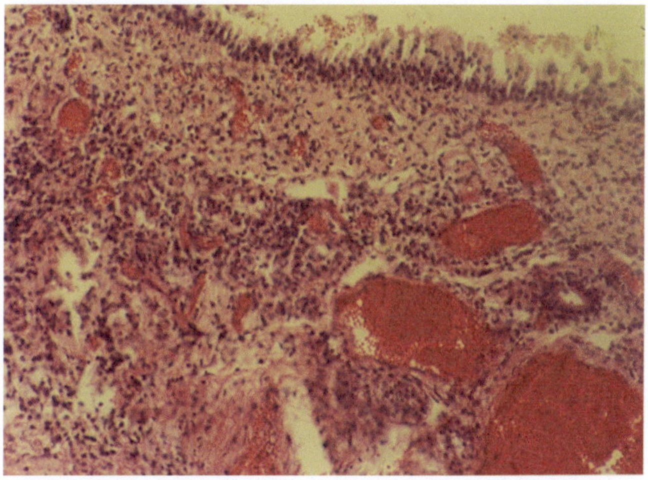

Fig. 7.1 Acute catarrhal rhinitis. Bovine acute catarrhal fever. Some of the nasal mucosal epithelium is necrotic and exfoliated. Some mucus and red blood cells are attached to the mucosal surface. The lamina propria is markedly congested, edematous with leukocyte infiltration. The vascular wall is necrotized with numerous lymphocytes and monocytes infiltrating around it. HE ×200. (Chen Huaitao)

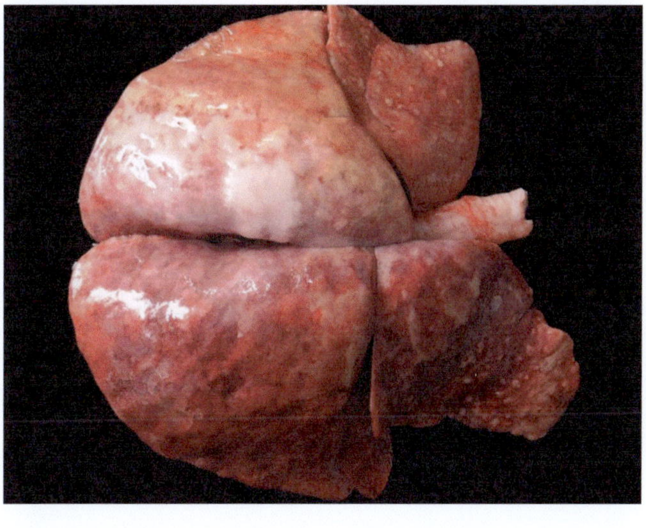

Fig. 7.2 Bronchopneumonia. There are yellowish-white lesions scattered in the apical and cardiac lobes of the lungs, with depressed areas and protruding emphysema areas on the lung surface. (Chen Huaitao)

H. Chen, *Color Atlas of Veterinary Pathology*, https://doi.org/10.1007/978-981-96-7617-0_7

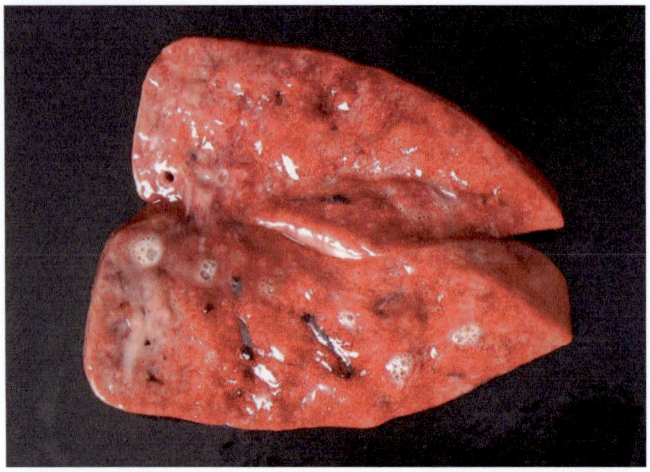

Fig. 7.3 Bronchopneumonia. Figure 7.2 Section of the lung lesion area: fluid with bubbles is flowing out of the bronchi, and small yellowish-white lesions are also observed. (Chen Huaitao)

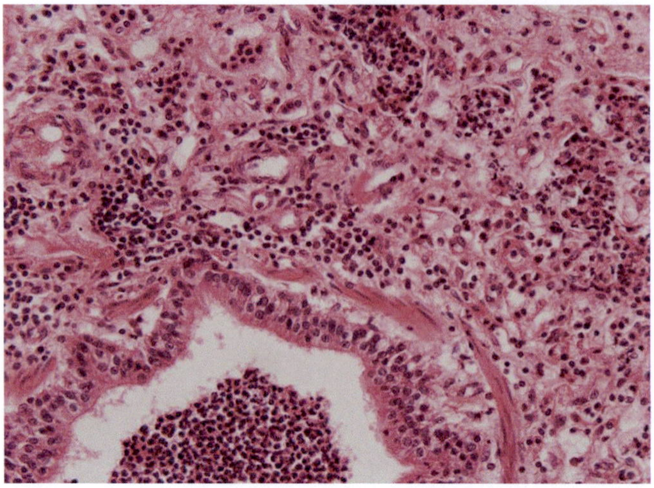

Fig. 7.5 Bronchopneumonia. The bronchiolar epithelium is degenerated with many neutrophils in the lumen. The peribronchial alveolar septa are congested with a number of inflammatory cells in the alveolar lumen. HE ×400. (Chen Huaitao)

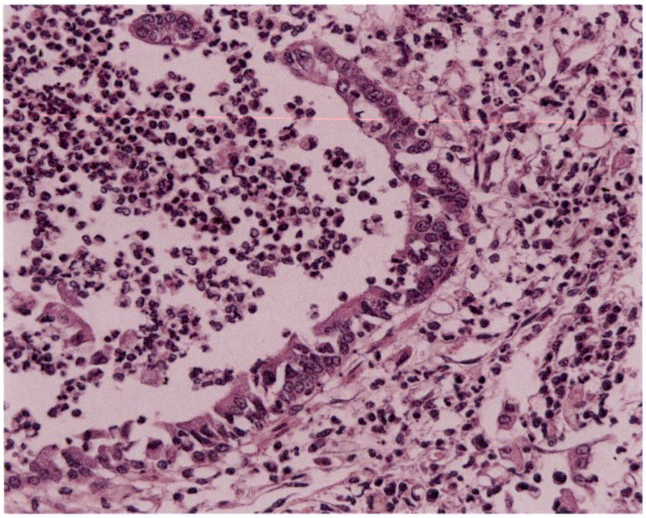

Fig. 7.4 Bronchopneumonia. The epithelium of the bronchiole is degenerated, necrotic, and exfoliated. Many neutrophils and exfoliated epithelial cells are present in the lumen. The lung tissue surrounding the bronchioles is also infiltrated by many inflammatory cells. HE ×400. (Wang Wenhui)

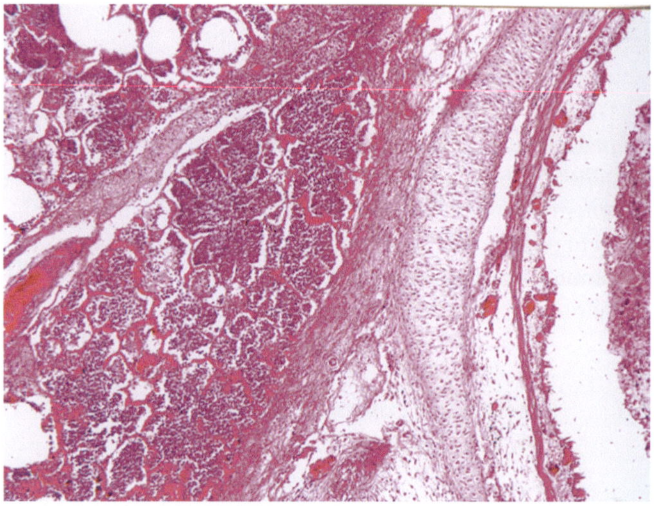

Fig. 7.6 Bronchopneumonia. Glanders. Septic bronchopneumonia: bronchial mucosa is congested, edematous, infiltrated by inflammatory cells, with severe degeneration, necrosis, and exfoliation of the mucosal epithelium. There area large amount of mucus, detached epithelial cells, neutrophils, and erythrocytes in the lumen. The alveolar septum is congested, with accumulation of a large number of neutrophils in the alveolar lumen. The interlobular tissue is edematous and widened. The lymphatic vessels are dilated with lymphatic thrombus formation. HE ×100. (Chen Huaitao)

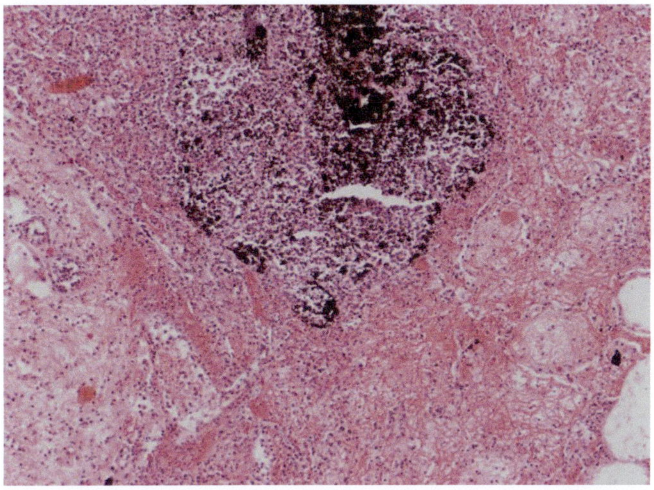

Fig. 7.7 Bronchopneumonia. Bovine foreign body pneumonia. Gangrenous pneumonia due to careless oral administration of medicinal solution: black amorphous foreign bodies and numerous pus cells are present in the bronchial lumen. The bronchial wall is necrotic and the epithelium is indistinct. The bronchial periphery is markedly congested, hemorrhagic, and edematous as well as infiltrated with inflammatory cells. HE ×200. (Chen Huaitao)

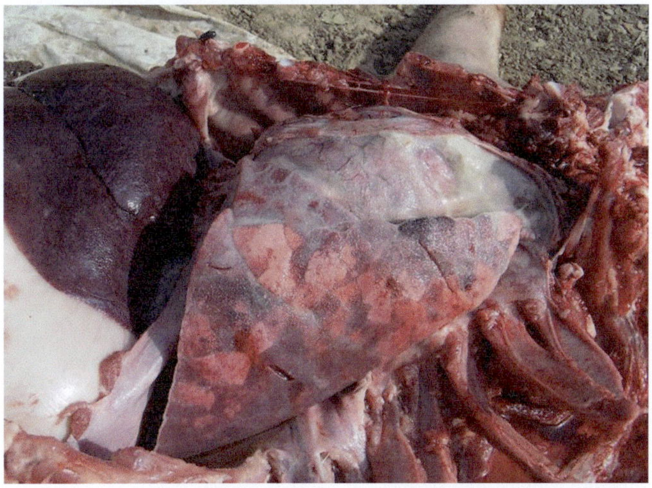

Fig. 7.8 Fibrinous pneumonia. Infectious pleuropneumonia in pigs: Lungs are enlarged with interstitium widened and texture hardened. The hepatization is obvious, and the pleura is attached with fibrinous membrane, which is yellowish white. (Liu Andian)

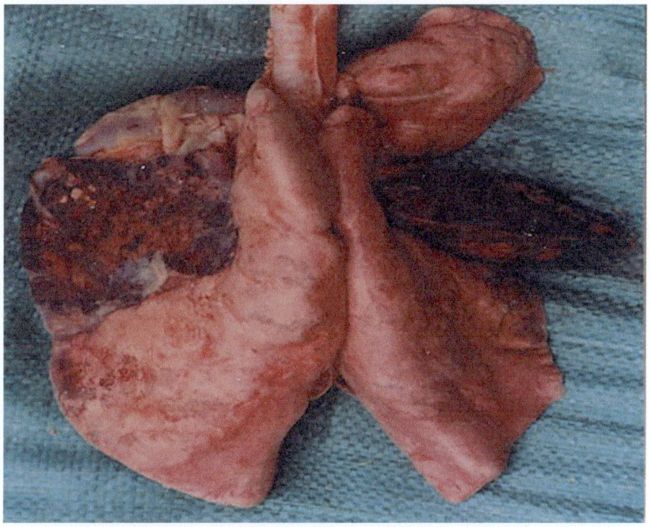

Fig. 7.9 Fibrinous pneumonia. Pasteurellosis in sheep: The cardiac lobes are red and hardened with fibrin attached to the pulmonary pleura (red hepatic changes). (Chen Huaitao)

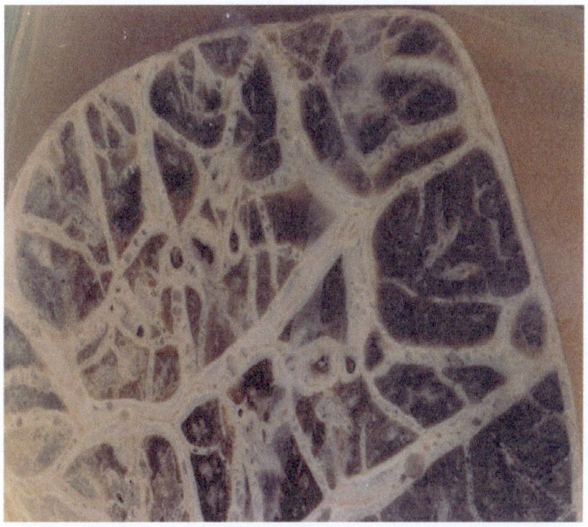

Fig. 7.10 Fibrinous pneumonia. Infectious pleuropneumonia in cattle: The red and gray hepatization of lung lobules is obvious on lung sections. The interstitium is edematous and widened with the lymphatic vessels expanded, so the lungs show typical marble-like scenes. (Veterinary Pathology Unit, Gansu Agricultural University)

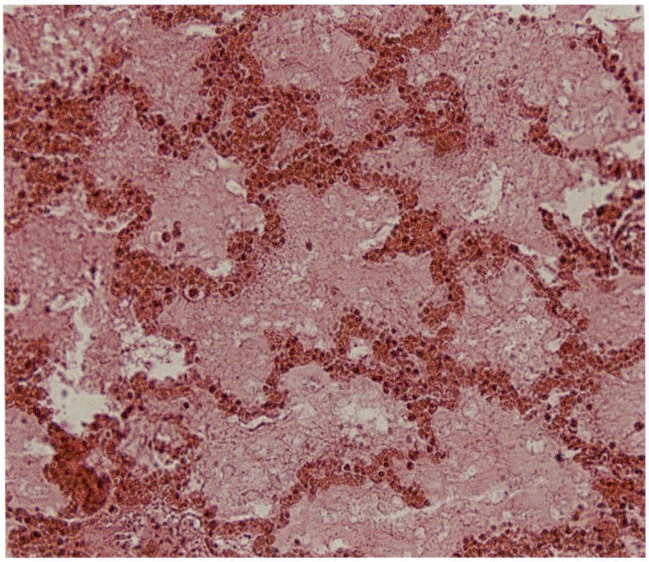

Fig. 7.11 Fibrinous pneumonia (congestive edematous phase). The alveolar septal capillaries are highly dilated and congested, and a large amount of serum, a few red blood cells, and leukocytes are present in the alveolar cavity. HE ×400. (Chen Huaitao)

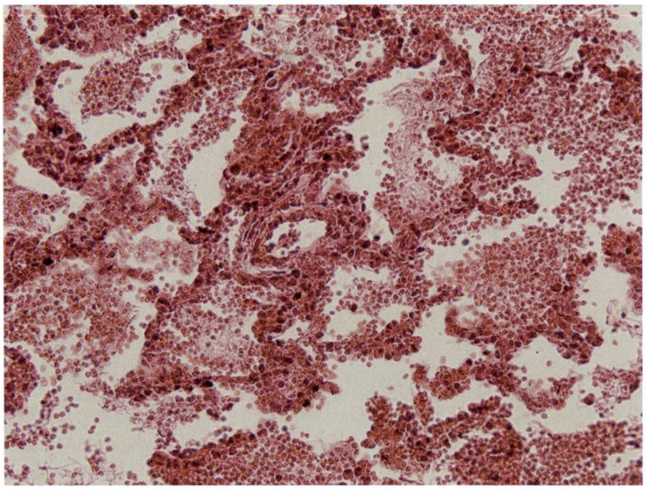

Fig. 7.12 Fibrinous pneumonia (red hepatization phase). The alveolar septal capillaries are highly dilated and congested, and the alveolar lumen contains a large number of erythrocytes, fibrin, inflammatory cells, and detached alveolar epithelial cells. HE ×400. (Chen Huaitao)

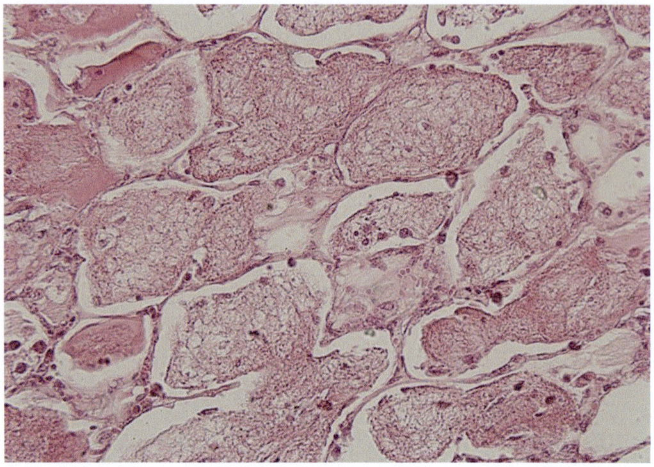

Fig. 7.13 Fibrinous pneumonia (gray hepatization phase). Atresia of alveolar septum capillaries, loss of congestion, large amount of fibrinous exudate, and small amount of neutrophils in the alveolar lumen; fibrin can cross the alveolar pores to connect with each other in the adjacent alveoli. HE ×400. (Chen Huaitao)

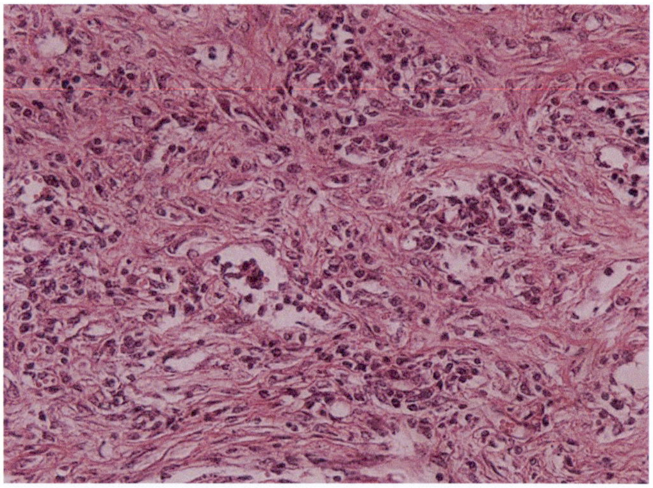

Fig. 7.14 Organization of pneumonia exudate. Exudates such as fibrin in the alveoli have been replaced by granulation tissue, and the lung structure is indistinguishable. HE ×400. (Chen Huaitao)

2.3 Interstitial Pneumonia (Figs. 7.16, 7.17, 7.18, 7.19, 7.20, 7.21, 7.22, 7.23, 7.24, 7.25, 7.26, 7.27, and 7.28)

Interstitial pneumonia is an inflammatory process that occurs in the lung interstitium. The lesions often originate from the alveolar wall and alveolar interstitium and subsequently spread to the interlobular, bronchial, and perivascular connective tissues.

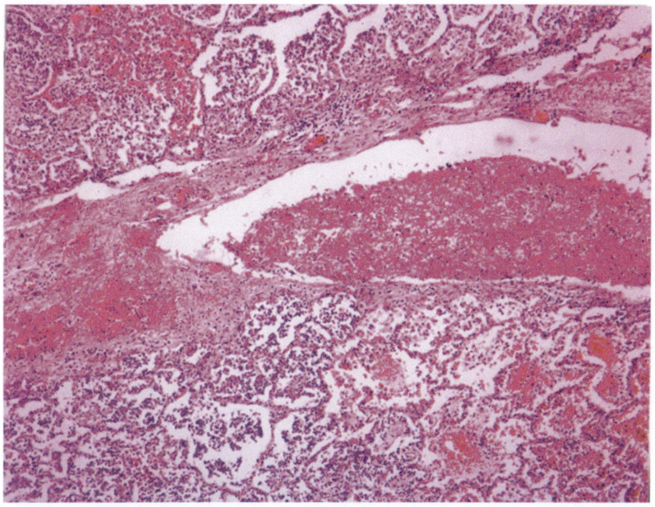

Fig. 7.15 Fibrinous pneumonia. Swine pasteurellosis. Fibrinohaemorrhagic pneumonia: The lobular interstitium is widened and edematous, with a large amount of fibrin, neutrophils, and erythrocytes in the interstitium and alveoli. The interlobular lymphatic vessels are dilated, in which lymph emboli are formed. HE ×100. (Chen Huaitao)

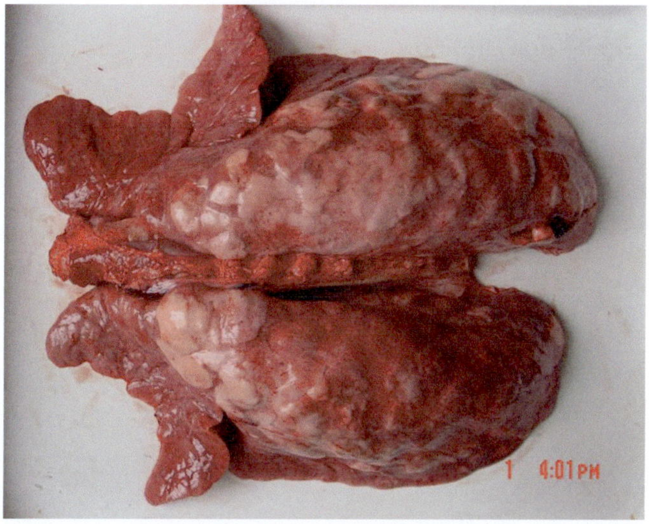

Fig. 7.17 Interstitial pneumonia. Mycoplasma pneumonia (porcine wheezing disease) in pigs: the area of pneumonia is located in the apical and cardiac lobes, with a solid texture, grayish-red color, pancreas-like appearance (pancreatic transformation), and emphysema being present in the diaphragmatic lobe. (Wu Bin)

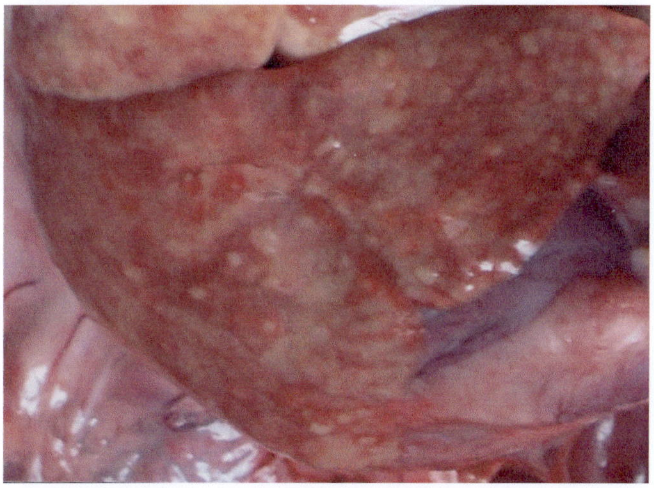

Fig. 7.16 Interstitial pneumonia. Canine distemper pneumonia: many foci of grayish-yellow pneumonia of varying sizes are present on a dark red background. (Chen Huaitao, Xu Xiaohong)

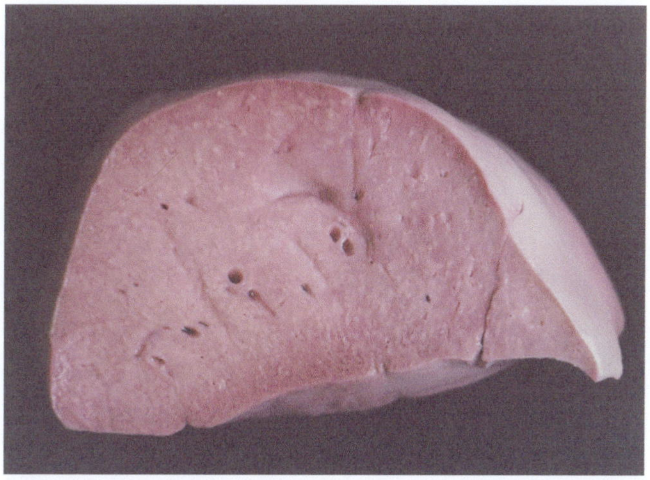

Fig. 7.18 Interstitial pneumonia. Chronic progressive pneumonia (Maedi-Visna disease) in sheep: The lungs are enlarged with numerous fine gray-white nodules scattered on cut surface. (Chen Huaitao)

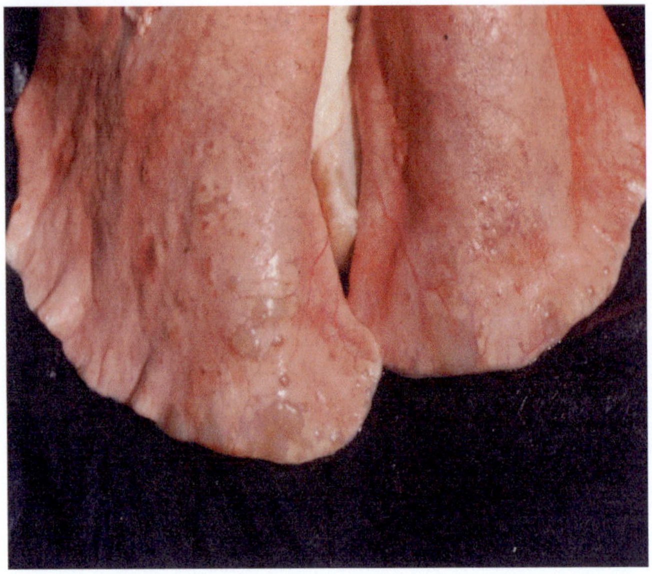

Fig. 7.19 Interstitial pneumonia. Pulmonary nematode pneumonia in sheep: Numerous grayish-yellow pulmonary nematode nodules and lamellar solid areas are present on the posterior margin of dorsal diaphragmatic lobe, around which are hemorrhagic spots and alveolar emphysema. (Chen Huaitao)

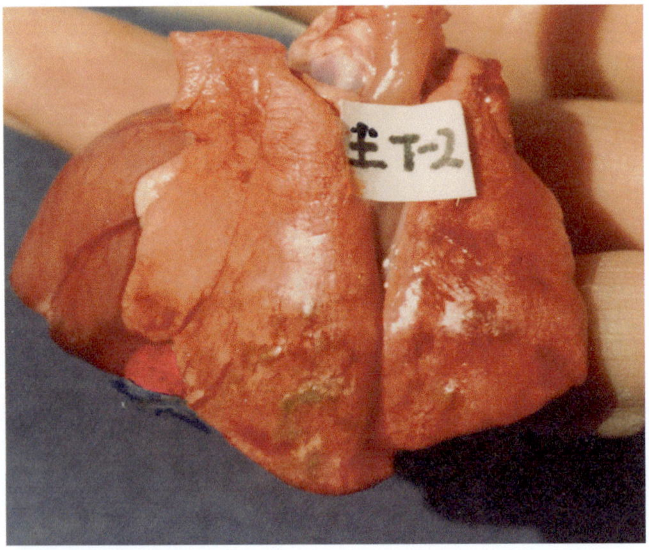

Fig. 7.20 Interstitial pneumonia. Rabbit pneumoconiosis: There are dark brownish-yellow areas of pneumonia of variable size at the dorsal posterior area of the diaphragic lobe of the lungs, with indistinct borders. (Li Xiaoming)

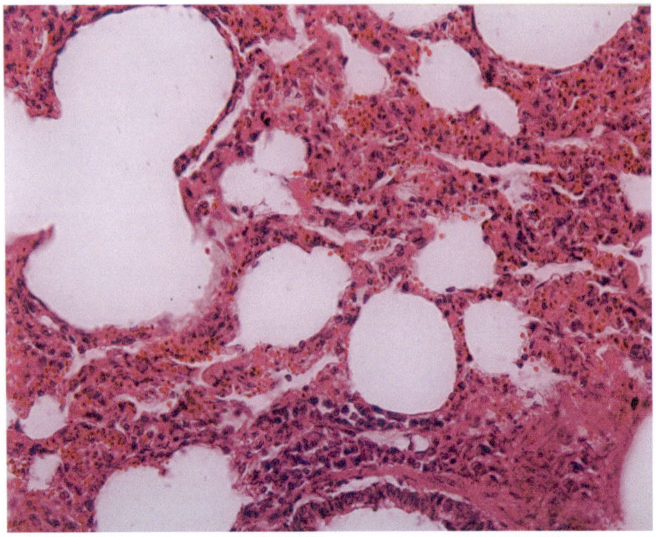

Fig. 7.21 Interstitial pneumonia. Acute interstitial pneumonia: alveolar septa is widened due to congestion, edema, and inflammatory cell infiltration. Many alveoli have shrunk or even disappeared, but some alveoli develop compensatory emphysema. HE ×400. (Wang Wenhui)

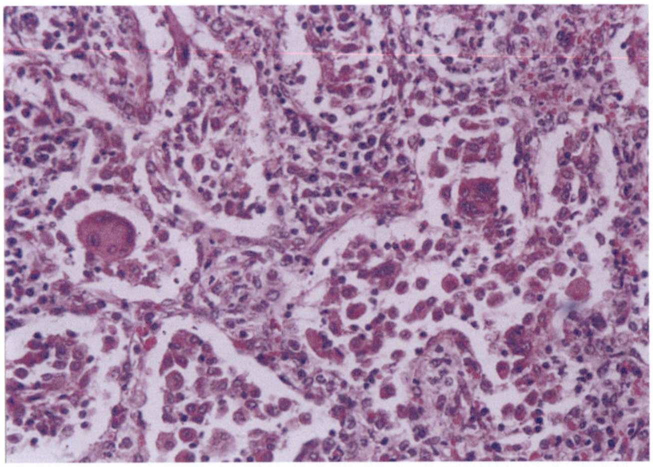

Fig. 7.22 Interstitial pneumonia. Equine asthma (allergic pneumonia). The alveolar septum is markedly widened, in which lymphocytes and monocytes infiltrate and connective tissue hyperplasia is observed. The alveolar epithelium is still somewhat proliferated and detached, and there are lymphocytes, monocytes, and detached epithelial cells in the alveolar lumen. HE ×400. (Chen Huaitao)

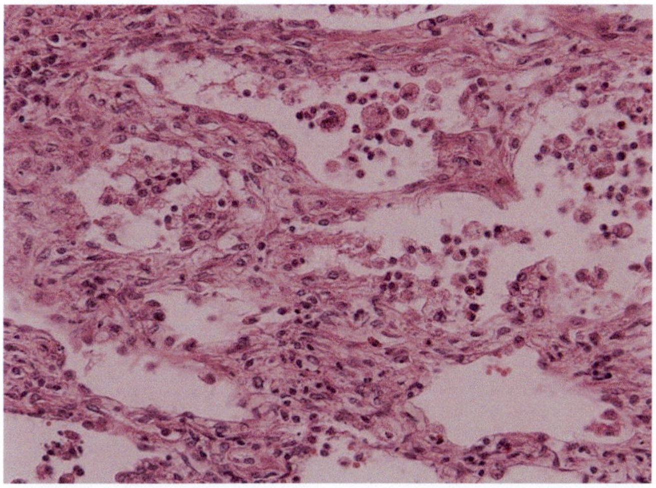

Fig. 7.23 Interstitial pneumonia. Canine distemper. The alveolar septal blood vessels are congested with cellular proliferation, so the alveolar septum is thickened and the alveolar epithelium is proliferated, and a few macrophages are present in some alveolar margins. HE ×400. (Chen Huaitao)

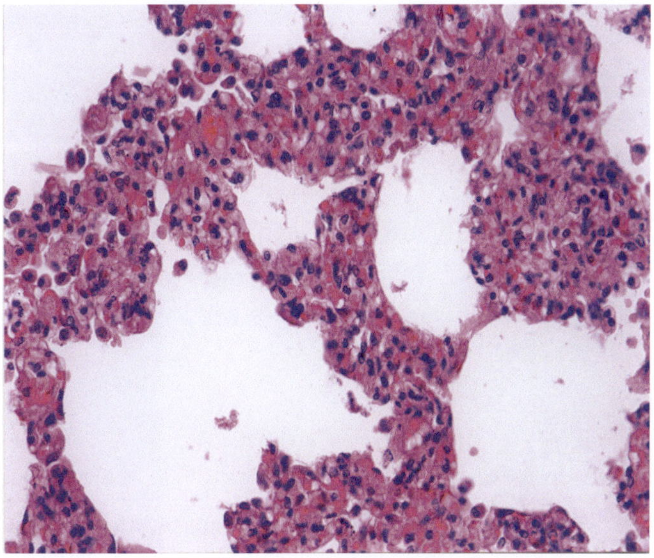

Fig. 7.24 Interstitial pneumonia. Canine distemper. The alveolar septal vessels are congested, the alveolar epithelium is hyperplastic and detached, and a large number of macrophages, shed epithelial cells and a few neutrophils and lymphocytes are present in alveolar cavity. The macrophages vary considerably, some are extremely large, and giant cells are also observed. HE ×400. (Chen Huaitao, Zhaxi Yingpai)

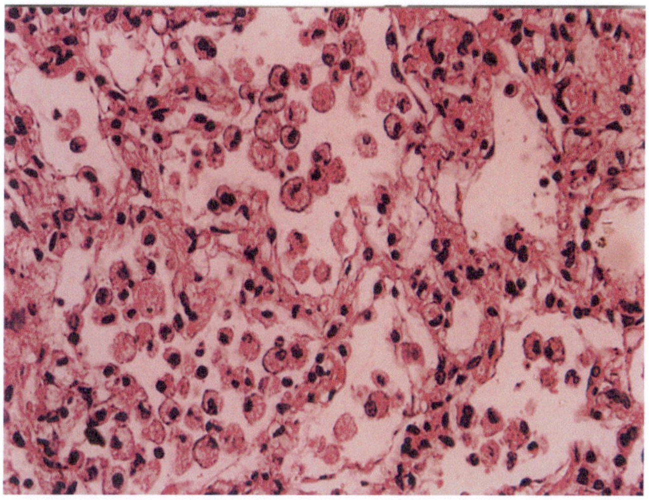

Fig. 7.25 Interstitial Pneumonia. Chronic progressive pneumonia in sheep. There is lymphoid follicles proliferation around the bronchioles, in the alveolar septa, and the surrounding bronchioles. The alveoli are compressed and deformed. HE×100. (Chen Huaitao)

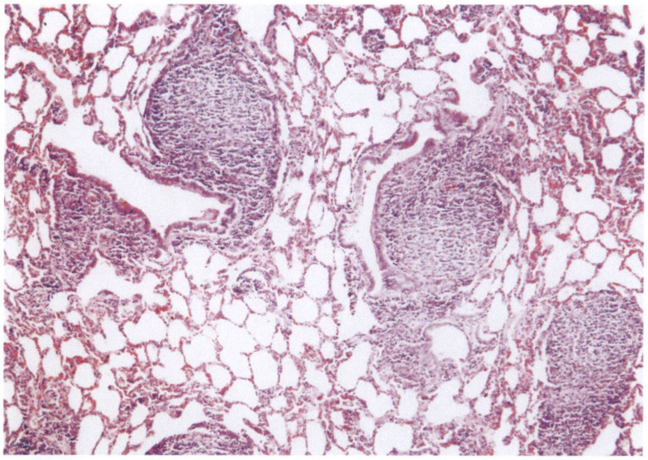

Fig. 7.26 Interstitial pneumonia. Porcine endemic pneumonia (porcine asthma). There is a massive infiltration of lymphocytes and monocytes around the bronchioles and blood vessels, resulting in the characteristic lesion of this pneumonia, the phenomenon of tubular condensation. The bronchioles are narrowed with increased wrinkles, a small number of exfoliated epithelial cells in the lumen, and many lymphocytes in the alveolar lumen and alveolar septum. HE ×100. (Chen Huaitao)

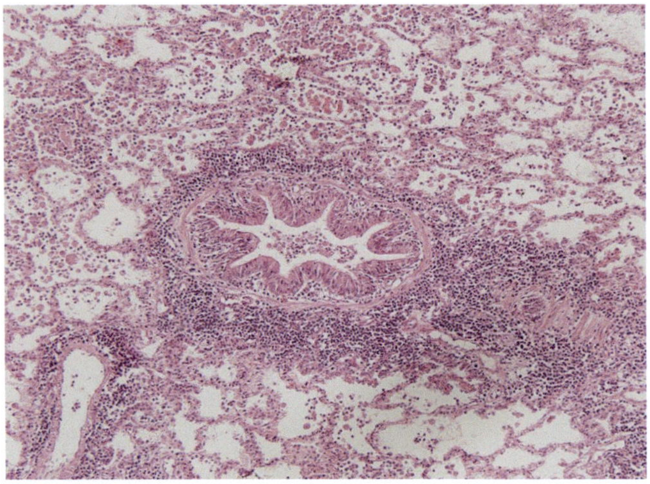

Fig. 7.27 Interstitial pneumonia. Lung nematodiasis. Many alveoli contain lung nematodes. The alveolar septa show obvious smooth muscle hyperplasia, fibroblast hyperplasia and a large number of lymphocyte infiltration. Therefore, the alveolar septa are thickened, the lung structure changed, and giant cells can be seen near the worm. HE×400. (Chen Huaitao)

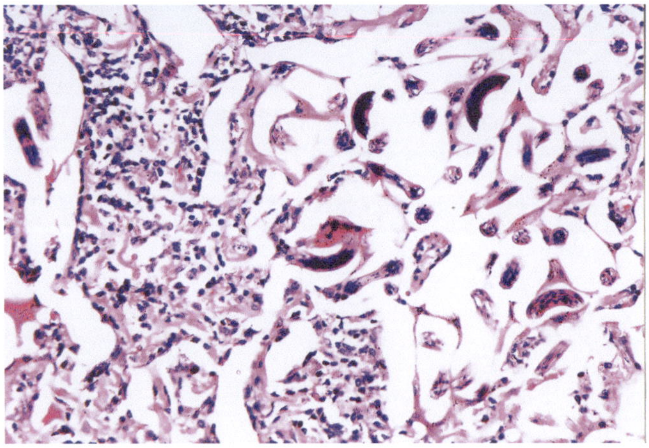

Fig. 7.28 Interstitial pneumonia. Equine pneumoconiosis. Interstitial hyperplasia is present with dust deposition, uneven thickening of alveolar septa, and marked dust nodule formation. Some alveoli show emphysema. HE ×100. (Wang Wenhui)

2.4 Granulomatous Pneumonia (Figs. 7.29, 7.30, and 7.31)

Granulomatous pneumonia is characterized by the formation of variable numbers of caseous or non-caseous granulomas consisting of specific cellular components in the lungs. On palpation, the lungs may be felt to have typical nodules that are well defined and vary in size with hard texture (especially when calcification occurs). Such granulomas in lungs may occasionally be confused with tumors in necropsy.

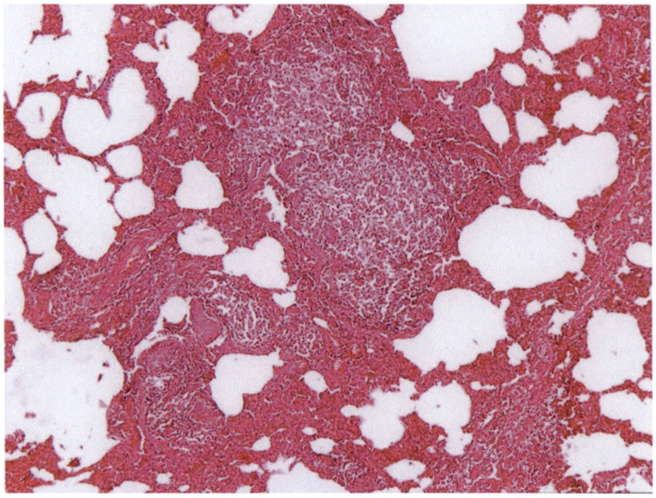

Fig. 7.29 Granulomatous pneumonia. Duck lung (duck tuberculosis). Plenty of yellowish-white nodules of tuberculosis of varying sizes are present on the surface of the lungs. (Zhou Shiqi, Hu Xueying)

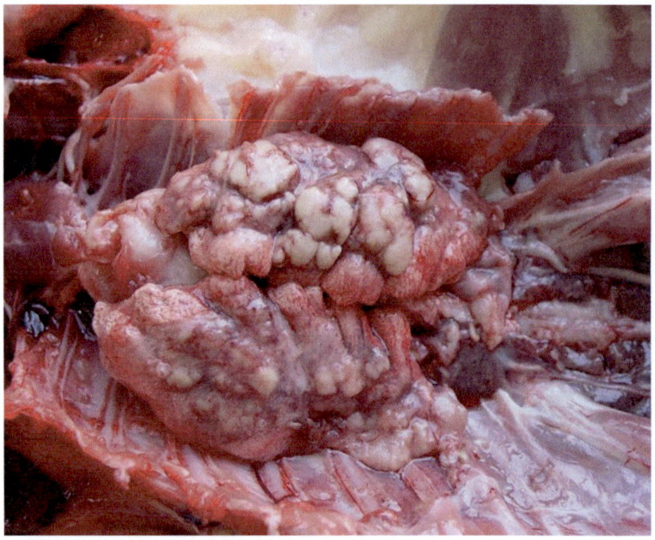

Fig. 7.30 Granulomatous pneumonia. Bovine tuberculosis. Tuberculosis nodules consist of epithelioid cells, giant cells, and encapsulating connective tissues. Caseous necrosis has not yet developed in the center of the lesion. HE ×100. (Wang Wenhui)

3 Pulmonary Emphysema (Figs. 7.32, 7.33, 7.34, 7.35, and 7.36)

Emphysema is the enlargement of the lungs due to increased air content. The increased air content in the alveoli is called alveolar emphysema; the expansion of the lung interstitium due to the rupture of the alveoli and the entry of air into the interstitium is called interstitial emphysema.

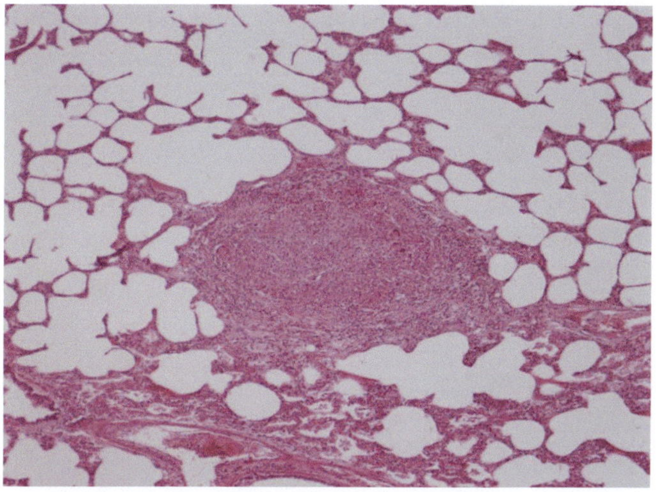

Fig. 7.31 Granulomatous pneumonia. Equine glanders. The figure shows several glanders nodules in the lung, which consists of epithelioid cells, giant cells, and peripheral connective tissue with many nuclear fragments of neutrophils in its center. HE ×100. (Wang Wenhui)

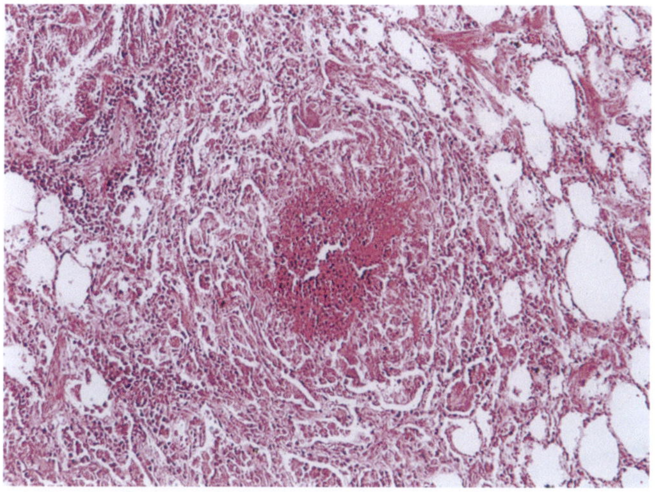

Fig. 7.32 Pulmonary emphysema. Swine lung nematode disease. Wedge-shaped areas of alveolar emphysema are present on the lateral and posterior margins of the lung diaphragm lobes. (Zhou Shiqi, Hu Xueying)

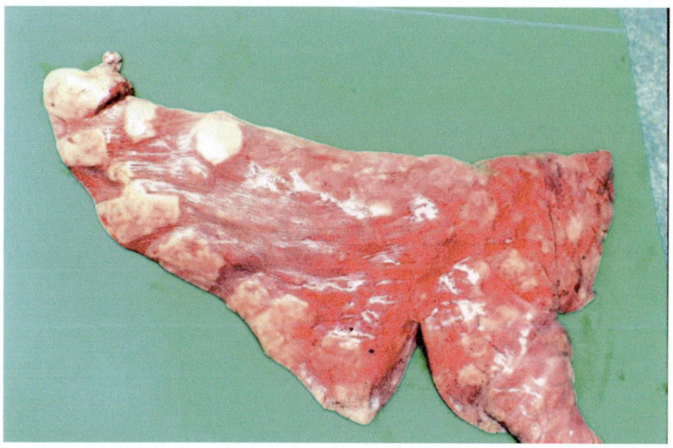

Fig. 7.33 Pulmonary emphysema. Bovine moldy sweet potato poisoning. The lung section is honeycombed and filled with bead-like bubbles of varying sizes between the lobules. (Qibao Min)

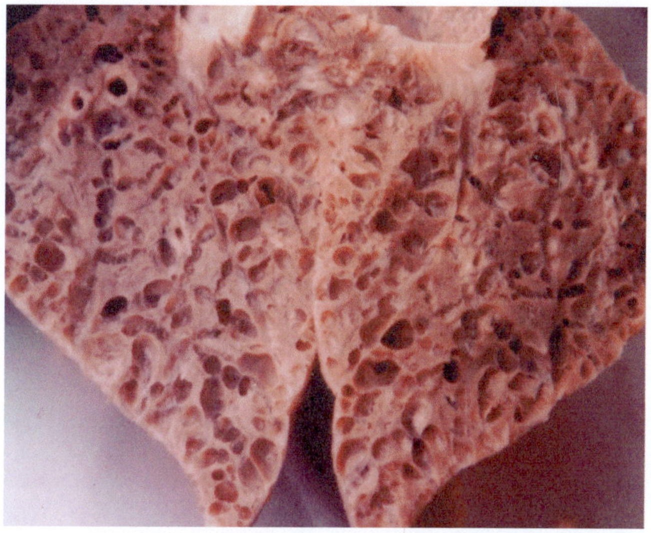

Fig. 7.34 Pulmonary emphysema. The inflammatory exudate is present in bronchioles with serous exudate in some alveoli, so compensatory emphysema have developed in some alveoli in the inflammatory zone. HE ×400. (Wang Wenhui)

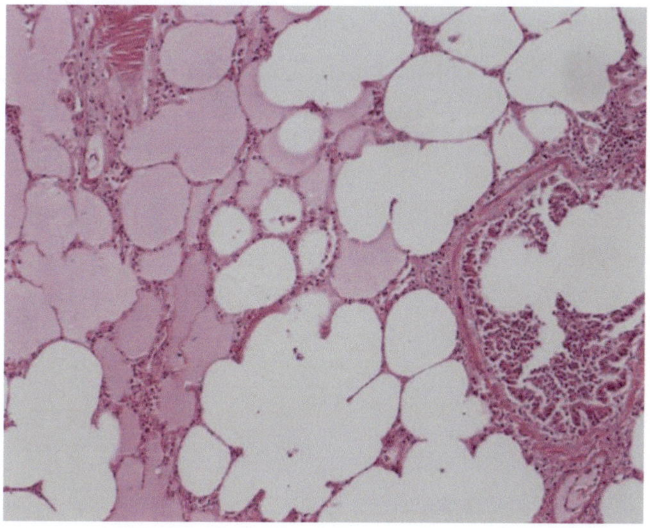

Fig. 7.35 Pulmonary emphysema. Equine pneumoconiosis. In the area of the pneumoconiosis lesion, alveoli are dilated, with thinning of the alveolar walls and some alveoli having ruptured into large cystic cavities. HEA ×400. (Chen Huaitao)

4 Collapse of Lung (Figs. 7.37 and 7.38)

Collapse of lung is a condition in which the alveoli are deflated due to a decrease in the amount of air in the alveoli. Collapse must be distinguished from congenital lung insufflation or atelectasis. Atelectasis is a congenital condition in which the lungs have never been expanded by air, whereas atrophy is a deflation of lung tissue that was once expanded and performed respiratory functions.

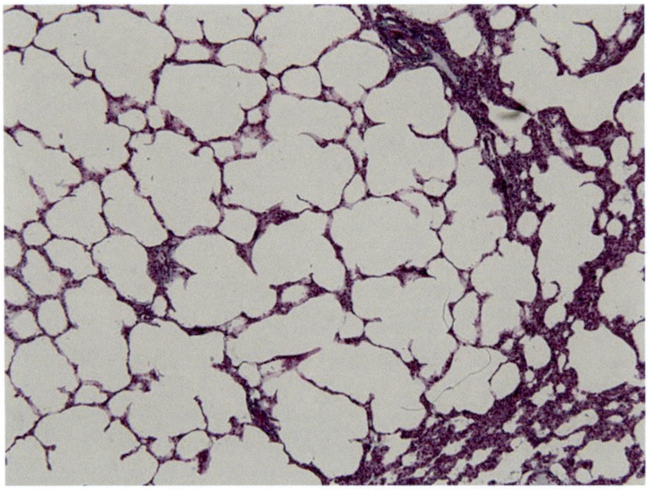

Fig. 7.36 Pulmonary emphysema. The interstitial and lymphatic vessels under the pleura of the lungs are highly dilated due to filling with gas and the alveoli become emphysematous. HE ×100. (Chen Huaitao)

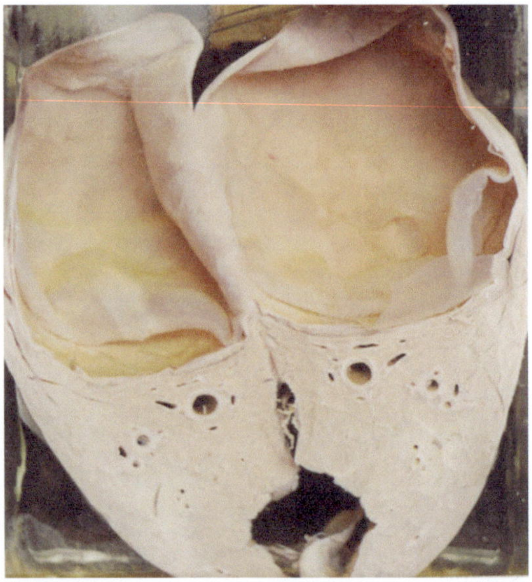

Fig. 7.37 Collapse of lung. The alveolar cavity becomes smaller, forming an elongated strip, with alveolar walls close together and arranged in parallel. HE ×100. (Chen Huaitao)

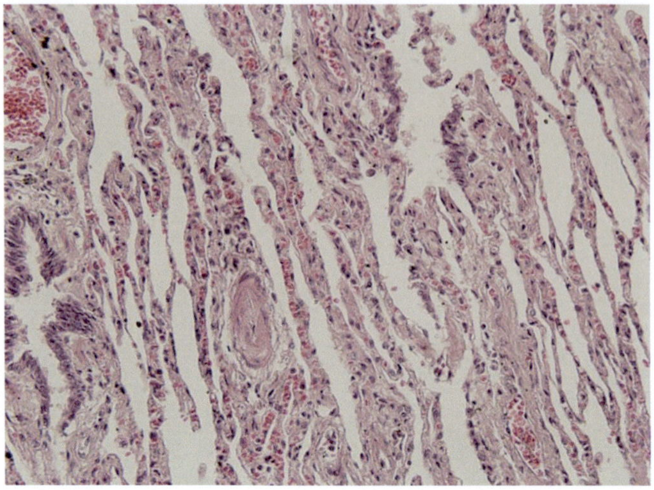

Fig. 7.38 Atelectasis. The alveolar epithelium is cuboidal, and the alveoli resemble acini. The alveolar walls are thick and curved, and the alveolar septal capillaries have not yet been passed by blood. HE×400. (Chen Huaitao)

Bibliography

1. Lirang Q, editor. Pathological anatomy of domestic animal systems. Beijing: China Agricultural Press; 1992.

8 Pathology of the Cardiovascular System

1 Pathological Changes of Heart

1.1 Cardiac Hypertrophy (Fig. 8.1)

Cardiac hypertrophy is an increase in the size and weight of the heart and a thickening of the heart wall. It is also called myocardium hypertrophy because the enlargement is based on the thickening of the heart muscle fibers.

Cardiac hypertrophy is caused by a variety of factors and usually occurs in the functionally enhanced atria or ventricles, either unilaterally or bilaterally in the heart, or in one ventricle or one atrium, but left ventricular hypertrophy is the most common case.

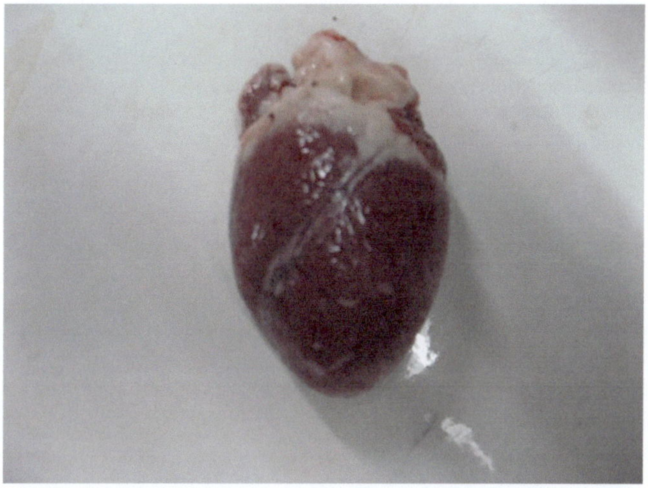

Fig. 8.1 Cardiac hypertrophy. Hypertrophy of the left heart in goats. The heart is increased in size with the change in shape, especially with the increase in longitudinal diameter. The heart increase in weight, and thickening of the left ventricular wall. (Wang Wenhui)

1.2 Cardiac Dilatation (Figs. 8.2, 8.3, and 8.4)

Cardiac dilatation is a pathological enlargement of the heart chamber volume, which is often secondary to cardiovascular disease. Cardiac dilatation is also a manifestation of cardiac insufficiency, which occurs usually due to the overload of blood in the heart, and generally develops chronically. The dilatation may occur in the entire heart or in one or two to three atria or ventricles, but right ventricular dilatation is the most common case.

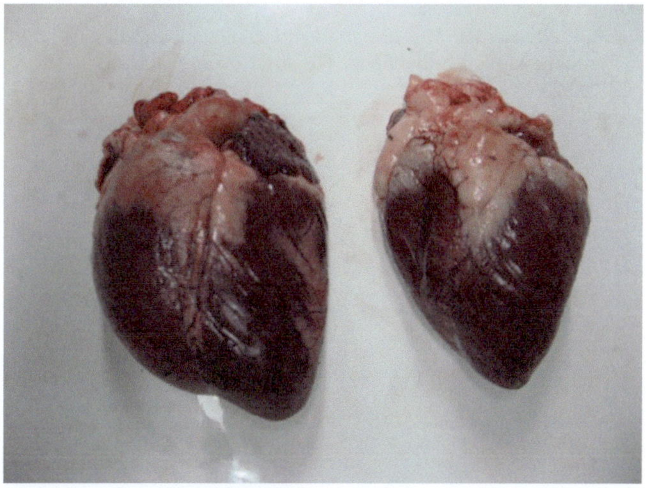

Fig. 8.2 Cardiac dilatation. The left one is a goat heart with dilated right ventricle. The heart is enlarged in volume, widened in transverse diameter, and blood clots accumulated in the right ventricle. The right one is a normal heart. (Wang Wenhui)

1.3 Endocarditis

1.3.1 Verrucose Thromboendocarditis (Figs. 8.5 and 8.6)

Verrucose thromboendocarditis is often caused by the infection of low virulent bacteria. It is characterized by the slow progression of the inflammatory process and mild damage to the heart valves. Thrombus and verrucose vegetations are usually present on the free edge of the atrial surface of the mitral valve and the ventricular surface of the aortic valve.

H. Chen, *Color Atlas of Veterinary Pathology*, https://doi.org/10.1007/978-981-96-7617-0_8

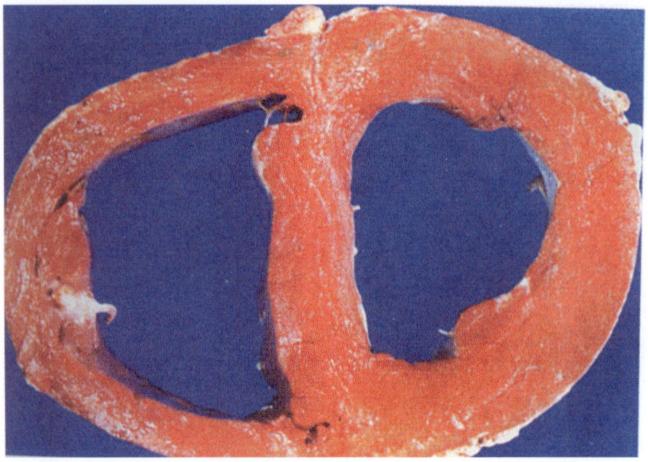

Fig. 8.3 Cardiac dilatation. Dairy cattle. Subcoronal cross-section. The left and right ventricles are highly dilated, with thinning of the ventricular walls and pale myocardium. (Zhang Xujing)

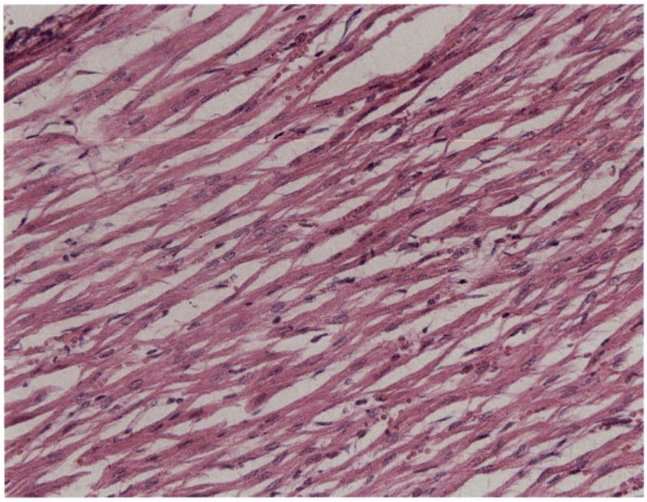

Fig. 8.4 Myocardial fiber atrophy. Cardiac dilatation leads to atrophy and thinning of myocardial fibers. HE ×100. (Wang Wenhui)

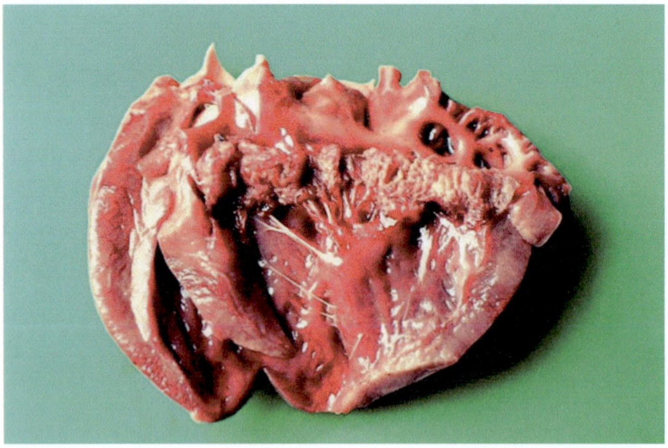

Fig. 8.5 Verrucose thromboendocarditis. Chronic porcine erysipelas. The cauliflower-like vegetations are present on the left mitral valve. (Hu Xueying, Zhou Shiqi)

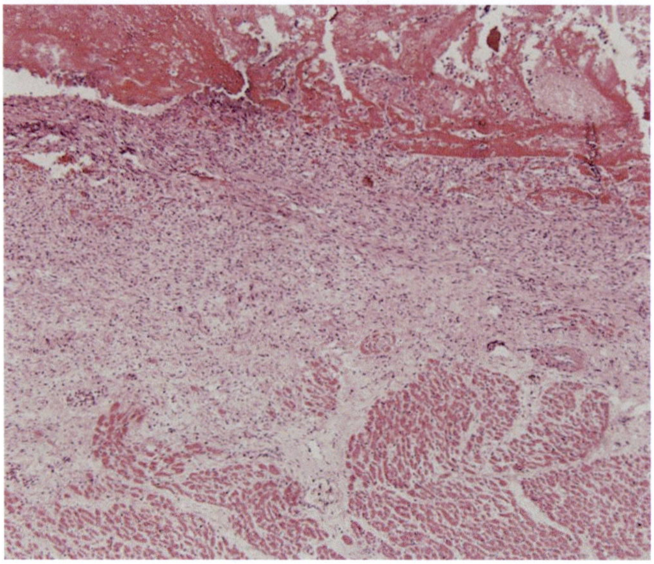

Fig. 8.6 Verrucose thromboendocarditis. The top is the thrombus, the middle is the part of organization, and the bottom is the myocardial fiber (cross-section). HE ×100. (Wang Wenhui)

1.3.2 Ulcerative Endocarditis (Figs. 8.7 and 8.8)

Ulcerative endocarditis is often associated with septic process; therefore, it is also known as septic endocarditis. It is usually caused by septic or high pathogenic bacterial infections. This disease shows an acute course with rapid progression of inflammation, severe damage to the valves, or other areas of the endocardium. It often spreads to deeper tissues, with a marked necrotic process and thrombotic verrucose vegetation formed on the surface.

1.4 Pericarditis

Pericarditis is an inflammation occurring on the parietal pericardium and visceral pericardium, which is primarily caused by bacterial infection or mechanical injury. This disorder is characterized by accumulation of a large amount of inflammatory exudate in the pericardial cavity and adherence of fibrinous or fibrinopurulent inflammatory exudate to the pericardium.

1.4.1 Infectious Pericarditis (Figs. 8.9 and 8.10)

Infectious pericarditis is caused by pathogenic microorganisms such as bacteria, mycoplasma, and viruses. It often takes an acute course, beginning as a serous inflammation, then progressing to serous fibrinous inflammation.

1.4.2 Traumatic Pericarditis (Fig. 8.11)

Traumatic pericarditis is caused by mechanical injury to the pericardium, which occurs frequently in cattle and occasionally in sheep. It usually shows the serous and fibrinous inflammation with a purulent putrefactive process.

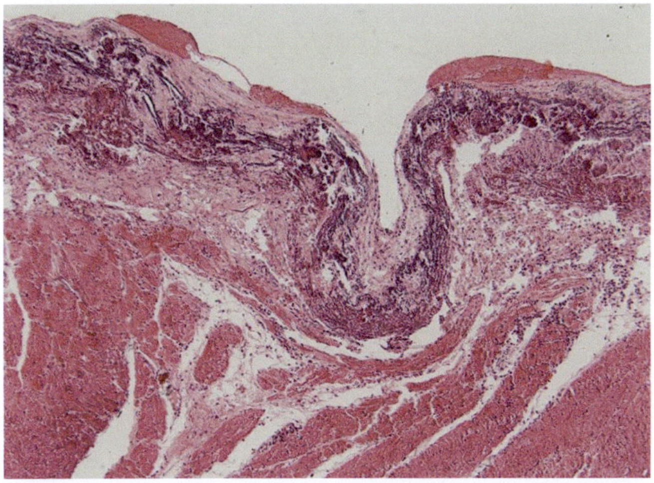

Fig. 8.7 Ulcerative endocarditis. The endocardium is necritized with inflammatory cell infiltration, localized endothelial exfoliation, and a small amount of thrombus attached to the surface. HE ×100. (Chen Huaitao)

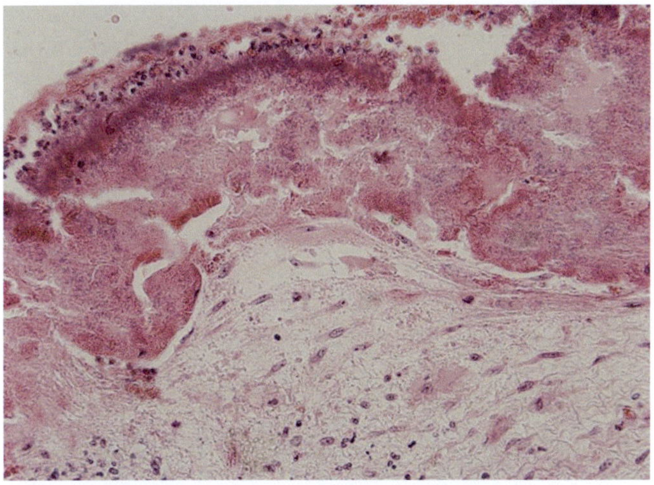

Fig. 8.8 Ulcerative endocarditis. Figure 8.7 Local magnification of the endocardium. The endocardial surface tissue is necrotized with thrombus attached and inflammatory cell infiltration. The underlying connective tissue is hyperplastic. HE ×400. (Chen Huaitao)

1.4.3 Parasitic Pericarditis (Fig. 8.12)

Porcine plasma membrane filarial epicarditis can be used as a representative. The adult worms are parasitic in the epicardial lymphatic vessels causing lymphatic vessel embolism and lymphangitis, which is manifested microscopically by massive eosinophil and lymphocyte infiltration and even granuloma formation around the lymphatic vessels obstructed by the worms.

1.5 Myocarditis

Myocarditis is an inflammation of the myocardium, and the alternative myocarditis is the most common one.

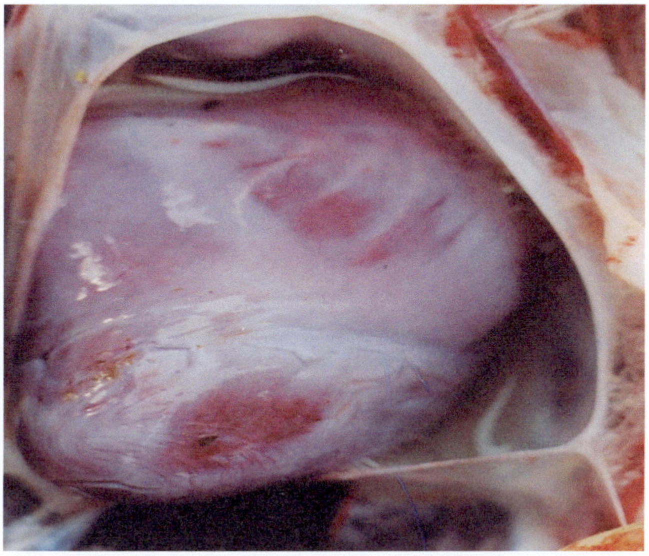

Fig. 8.9 Infectious pericarditis. Colibacillosis in ostriches: the pericardium is dilated with a large amount of serous exudate. (Chen Huaitao)

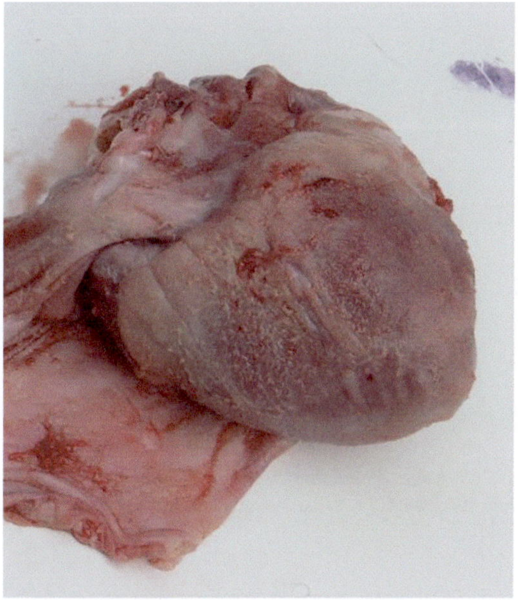

Fig. 8.10 Infectious pericarditis. The epicardium is attached by a large amount of fibrin exudate, resulting in the appearance of cor villosum. (Wu Bin)

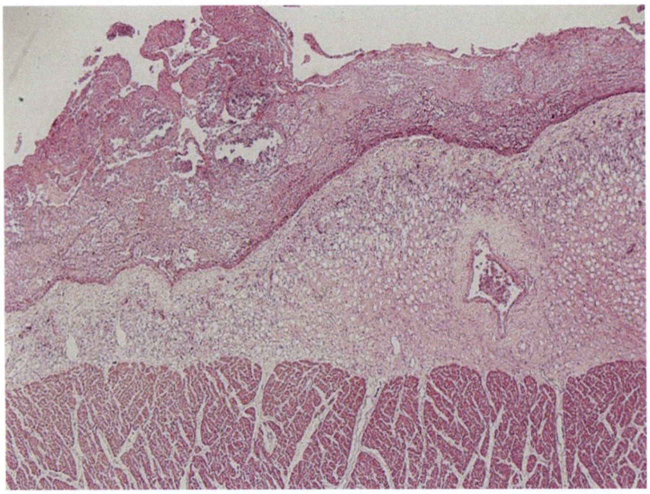

Fig. 8.11 Traumatic pericarditis. Bovine traumatic pericarditis: A thick layer of inflammatory exudate adheres to the epicardium, with infiltration of a large number of neutrophils and pus cells in the exuding fibrin strips. The surface of the exudate is uneven, with hyperplasia of the epicardial connective tissue. HE ×40. (Chen Huaitao)

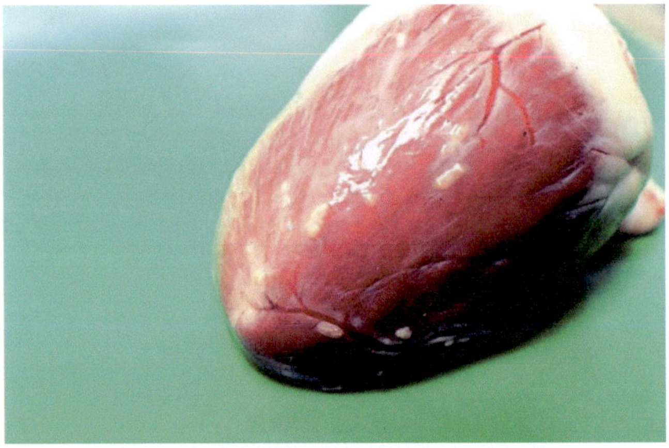

Fig. 8.12 Parasitic pericarditis. Porcine serosa filariasis: There are milk-white blister-like, rod-like, or striated lesions in the epicardium. (Zhou Shiqi)

1.5.1 Parenchymatous Myocarditis (Figs. 8.13, 8.14, and 8.15)

Inflammation mostly takes an acute course, with marked myocardial fibrous degeneration and necrosis, and it is commonly associated with viral infectious diseases, acute sepsis, and toxic diseases.

1.5.2 Interstitial Myocarditis (Fig. 8.16)

The inflammatory changes in the interstitium are more obvious, mainly with exudative and proliferative changes, while the alteration and necrosis of the myocardial fibers are less severe. It commonly occurs in viral or bacterial infectious diseases and poisoning diseases.

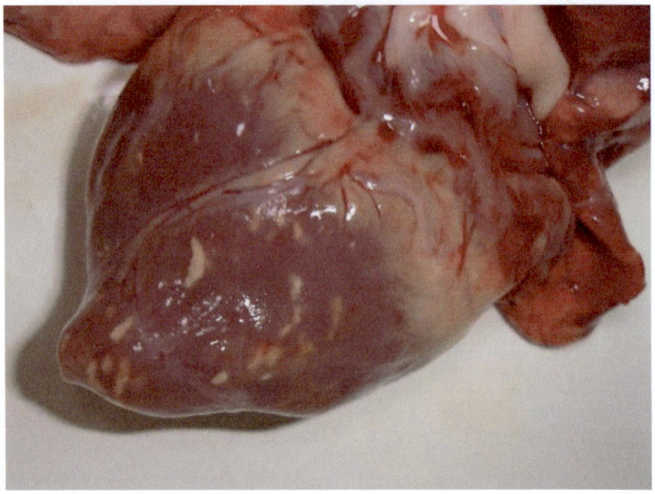

Fig. 8.13 Parenchymatous myocarditis. Malignant foot-and-mouth disease in pigs: numerous grayish or grayish-yellow spotty and streaky lesions are present on the epicardium. (Wu Bin)

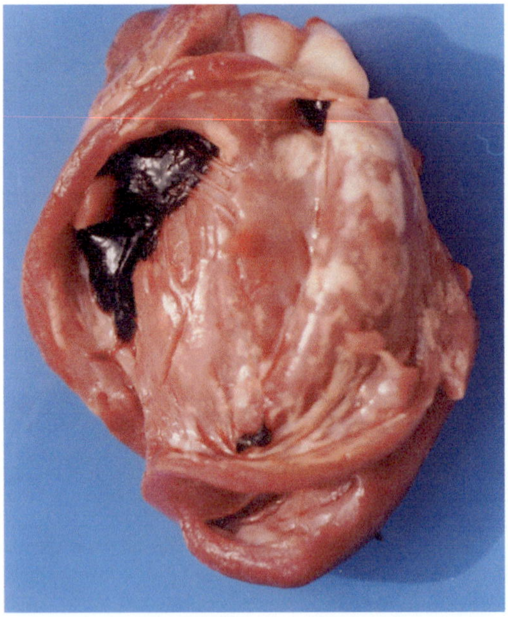

Fig. 8.14 Parenchymatous myocarditis. Sheep heart: many spots and patches of grayish-white lesions of varying sizes are present on the endocardium. (Chen Huaitao, Jia Ning)

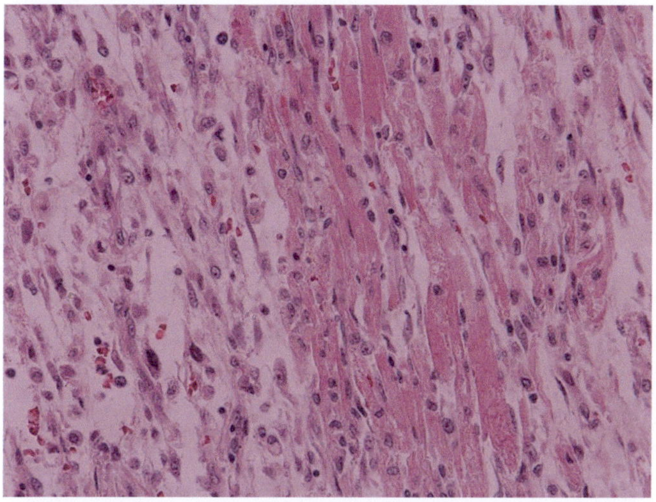

Fig. 8.15 Parenchymatous myocarditis. Myocardial fibers are degenerated and necrotized with interfibrillar neutrophil and monocyte infiltration. HE ×400. (Chen Huaitao)

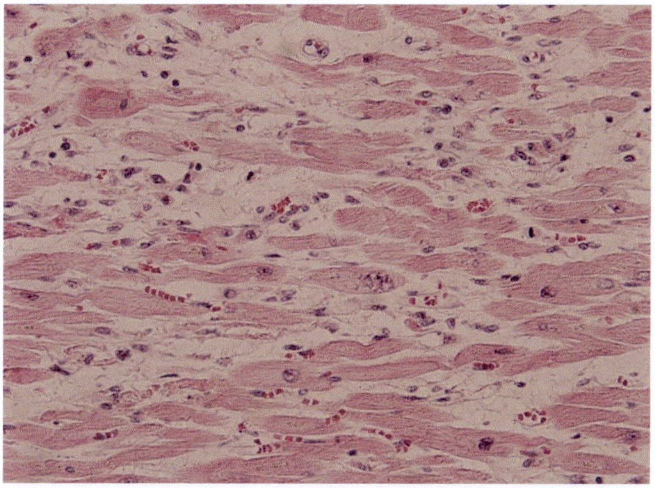

Fig. 8.16 Interstitial myocarditis. Mononuclear cell infiltration and connective tissue hyperplasia are observed between myocardial fibers, with atrophy and necrosis of some fibers. HE ×400. (Chen Huaitao)

The gross changes in interstitial myocarditis are very similar to those in parenchymal myocarditis and are difficult to distinguish, so they are often identified by microscopic examination.

1.6 Cardiomyopathy (Figs. 8.17 and 8.18)

Cardiomyopathy is a group of acute or chronic disorders in which the myocardial fibers are directly damaged, with the common feature of diffuse or multifocal degeneration and necrosis of the myocardial fibers, often without an inflammatory response.

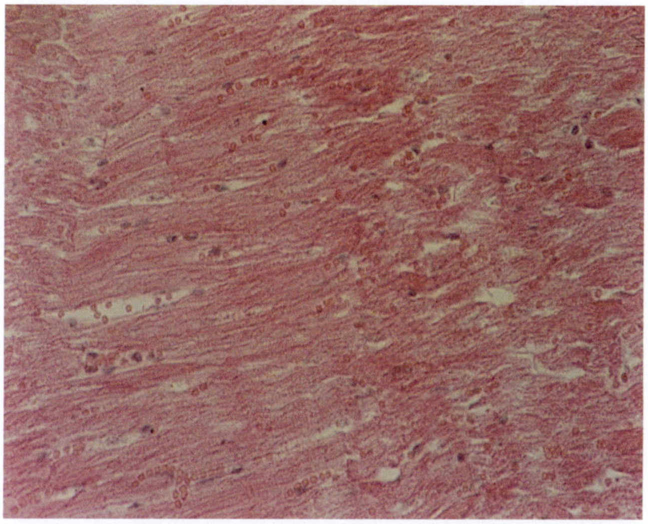

Fig. 8.17 Cardiomyopathy. Bovine moldy sweet potato poisoning: Diffuse granular degeneration of myocardial fibers is observed with necrosis of many fibers, and interfibrillary congestion, but no obvious inflammatory cell infiltration. HE ×400. (Yang Mingqi, Chen Huaitao)

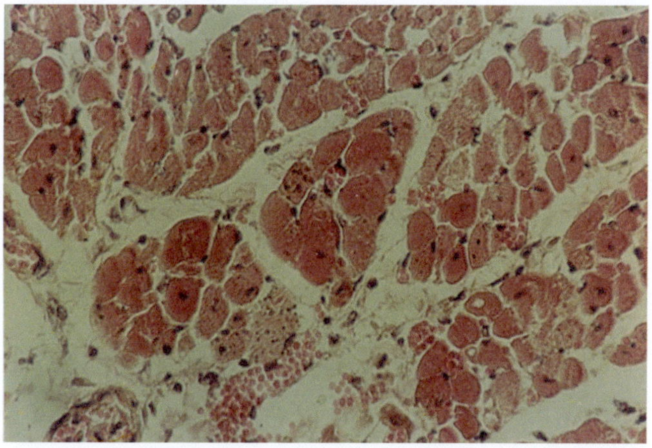

Fig. 8.18 Cardiomyopathy. Bovine enterotoxemia: Diffuse necrosis of myocardial fibers is observed, in which myofiber cross-section is unevenly stained with deep staining of some coagulation spots. The nuclei are mostly disintegrated, and some are concentrated. Edema, congestion, and light hemorrhage are observed among fibers, but inflammatory cells are rare. HE ×400. (Chen Huaitao, Lian Can)

2 Pathological Changes of Blood Vessel

2.1 Arteritis (Figs. 8.19, 8.20, 8.21, 8.22, and 8.23)

Arteritis is an inflammation of the walls of the arteries. The three common types of arteritis are acute arteritis, chronic arteritis, and periarteritis nodosa.

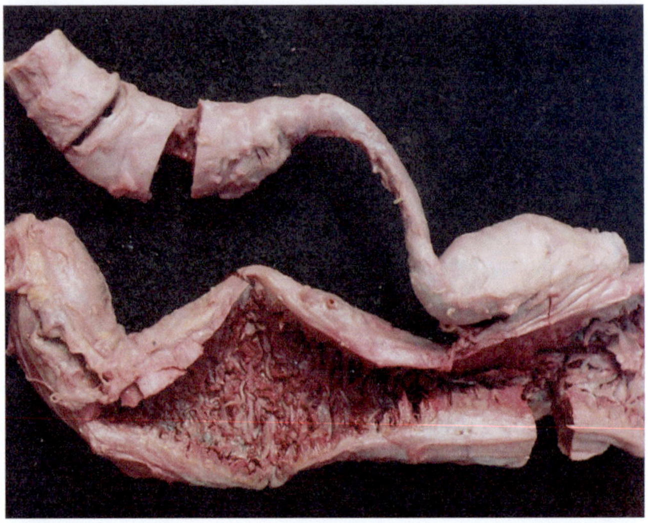

Fig. 8.19 Arteritis. Chronic arteritis in equine round nematode disease: the arterial wall of the anterior mesenteric artery is locally thickened and coarsened due to connective tissue hyperplasia, which resembles an aneurysm in appearance, with a rough inner lining, thrombosis, and attachment of worms. (Chen Huaitao)

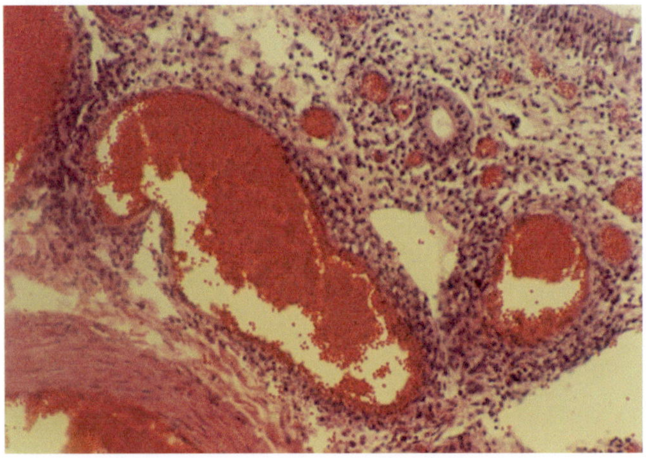

Fig. 8.20 Vasculitis. Bovine malignant catarrhal fever. Vasculitis of the nasal mucosa: acute necrotizing vasculitis of small arteries, veins, and capillaries is observed, with indistinct wall structure and many lymphocytes as well as monocytes infiltrating around them. HE ×200. (Chen Huaitao)

2.2 Phlebitis (Figs. 8.24, 8.25, and 8.26)

Phlebitis is an inflammation of the veins, often accompanied by thrombosis, while bleeding occurs less frequently. Based on the inflammatory process, phlebitis can be classified into two types: acute and chronic.

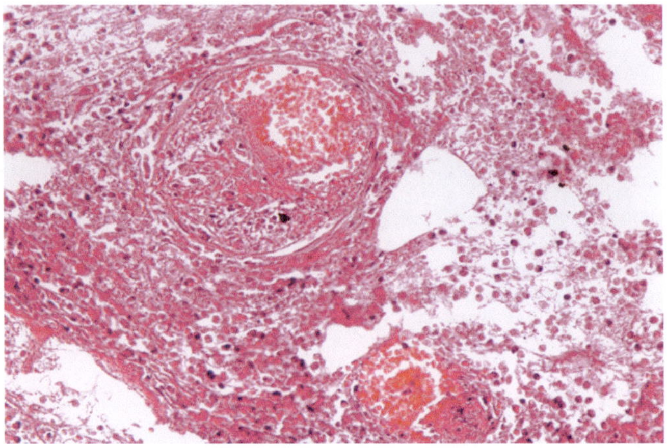

Fig. 8.21 Vasculitis. Porcine pharyngeal anthrax. Vasculitis in subcutaneous tissue: fibrinoid necrosis of both small arterial and small venous blood vessel walls is observed with structural destruction and thrombosis in the lumen. HE ×400. (Chen Huaitao)

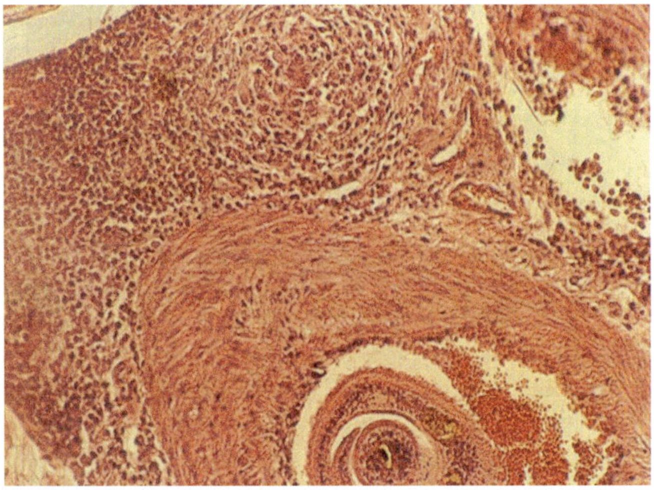

Fig. 8.22 Arteritis. Schistosomiasis in sheep. Arteritis of the intestinal wall: two schistosomes of both sexes are present in the artery. Endothelial cells show marked proliferation and necrosis with extravascular eosinophilic infiltration, and proliferation of connective tissue. HE ×200. (Chen Huaitao)

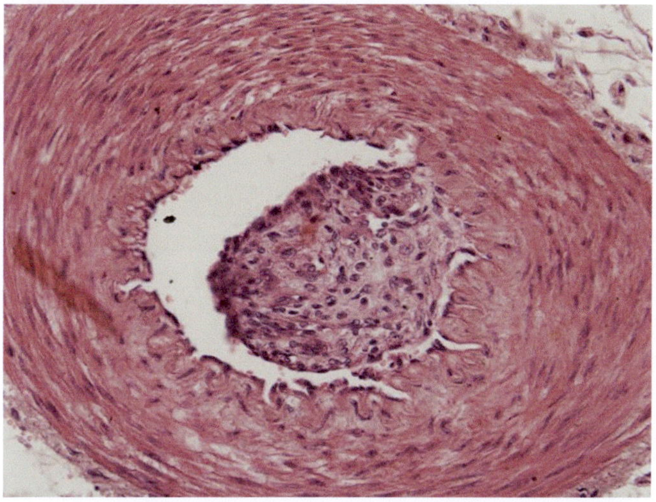

Fig. 8.23 Arteritis. Endarteritis of the renal artery: The intima is locally hyperplastic which is like a nodule protruding into the lumen, resulting in the narrowing and deformation of the lumen. HE ×400. (Chen Huaitao)

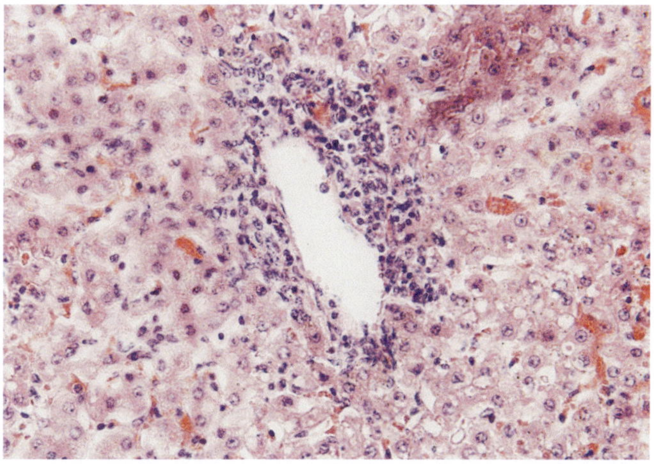

Fig. 8.24 Phlebitis. Acute endophlebitis in porcine liver: Inflammation of interlobular veins in portal area is observed, which results in rough intima, visible neutrophil adherence, as well as neutrophil infiltration around the veins. HE ×400. (Wang Wenhui)

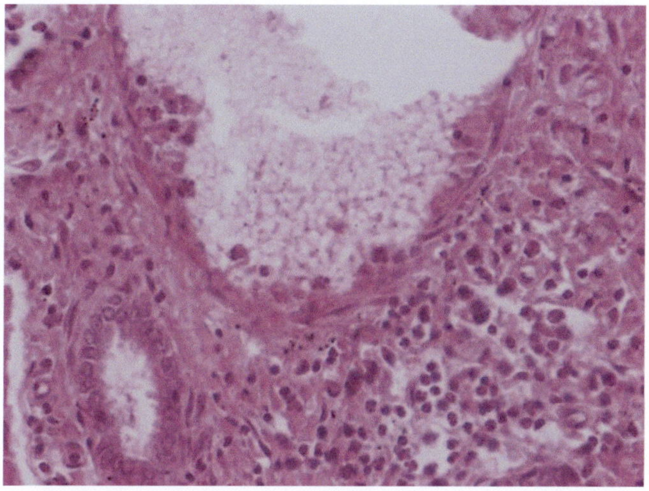

Fig. 8.25 Phlebitis. Schistosomiasis in sheep. Chronic phlebitis of the intestinal wall: schistosome parasitizes in the veins. Vascular endothelial cells are obviously proliferative. The connective tissue in the vessel wall proliferates and protrudes into the lumen, and there are a large number of eosinophils infiltrating in and around the vessel wall. HE ×200. (Chen Huaitao)

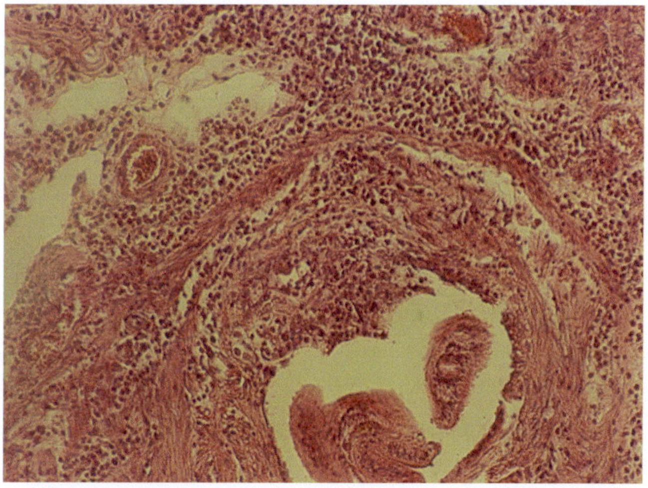

Fig. 8.26 Phlebitis. Acute endophlebitis in piglet salmonellosis. There is a severe infiltration of inflammatory cells beneath the central venous intima, along with granular degeneration and fatty degeneration of liver cells. HE ×400. (Chen Huaitao)

Bibliography

1. Baoyan L, Zhendong Q, editors. Color atlas of animal pathology and histology. Changchun: Jilin Science and Technology Press; 1990.
2. James F, Zachary M, McGavin D, editors. (Zhao Deming etc.tr.) Pathologic basis of veterinary disease. 5th ed. Beijing: Chemical Industry Press; 2015.

Pathology of the Immune System and Blood

9

1 Lymphadenitis

1.1 Acute Lymphadenitis

There are several common types of acute lymphadenitis.

1.1.1 Simple (Serous) Lymphadenitis (Figs. 9.1, 9.2, 9.3, 9.4, 9.5, 9.6, and 9.7)

Simple lymphadenitis often occurs in the early stages of acute infectious disease, especially in lymph nodes with acute inflammation of adjacent tissues.

1.1.2 Hemorrhagic Lymphadenitis (Figs. 9.8, 9.9, and 9.10)

It usually develops from simple lymphadenitis and is commonly associated with infectious diseases such as swine fever, swine pasteurellosis, and swine erysipelas.

1.1.3 Necrotizing Lymphadenitis (Figs. 9.11 and 9.12)

Necrotizing lymphadenitis is an inflammatory disease characterized by necrosis of lymphoid tissue and occurs often in infectious and parasitic diseases such as anthrax, swine salmonellosis, toxoplasmosis, and necrotizing fungal disease.

1.1.4 Hemorrhagic Necrotizing Lymphadenitis (Figs. 9.13 and 9.14)

Hemorrhagic necrotizing lymphadenitis is a mixed lymphadenitis, which is characterized by hemorrhagic lymphadenitis with marked necrosis of lymphoid tissue.

1.1.5 Suppurative Lymphadenitis (Figs. 9.15 and 9.16)

Suppurative lymphadenitis usually occurs in the presence of purulent inflammation of the organ or tissue to which it belongs to, and it is characterized by massive neutrophil infiltration and purulent lysis of the tissue.

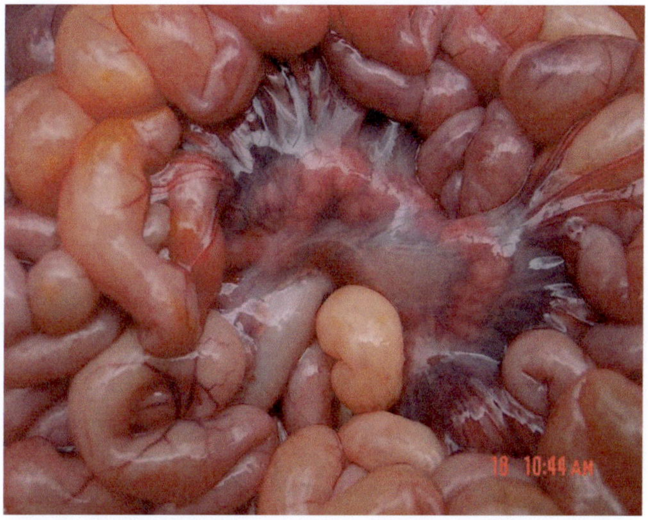

Fig. 9.1 Serous lymphadenitis. Swine edematous disease. Porcine mesentery: lymph nodes are enlarged, congested with red color, soft texture, moist and light red in cut surface. The mesentery is edematous. (Cheng Guofu)

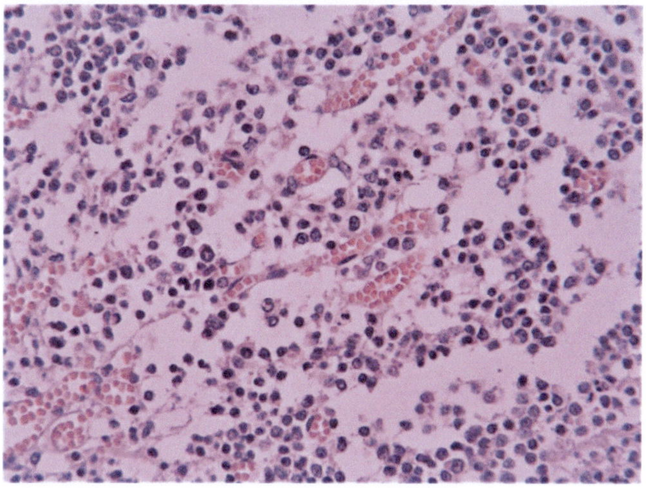

Fig. 9.2 Serous lymphadenitis. Lymphatic sinus is dilated, filled with serum and numerous neutrophils. HE ×400. (Liu Sidang)

H. Chen, *Color Atlas of Veterinary Pathology*, https://doi.org/10.1007/978-981-96-7617-0_9

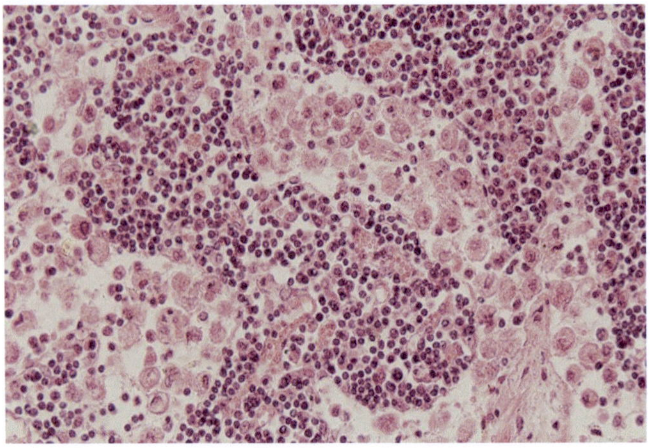

Fig. 9.3 Serous lymphadenitis. Catarrhal lymphadenitis (sinus catarrhal): The dilated lymphatic sinuses are filled with serum and numerous macrophages, white blood cells, and lymphocytes. HE ×400. (Chen Huaitao)

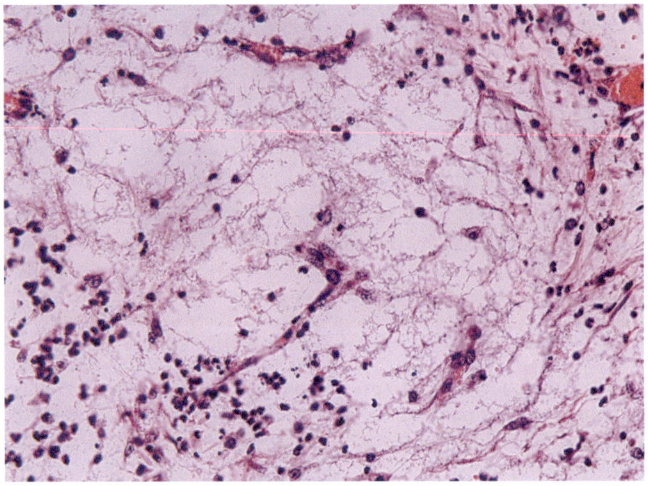

Fig. 9.4 Serous lymphadenitis. Streptococcal disease in sheep. The lymphocytes in the lymph nodes almost disappeared. The local tissue is loose and in reticular or luminal patterns. The lymph sinuses are dilated and filled with serum and bacterial capsular polysaccharide, and the neutrophils are markedly infiltrated with necrosis. HE ×400. (Chen Huaitao)

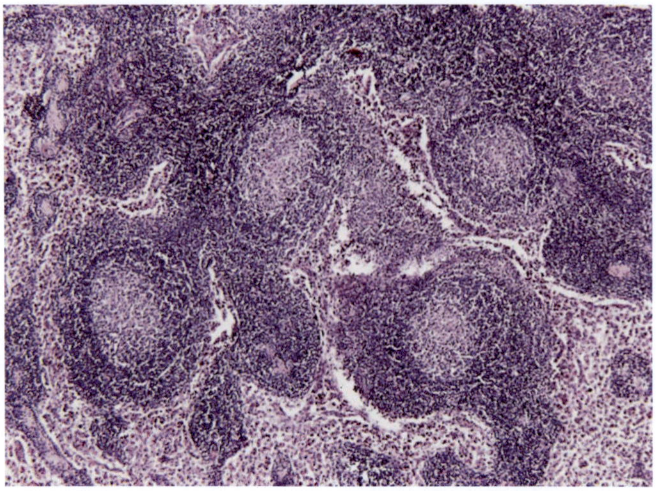

Fig. 9.5 Acute proliferative lymphadenitis. Red deer lymph nodes. The lymphoid nodules are markedly enlarged and increased in number. The germinal center is obvious with plenty of reticulocytes and macrophages within them, and a lot of macrophages in the lymphatic sinus. There are a large number of lymphocytes in the outer layer of the lymph nodules with many plasma cells and monocytes in their periphery and medullary cords. There is some immune response to the proliferation of lymphoid nodules. HE ×200. (Meng Qingling)

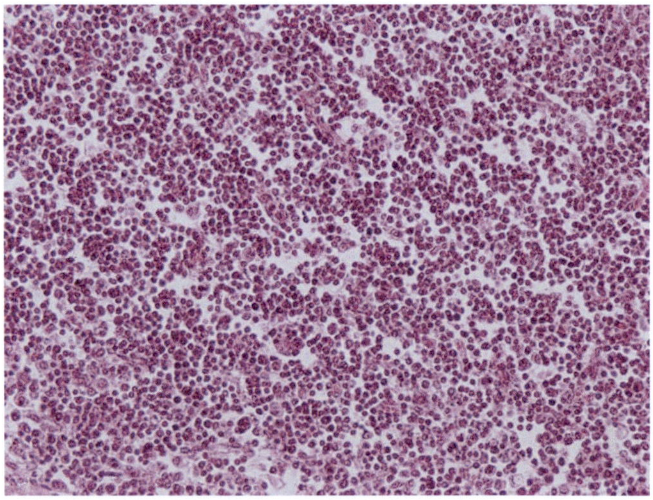

Fig. 9.6 Acute proliferative lymphadenitis. Mycoplasma pneumonia in pigs. Bronchial lymph nodes: The lymphocytes and reticulocytes diffusely proliferate with the presence of plasma cells and macrophages. The lymph nodules are indistinguishable from medullary cords, which indicates both inflammatory and immune response. HE ×400. (Chen Huaitao)

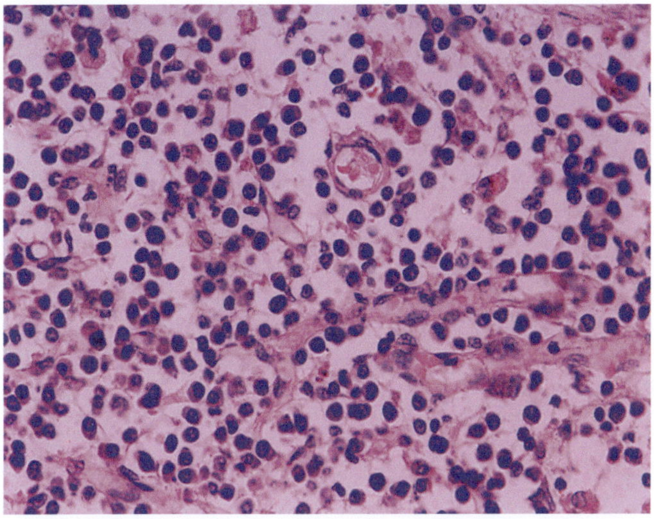

Fig. 9.7 Acute proliferative lymphadenitis. There are a large number of plasma cell infiltrating in lymph nodule peripheral area and medullary cord, and the reticulocytes as well as endothelial cells are hyperplastic with neutrophils scattered. HE ×400. (Chen Huaitao)

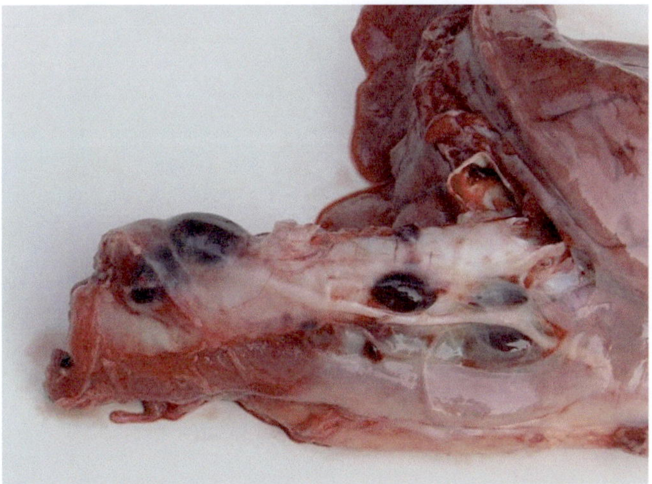

Fig. 9.8 Hemorrhagic lymphadenitis. The bronchial lymph nodes of the pig are severely hemorrhaged and almost became red. (Wu Bin)

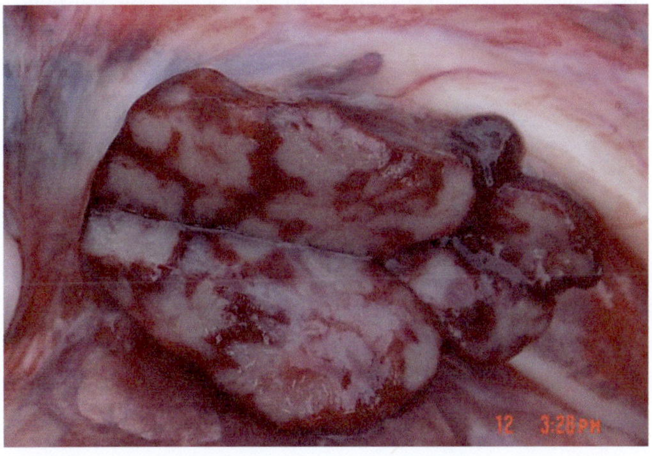

Fig. 9.9 Hemorrhagic lymphadenitis. Swine fever. The periphery and trabeculae of lymph node section are obviously hemorrhagic with marble-like changes. (Wu Bin)

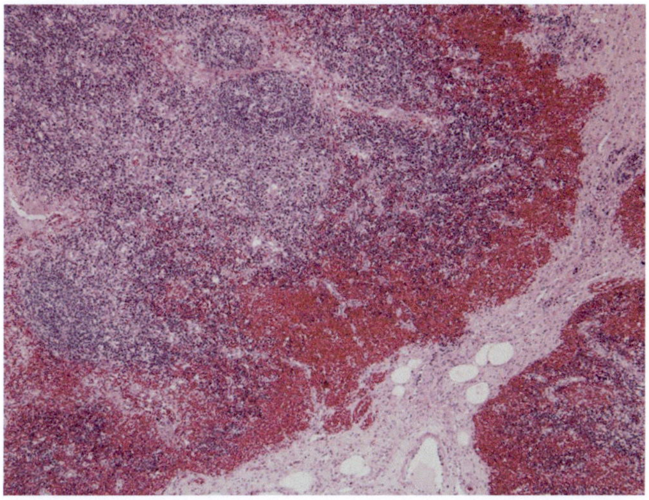

Fig. 9.10 Hemorrhagic lymphadenitis. Swine fever. Diffuse hemorrhage is present in the cortical lymph sinus and nearby lymphoid tissue of the lymph node with few lymphocytes. However, there are no hemorrhagic changes in the medulla. HE ×100. (Chen Huaitao)

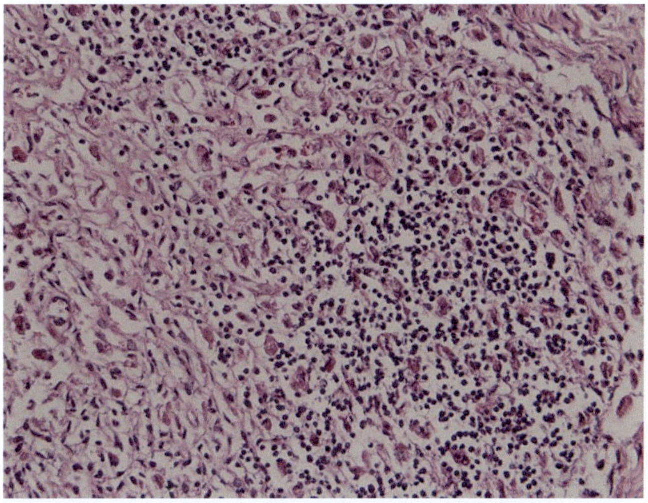

Fig. 9.11 Necrotizing lymphadenitis. Canine lymph node. Reticulocytes proliferation and lymphocytes necrosis are present, resulting in the reduction of lymphoid nodule size with only some lymphocytes remaining. HE ×400. (Wang Wenhui)

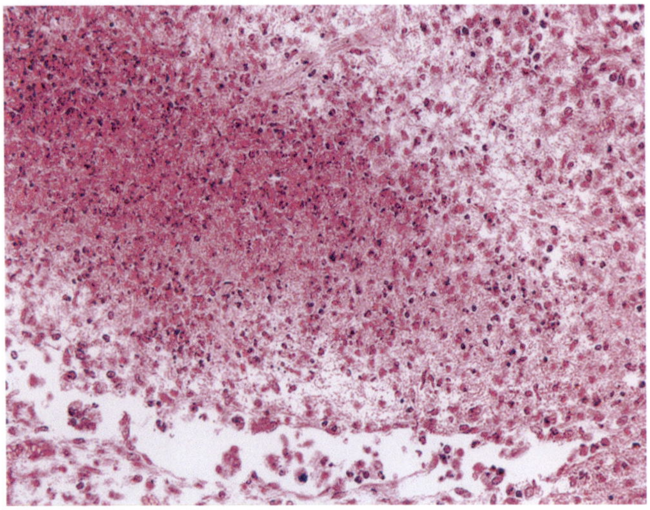

Fig. 9.12 Necrotizing lymphadenitis. Salmonellosis in pigs. The figure shows a focus of necrosis in a mesenteric lymph node, in which the lymphoid tissue is necrotically disintegrated, and many nuclear fragments are present. The necrotic material is red stained and some inflammatory cells are found infiltrating near the necrotic focus and in the lymphatic sinus. HE ×400. (Chen Huaitao)

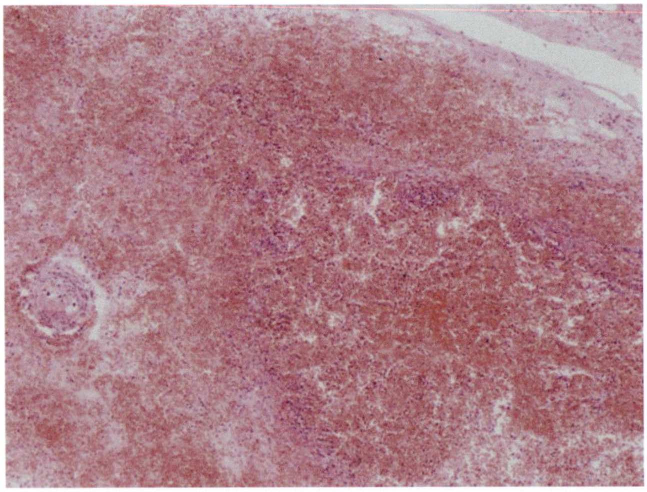

Fig. 9.13 Hemorrhagic necrotizing lymphadenitis. Porcine anthrax. The structure of the submandibular lymph node is severely disrupted, with almost the entire lymphoid tissue necrotized and disappeared and only a few lymphocytes remaining. Congestion, hemorrhage, and neutrophil infiltration are obvious. HE ×100. (Wang Wenhui)

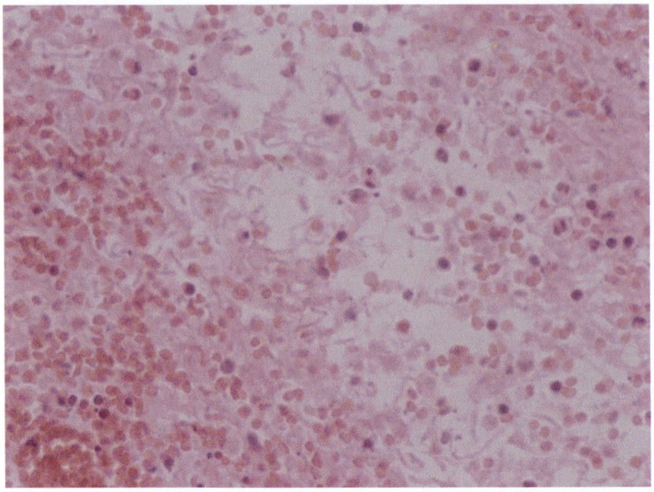

Fig. 9.14 Hemorrhagic necrotizing lymphadenitis. Porcine anthrax. Lymphoid tissue in the submandibular lymph node is necrotized with markedly reduced lymphocytes, numerous erythrocytes, and rod-like or short chain-like *Bacillus anthracis* in the lesion. HE ×400. (Wang Wenhui)

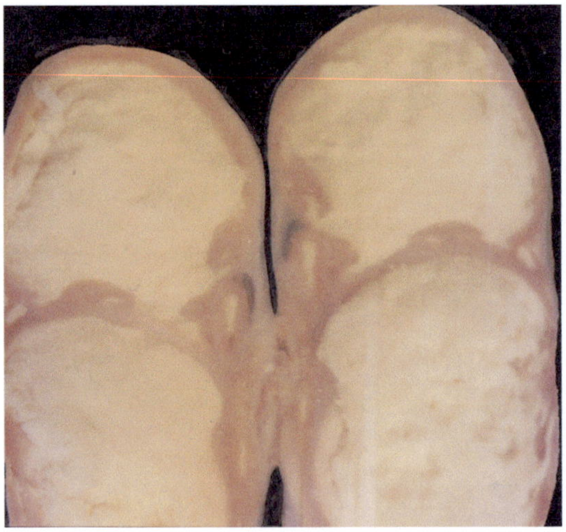

Fig. 9.15 Suppurative lymphadenitis. Pseudotuberculosis in sheep. The lymph node section shows purulence of the entire lymphoid tissue, which is like thick caseous substance. The abscess is encapsulated with thick connective tissue. (Veterinary Pathology Unit, Gansu Agricultural University)

1.2 Chronic Lymphadenitis

Chronic lymphadenitis are often from acute lymphadenitis or caused by the persistent infection of pathogenic factors. It is common in local lymph nodes of chronic diseases, such as tuberculosis, paratuberculosis, and pneumoconiosis.

Chronic lymphadenitis can be classified into fibroproliferative lymphadenitis and granulomatous lymphadenitis.

1.2.1 Fibroproliferative Lymphadenitis (Fig. 9.17)

Fibroproliferative lymphadenitis, also known as fibrous lymphadenitis, is characterized by proliferation of connective tissue and collagenization of reticular fibers within the lymph nodes.

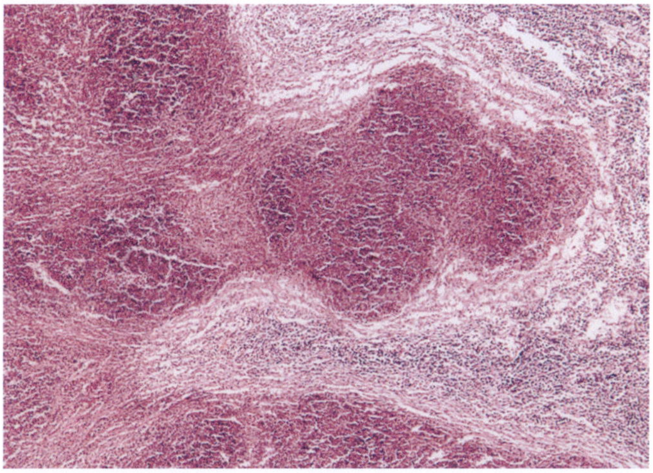

Fig. 9.16 Suppurative lymphadenitis. Porcine streptococosis. The submandibular lymph nodes are suppurative, and the local lymphoid tissue structure has been completely destroyed, which is filled with dense pus cells, and the abscess is bordered by a proliferating connective tissue capsule. HE ×100. (Chen Huaitao)

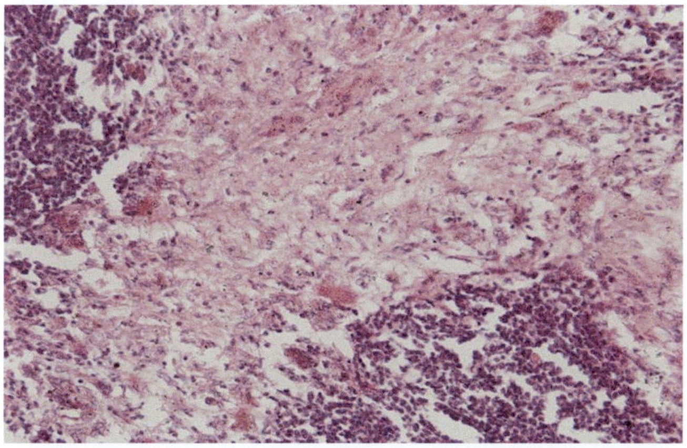

Fig. 9.17 Fibroproliferative lymphadenitis. Equine pneumoconiosis. The connective tissue in the bronchial lymph nodes is hyperplastic, while the lymphoid tissue is atrophied or reduced. HE ×400. (Chen Huaitao)

1.2.2 Granulomatous Lymphadenitis (Fig. 9.18)

Granulomatous lymphadenitis mainly occurs in diseases with granuloma formation such as tuberculosis, brucellosis, actinomycosis, glanders, and mycosis.

2 Splenitis (Figs. 9.19, 9.20, 9.21, 9.22, 9.23, 9.24, 9.25, and 9.26)

There are several types of splenitis with inconsistent classification. The common ones are acute splenitis (acute inflammatory splenomegaly, septic spleen), necrotizing splenitis, and chronic splenitis.

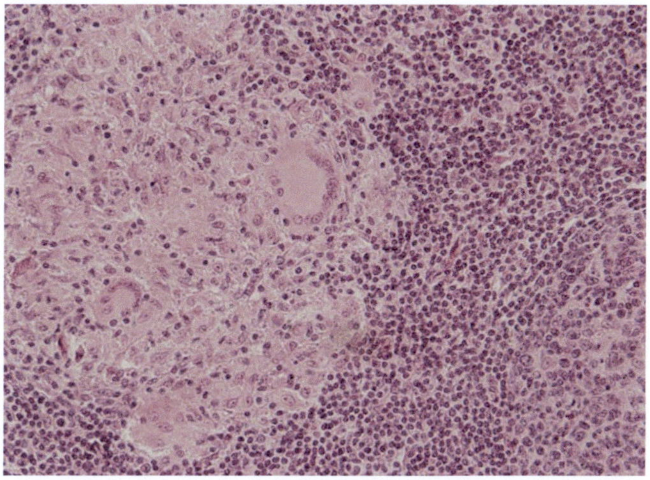

Fig. 9.18 Granulomatous lymphadenitis. There is a lightly stained area in the tissue of the lymph node, which is the granuloma. The granuloma is composed of a large number of epithelioid cells and a few Langhans giant cells. HE ×400. (Chen Huaitao)

3 Bursitis of Fabricius (Fig. 9.27)

Bursitis of Fabricius occurs mainly in the course of various infectious diseases. It can be exudative, necrotic, or proliferative process. In many immunocompromised infectious cases, necrotic bursitis of Fabricius often occurs. In addition, in some neoplastic infectious diseases, the lymphoid follicles of the bursa Fabricius may be enlarged by primary tumor cell proliferation (e.g., chicken lymphosarcoma) or the lymphoid follicles may be compressed and atrophied by infiltration of tumor cells (e.g., chicken Marek's disease) .

4 Thymitis (Figs. 9.28 and 9.29)

In addition to the general pathological changes observed in the thymus, a number of infectious processes are often accompanied by inflammatory changes, especially necrotizing thymitis.

5 Osteomyelitis (Figs. 9.30 and 9.31)

Osteomyelitis is mostly caused by infection and can be classified into acute osteomyelitis and chronic osteomyelitis, both of which can present as purulent and non-purulent osteomyelitis. Purulent osteomyelitis is mainly caused by purulent bacteria, and nonsuppurative osteomyelitis occurs in the course of certain infectious diseases (e.g., equine

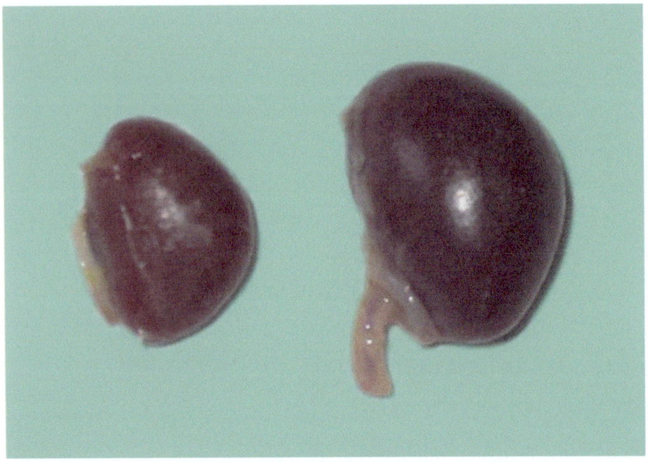

Fig. 9.19 Acute splenitis. Chicken spleen. The right one is the spleen of the diseased chicken, which is enlarged with soft texture and dark red color; the left one is the spleen from normal control chicken. (Wang Wenhui)

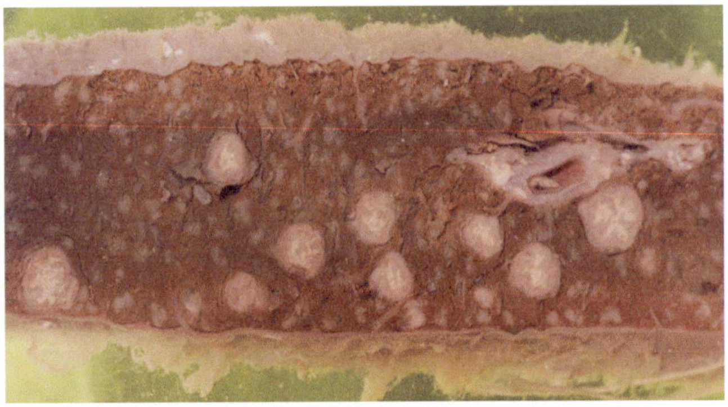

Fig. 9.20 Chronic splenitis. Bovine tuberculosis. The spleen is slightly enlarged, firm in texture, light reddish-brown in section, with obvious grayish-white granules and large round hyperplastic tuberculous nodules containing caseous necrotic material. (Veterinary Pathology Unit, Gansu Agricultural University)

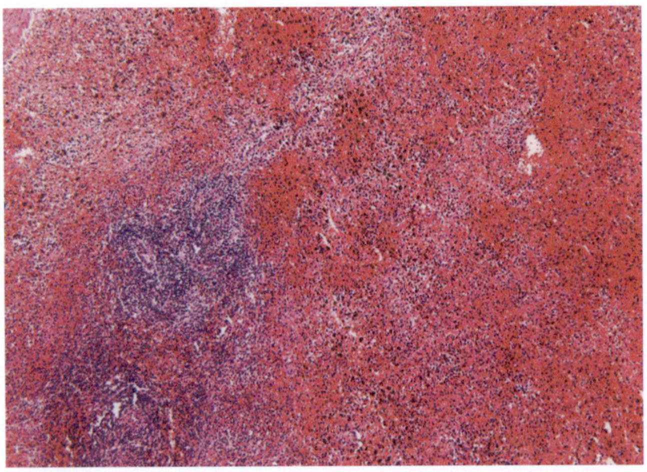

Fig. 9.21 Acute splenitis. Bovine malignant catarrhal fever. The spleen is congested and hemorrhagic, and the splenic tissue is almost occupied by red blood cells. The walls of small vessels are necrotic, and there are only a few lymphocytes and monocytes around the central artery. HE ×100. (Chen Huaitao)

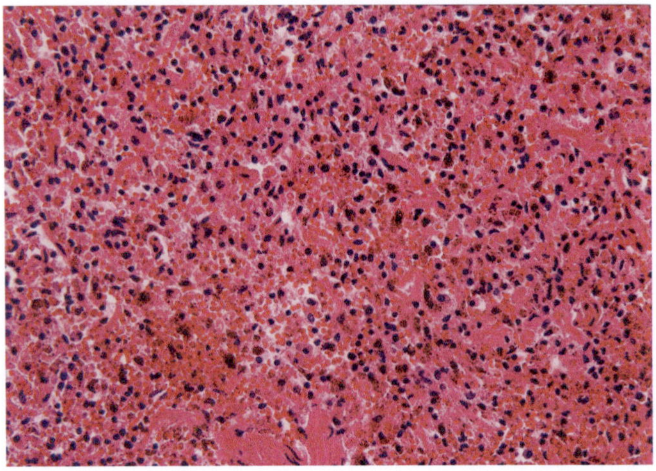

Fig. 9.22 Acute splenitis. Figure 9.21 Local magnification. The red blood cells are almost present in the entire splenic pulp, with scattered neutrophils and lymphocytes. The splenic red pulp is poorly defined, and the splenic trabecular smooth muscle is loose and degenerated. There are scattered deposition of hemosiderin. HE ×400. (Chen Huaitao)

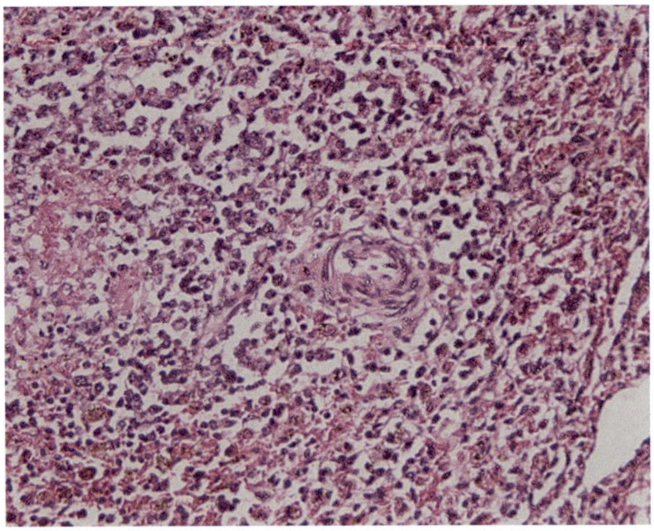

Fig. 9.23 Necrotizing splenitis. The spleen is congested with obvious reduction in lymphocytes due to necrosis. The neutrophil infiltration is observed. HE ×400. (Wang Wenhui)

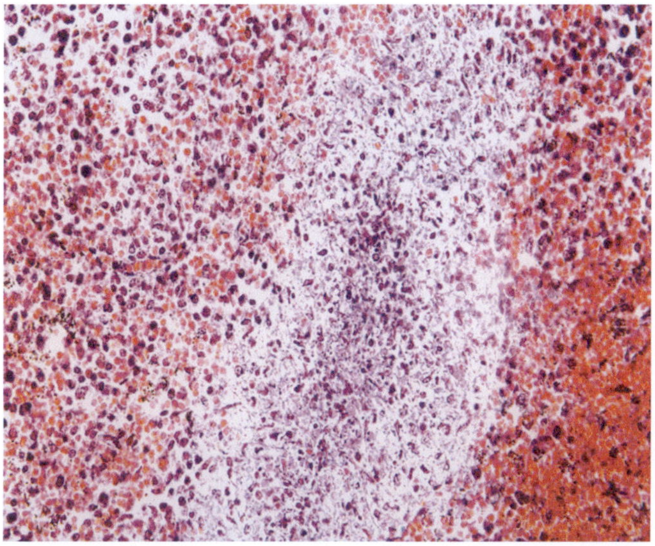

Fig. 9.24 Necrotizing splenitis. Salmonellosis in a piglet. There is a distinct focus of necrosis in the spleen tissue with local histiocyte necrosis and disintegration, neutrophil infiltration, and reticulocytosis. HEA ×400. (Chen Huaitao)

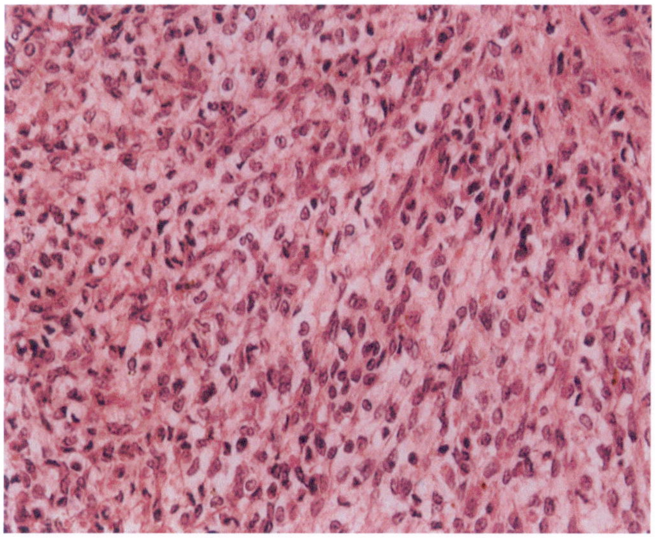

Fig. 9.25 Chronic splenitis. The reticular cells of the spleen are hyperplastic in large numbers, and lymphocytes are still present in some areas. HE ×400. (Chen Huaitao)

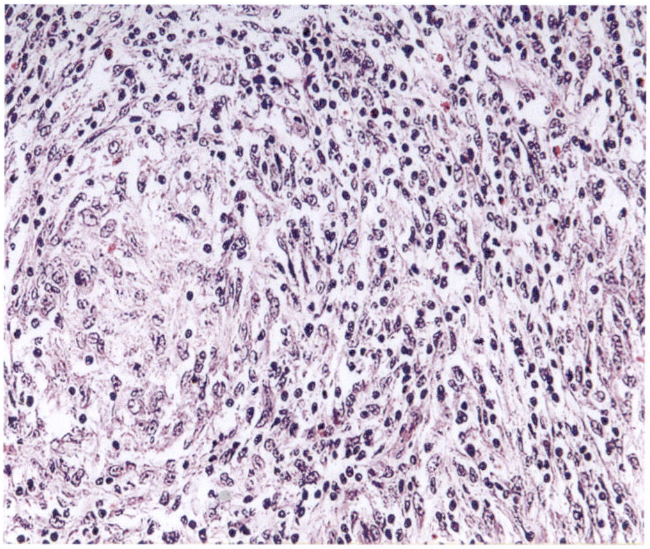

Fig. 9.26 Chronic splenitis. Splenic reticuloendothelial cells are hyperplastic, which formed an oval nodule. Connective tissue in the periphery of the nodule and in the splenic parenchyma is markedly hyperplastic, while lymphocytes are reduced and splenic corpuscles and cords are atrophied. HE ×400. (Chen Huaitao)

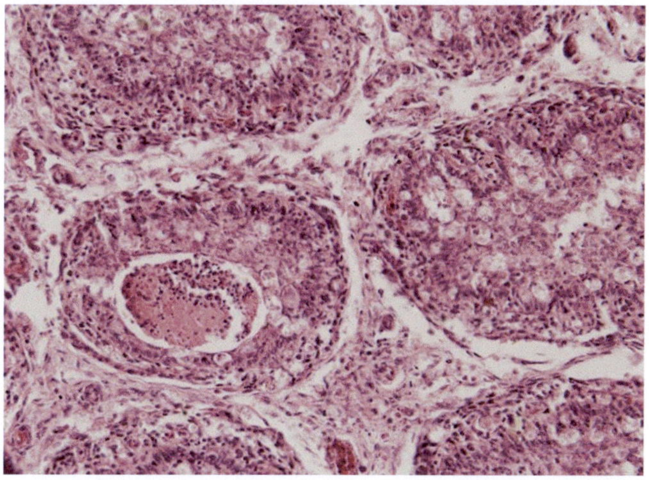

Fig. 9.27 Necrotizing bursitis of Fabricius. Infectious bursa Fabricius disease in chicken. The medulla and cortical cells of lymphoid follicles in bursa of Fabricius are necrotic, their boundaries are indistinct, and the medulla of some follicles is necrotic, whereas cyst containing necrotic cells, heterophilic granulocytes, and homogeneous proteinaceous material is formed. Edema and inflammatory cell infiltration can be observed in interfollicular tissue. HE ×400. (Chen Huaitao)

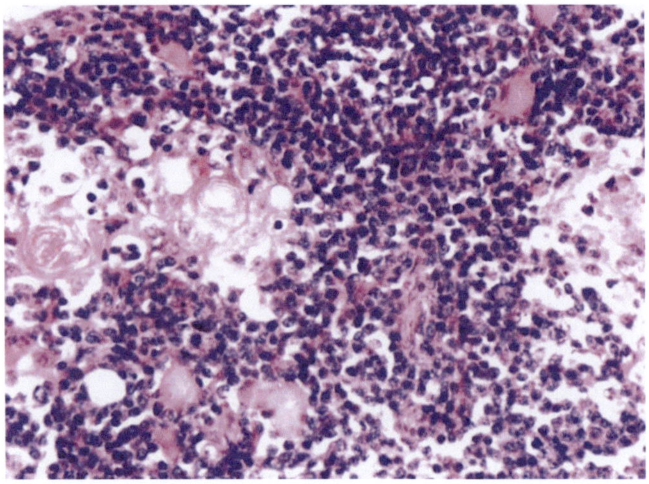

Fig. 9.28 Necrotizing thymitis. Infectious bursa Fabricius disease in chicken. Spotty necrosis of lymphocytes and reticulocytes is present in the medulla of the thymus. HE ×400. (Liu Sidang)

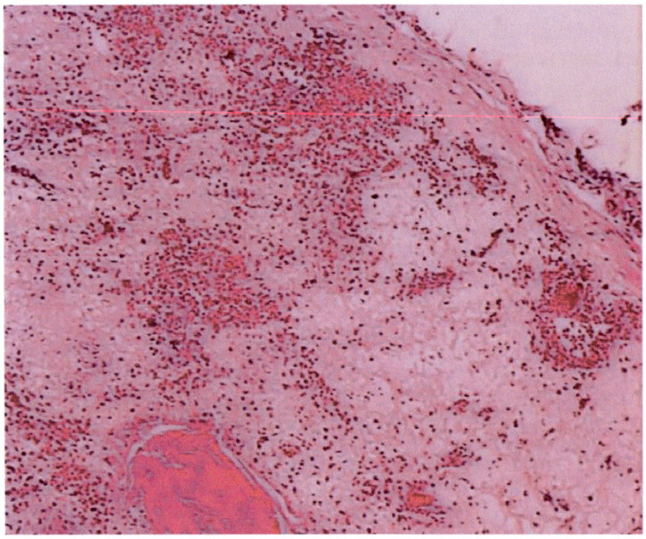

Fig. 9.29 Hemorrhagic necrotizing thymitis. Duck plague. Thymic tissue is markedly hemorrhagic and edematous. Lymphocytes reduced in number due to necrosis. HE ×100. (Hu Xueying)

infectious anemia). In addition, some pathological changes associated with aplastic anemia, such as bone marrow atrophy, are also present.

6 Pathological Red Blood Cells (Abnormal Red Blood Cells) (Figs. 9.32, 9.33, 9.34, 9.35, and 9.36)

Each species shows a certain morphology and staining characteristics of red blood cells. Hematological changes in red blood cells, or pathological red blood cells, occur in many diseases such as anemia. The pathological erythrocytes can manifest themselves in a variety of ways, including changes in their size, morphology, and staining features. Reticulocytes, nucleated erythrocytes, Joily's vesicles, and Cabot's rings can also be observed.

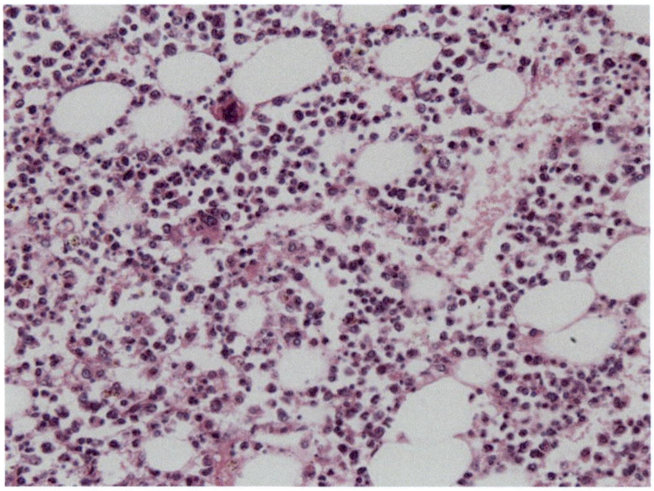

Fig. 9.30 Acute nonsuppurative osteomyelitis. Acute equine infectious anemia. Necrotizing osteomyelitis: Red bone marrow cells reduced in number with marked necrosis and disintegration of cells of the erythrocyte, granulocyte, and megakaryocyte lineages, as the reduction of later-stage cells in each of these lineages is obvious. Monocytes is focally hyperplastic, and hemorrhage as well as serous exudate can still be observed. HE ×400. (Veterinary Pathology Unit, Gansu Agricultural University)

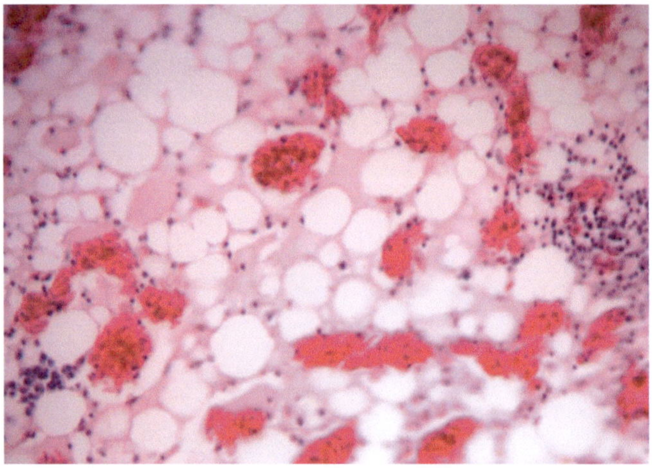

Fig. 9.31 Bone marrow atrophy. Infectious anemia in chicken. The red bone marrow of the femur is markedly atrophied and reduced, which is replaced by a large amount of fatty tissue (yellow bone marrow). (Xinhua Wang)

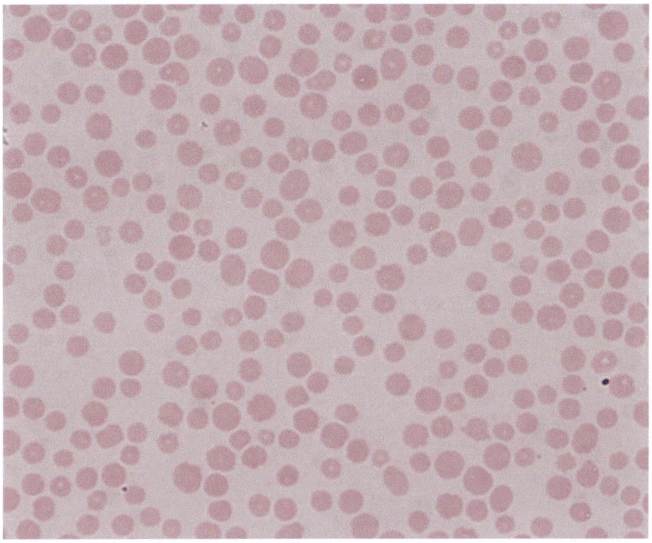

Fig. 9.32 Pathological red blood cells. Erythrocytes vary in size: The erythrocytes show significant difference in size. Some cells are larger than normal erythrocytes, which are called large erythrocytes; some cells are smaller than normal erythrocytes, which are called small erythrocytes. Wright-Giemsa ×1000. (Wang Qiuchan)

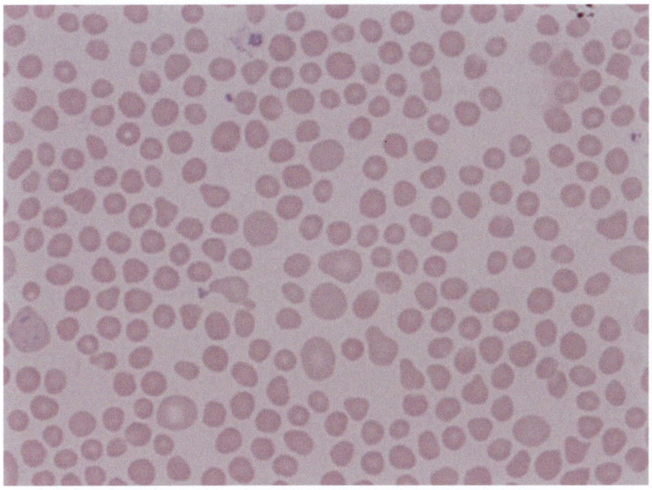

Fig. 9.33 Pathological red blood cells. Erythrocytes are morphologically diverse: The cells show oval, oblate, triangular, star-shaped, gourd-shaped, and irregular shapes. Wright-Giemsa ×1000. (Wang Qiuchan)

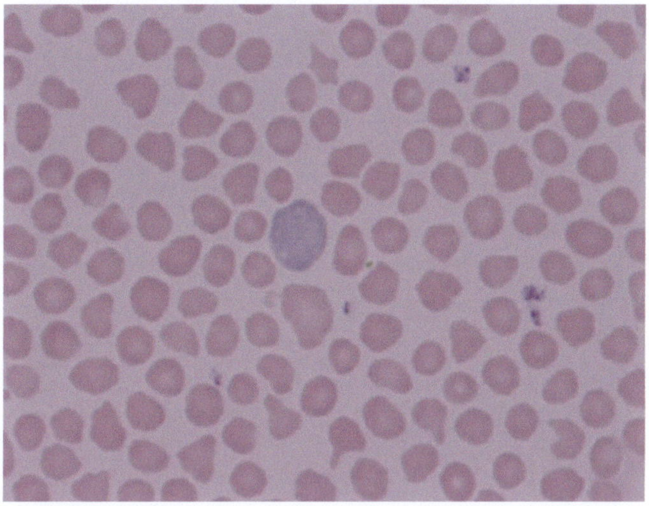

Fig. 9.34 Pathological red blood cells. Staining feature changes of erythrocytes: The normal erythrocytes are stained pale red, while the pathological red blood cells show changed staining features. This figure shows a pale blue stained erythrocyte in the center. Wright-Giemsa ×1000. (Wang Qiuchan)

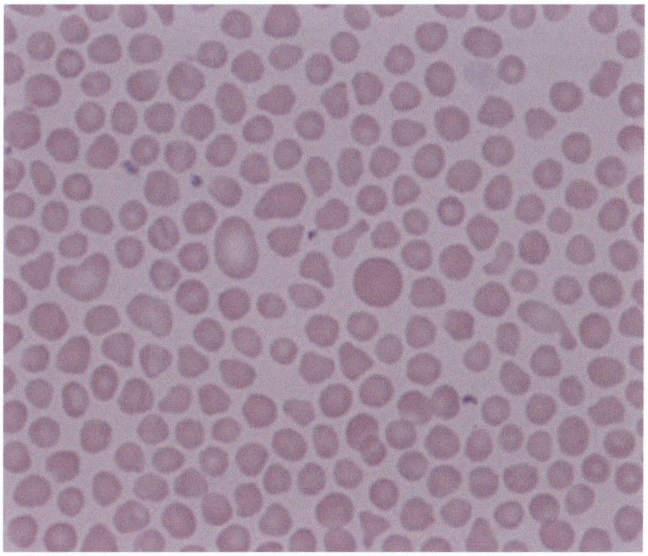

Fig. 9.35 Pathological red blood cells. Uneven erythrocyte staining: Normal erythrocytes are stained evenly with the periphery stained light red and the center stained pale. However, the hemoglobin content is altered in anemia, so some cells contain less protein, which are stained lightly with an enlarged ring-like central area, while others contain more protein and are stained darker. In the middle of this figure, there are two larger red blood cells with significantly different staining. Wright-Giemsa ×1000. (Wang Qiuchan)

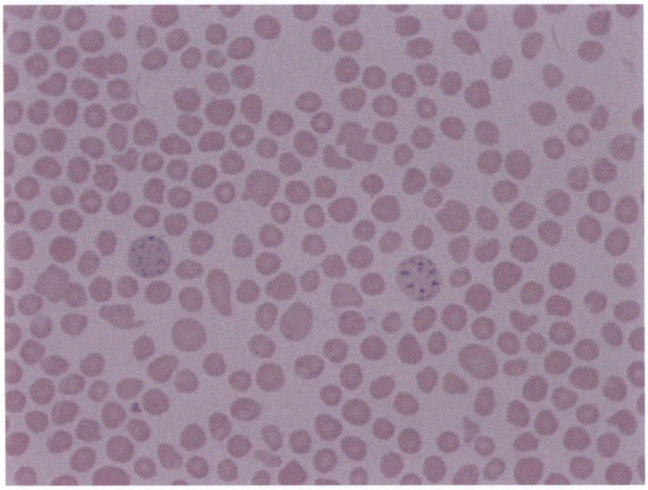

Fig. 9.36 Pathological red blood cells. Basophilic dot-colored erythrocytes: this image shows two basophilic dot-colored erythrocytes with some very distinct basophilic granules. Wright-Giemsa ×1000. (Wang Qiuchan)

Bibliography

1. Jiye S, editor. Pathology. Beijing: Science Press; 2000.
2. Jingquan S, Yisheng C, Xiuwu B, editors. Ultramicropathology. Beijing: Chemical Industry Press; 2005.

10 Pathology of the Urinary and Reproductive Systems

1 Nephritis

Nephritis is a group of diseases characterized by inflammatory changes in the glomeruli, tubules, and interstitium of the kidney. It is classified as glomerulonephritis, interstitial nephritis, and purulent nephritis.

1.1 Glomerulonephritis (Glomerular Nephritis)

Glomerulonephritis is a group of allergic diseases with predominantly glomerular damage, which manifests with both immune complex production and alteration, exudation as well as hyperplasia, the basic lesions of inflammatory response.

The types of glomerulonephritis are numerous and complex, and only a few of the major types are shown below.

1.1.1 Acute Exudative Glomerulonephritis (Figs. 10.1 and 10.2)

Inflammation occurs primarily in the glomerular vascular plexus and the glomerular capsule. Inflammatory exudate and inflammatory cells are present in the capsule lumen.

1.1.2 Acute Proliferative Glomerulonephritis (Fig. 10.3)

Acute proliferative glomerulonephritis, also known as endocapillary proliferative glomerulonephritis, is a condition in which the proliferating cells are predominantly mesangial cells and endothelial cells of the capillary tufts.

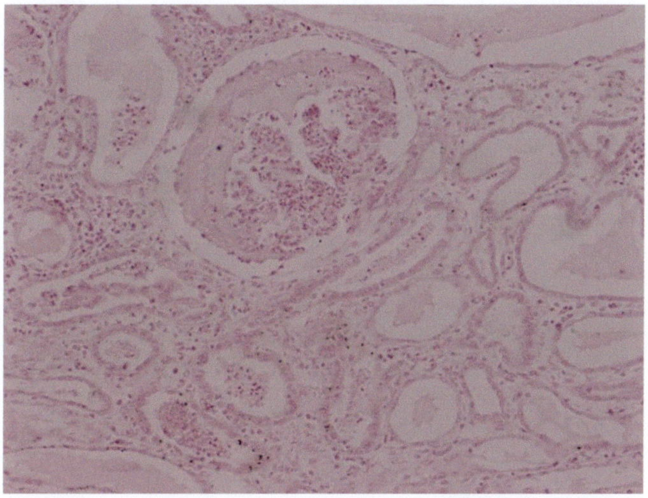

Fig. 10.1 Acute exudative glomerulonephritis. Serous glomerulonephritis: Plenty of neutrophils, fibrin, serum, and red blood cells are present in glomerular capsule lumen and glomerular capillary interstitium. The volume of the papillary tuft is reduced with papillary anemia. The renal tubular epithelium is degenerated with some tubular lumen dilatation, containing protein and neutrophils. HE ×200. (Veterinary Pathology Unit, Gansu Agricultural University)

1.1.3 Membranous Glomerulonephritis (Figs. 10.4 and 10.5)

Membranous glomerulonephritis is a disease of immune complex deposition characterized by diffuse thickening of capillary basement membrane and subepithelial electron microscopic deposits of immune complexes. This type of nephritis can be observed in swine fever, rabbit viral hemorrhagic disease, mink Aleutian disease, and some drug poisoning. Prognosis is characterized by massive proteinuria and nephrotic syndrome.

H. Chen, *Color Atlas of Veterinary Pathology*, https://doi.org/10.1007/978-981-96-7617-0_10

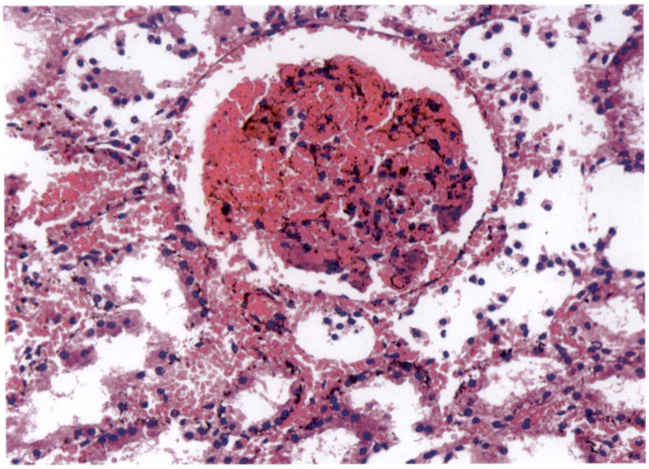

Fig. 10.2 Acute exudative glomerulonephritis. Acute swine erysipelas. Hemorrhagic glomerulonephritis: Glomerular capillaries are congested, and there are a large number of erythrocytes as well as neutrophils are present in the capsule. The glomeruli are enlarged. The interstitial vessels are obviously congested, and the tubular epithelium is deformed and detached. HE ×400. (Chen Huaitao)

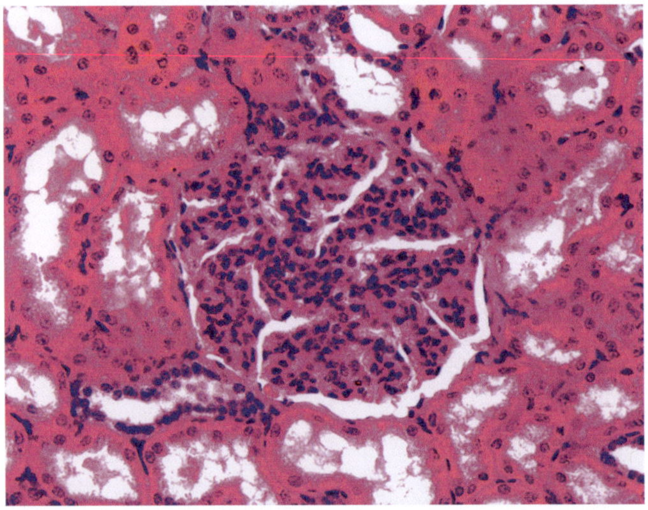

Fig. 10.3 Acute proliferative glomerulonephritis. The glomerulus is enlarged with increased cell numbers. The glomerular capillary endothelial cells and mesangial cells are hypertrophic and hyperplastic. Individual neutrophils and monocytes are present and the glomerular capsule lumen is narrowed in a fissure shape. Tubular epithelial cells are degenerated. HE ×400. (Chen Huaitao)

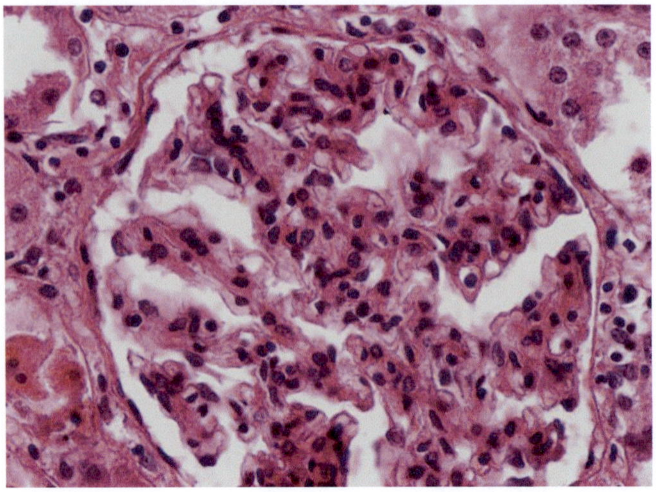

Fig. 10.4 Membranous glomerulonephritis. The glomerulus becomes larger in volume and the capillary wall is thickened. HE ×400. (Wang Wenhui)

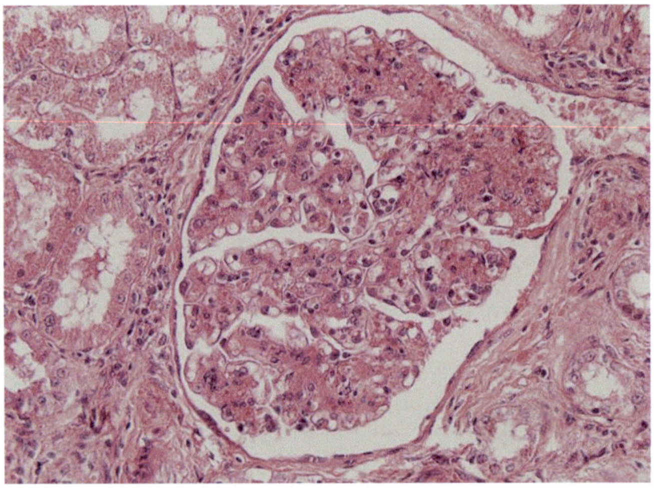

Fig. 10.5 Membranous glomerulonephritis. The glomerulus is enlarged, and the capillary wall is diffusely thickened with marked annularity in cross-section of blood vessels. The tubular epithelium is obviously degenerated, and a large amount of proteinaceous substance are present in the lumen. HE ×400. (Chen Huaitao)

1.1.4 Subacute Glomerulonephritis (Figs. 10.6 and 10.7)

The pathology of subacute glomerulonephritis is characterized by proliferation of most epithelial cells on glomerular capsule wall, forming crescent or ring bodies.

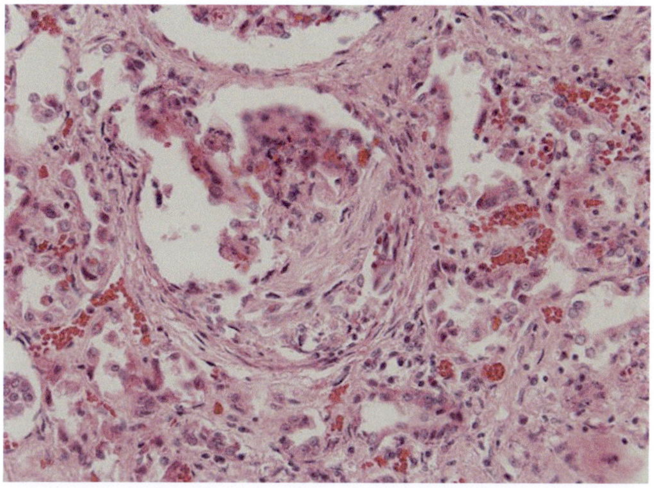

Fig. 10.6 Subacute glomerulonephritis. The epithelial cells of the glomerular capsule wall overlap and form a "crescent" on the lower right side (the urethral side of the capsule wall layer). The capillary tuft is compressed and the glomerulus adheres to the capsule. The epithelium of the renal tubule is degenerated and the interstitial inflammatory cells are infiltrated. HE ×400. (Chen Huaitao)

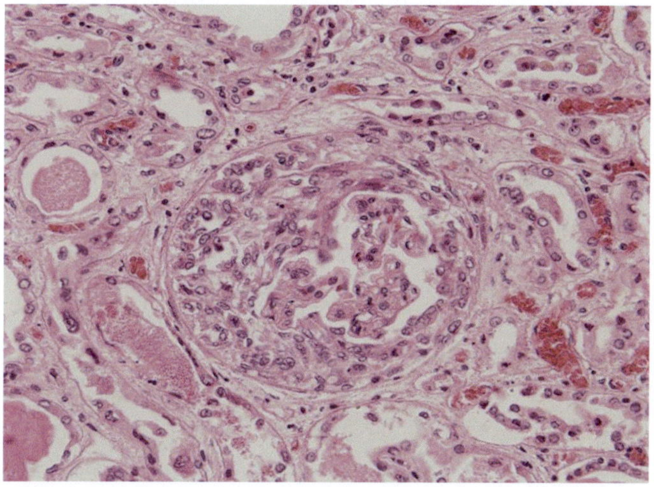

Fig. 10.7 Subacute glomerulonephritis. The epithelial cells in the glomerular capsule wall are obviously proliferated, forming "ring body," and the glomerular capillaries are compressed and atrophied. The tubular epithelium is degenerated, with plenty of proteinaceous substance in the lumen and interstitial inflammatory cells infiltration. HE ×400. (Chen Huaitao)

1.1.5 Chronic (Sclerosing) Flomerulonephritis (Figs. 10.8 and 10.9)

This is the final stage of pathology in the development of different types of nephritis, which is characterized by fibrosis or even hyaline changes in a large number of glomeruli and compensatory hypertrophy of the remaining glomeruli, resulting in a consolidated kidney with a granular surface, hence it is termed contracted kidney.

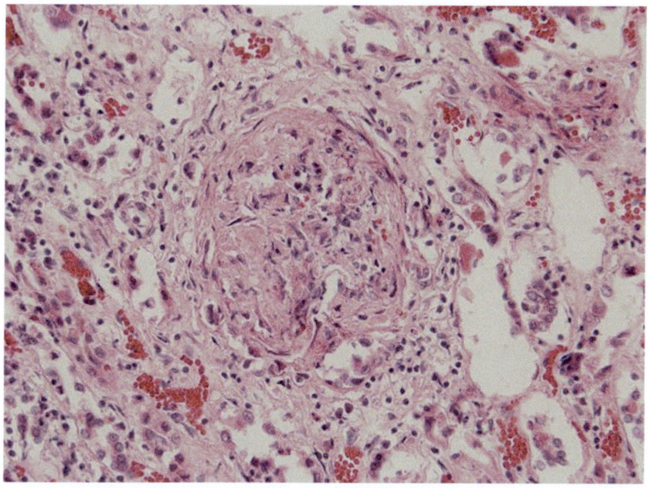

Fig. 10.8 Chronic glomerulonephritis. The glomerulus is markedly fibrotic, becoming a mass of fibrous connective tissue. The capillaries disappeared, and the glomerular capsule is completely occluded. HE ×400. (Chen Huaitao)

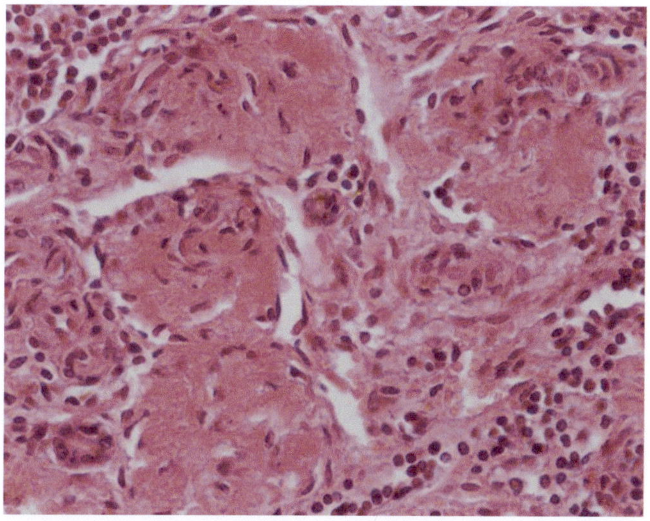

Fig. 10.9 Chronic glomerulonephritis. Hyaline changes have occurred in the glomeruli, which appear as a mass of structureless homogeneous material. Several glomeruli with hyaline change are present in this picture, which appear to have increased glomeruli. Connective tissue hyperplasia and lymphocyte infiltration are observed in the interstitium. HE ×400. (Chen Huaitao)

1.2 Interstitial Nephritis

Interstitial nephritis is a primary inflammatory disease of the renal interstitium characterized by lymphocyte and monocyte infiltration as well as connective tissue hyperplasia. It can be classified into acute interstitial nephritis and chronic interstitial nephritis according to the course of the disease.

1.2.1 Acute Interstitial Nephritis (Fig. 10.10)

1.2.2 Chronic Interstitial Nephritis (Fig. 10.11)

1.3 Suppurative Nephritis (Fig. 10.12)

Suppurative nephritis is a purulent inflammation of the renal parenchyma and renal pelvis due to infection with purulent bacteria. It can be classified into two types, embolic purulent nephritis and pyelonephritis, based on the route of infection.

1.3.1 Embolic Suppurative Nephritis

Embolic suppurative nephritis results from a hematogenous (downward) infection in which suppurative bacteria enter the kidney via the bloodstream and first form bacterial emboli in the glomerular capillary tufts, followed by the formation of suppurative foci in the glomerulus and gradual spreading around the glomerulus.

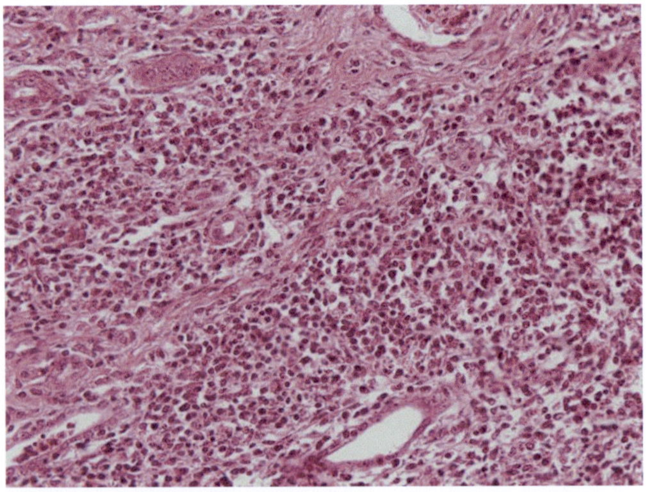

Fig. 10.10 Acute interstitial nephritis. The distance between renal tubules and between tubules and glomeruli is widened; there is a large infiltration of inflammatory cells, mainly lymphocytes; and the tubules are mostly atrophied and a few are dilated. HE ×400. (Chen Huaitao)

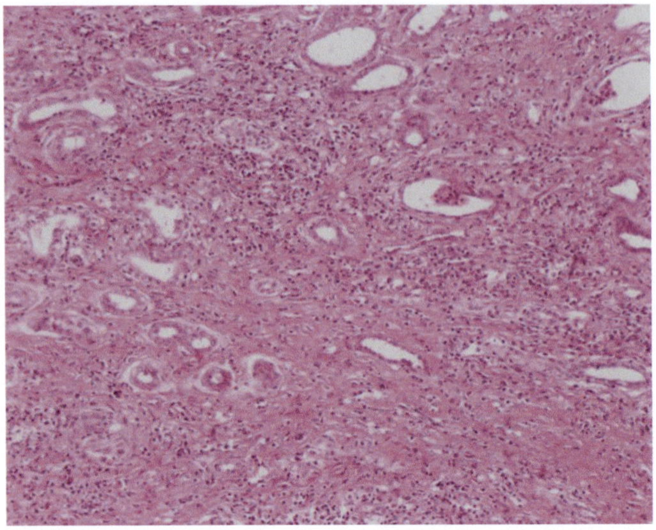

Fig. 10.11 Chronic interstitial nephritis. There is massive connective tissue hyperplasia in the interstitium with lymphocytic and plasma cell infiltration. Most of the tubules are atrophied or disappeared, but some are dilated. The glomeruli are also mostly atrophied and small, but some renal capsules are dilated. HE ×100. (Wang Wenhui)

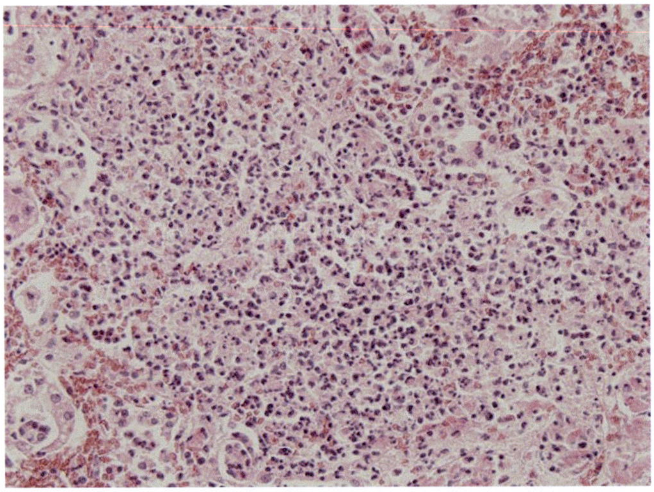

Fig. 10.12 Embolic suppurative nephritis. A large number of neutrophils and pus cells are in the glomerulus and its surrounding interstitium, with the local tissue structure being destroyed. HE ×400. (Chen Huaitao)

1.3.2 Pyelonephritis (Fig. 10.13)

Pyelonephritis is a purulent inflammation that occurs in the mucosa of the renal pelvis and the interstitium of the kidney. The common route of infection is urogenital (upward). When an infection occurs in the lower urinary tract (urethritis, cystitis), the suppurative bacteria can travel up the ureter to the renal pelvis, causing pyelonephritis first, where suppurative foci form, and further by the renal papillae and collecting ducts reaching the renal parenchyma, resulting in suppurative nephritis.

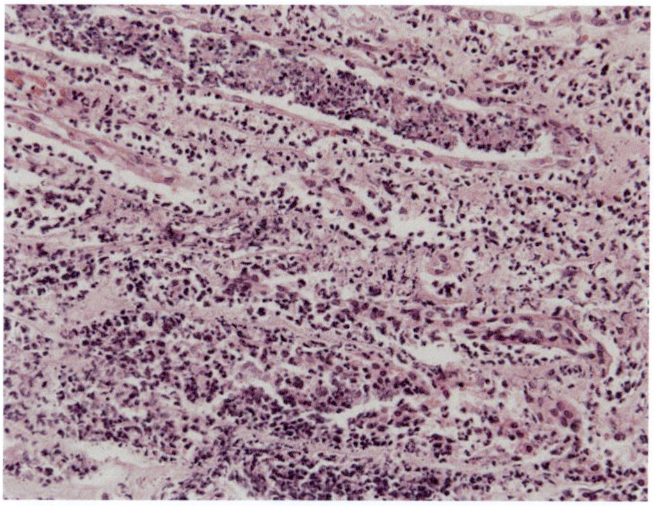

Fig. 10.13 Pyelonephritis. A large number of neutrophils and pus cells are present in the renal tubules and the local interstitium. Some tubules are necrotic and their boundaries are indistinct. HE ×400. (Chen Huaitao)

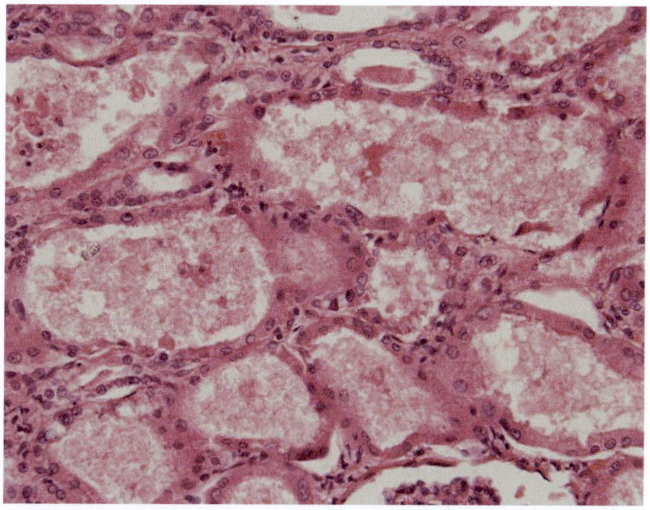

Fig. 10.14 Nephrosis. The renal tubular epithelium is degenerated and necrotic, and the tubules are filled with proteinaceous substance, but no inflammatory reaction is observed. HE ×400. (Chen Huaitao)

2 Nephrosis (Nephropathy) (Figs. 10.14, 10.15 and 10.16)

Nephrosis is a disease in which renal tubules undergo degeneration and necrosis without inflammatory changes. With the exception of amyloidosis, the most significant lesions are in the renal tubules, especially the proximal tubules.

3 Cystic Kidney (Figs. 10.17 and 10.18)

A cystic kidney refers to the formation of cystic cavities of variable sizes containing fluid in the kidney. Cysts of the kidney are common in domestic animals, and it occurs most often in pigs, followed by cattle and rabbits.

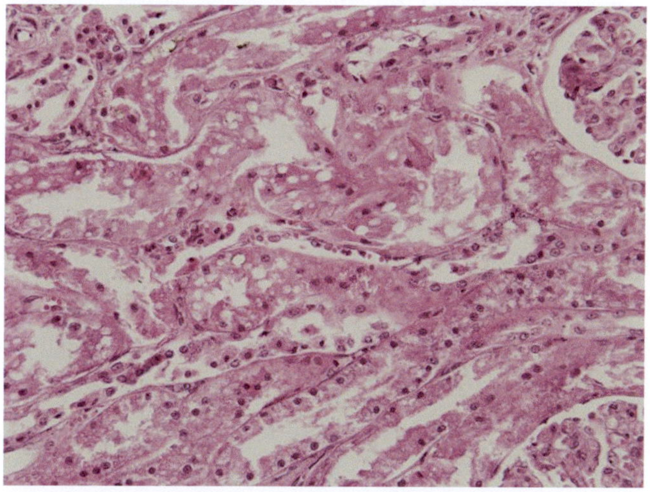

Fig. 10.15 Nephrosis. Fatty degeneration and necrosis are observed for the renal tubular epithelium, and many proximal tubules are filled with proteinaceous substance, but no inflammatory cell infiltration is observed inside or outside of the tubules. HE ×400. (Chen Huaitao)

4 Endometritis

Endometritis can be classified into acute and chronic inflammation according to the course of the disease and the nature of the inflammation. Acute endometritis mainly manifests as acute catarrhal inflammation, while chronic endometritis is further classified into chronic catarrhal and chronic suppurative endometritis, which is one of the major causes of infertility in female animals.

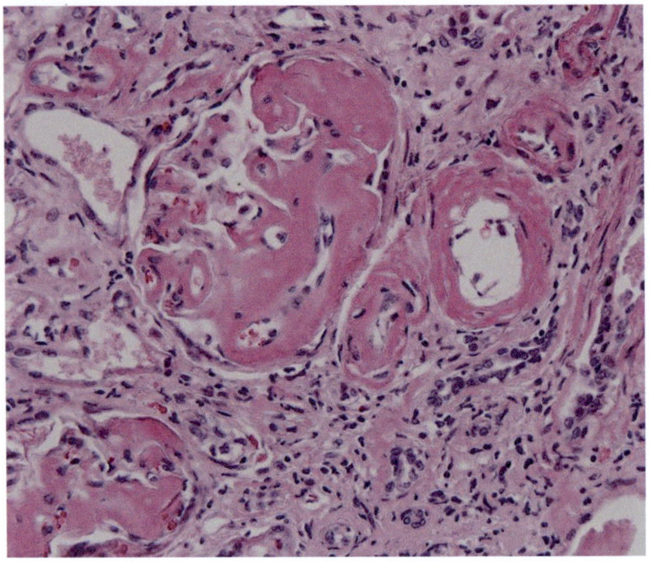

Fig. 10.16 Nephrosis. Amyloidosis nephropathy: amyloid substance is reddish in color and can be deposited in the glomerular mesangial areas as well as capillary basement membrane, so the basement membrane is diffusely thickened and the lumen is narrowed or occluded; amyloid substance is also deposited in the walls of small renal arteries and arterioles, so their walls are thickened and homogeneous. HE ×400. (Chen Huaitao)

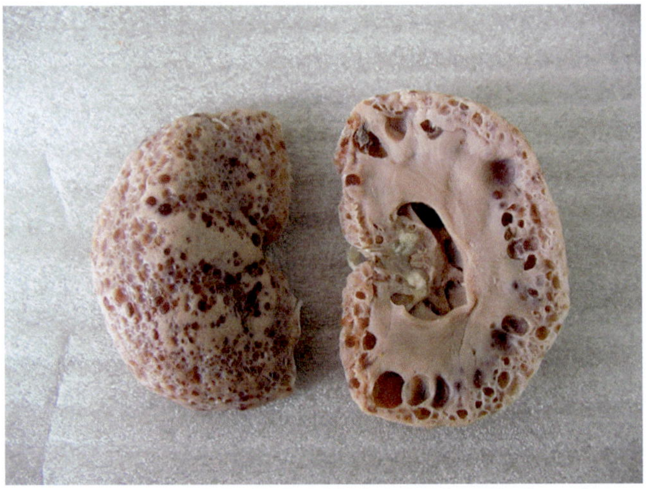

Fig. 10.17 Cystic kidney. Rabbit kidney. Numerous vesicles of variable size containing translucent fluid are densely distributed on the surface and in the cut surface of the renal cortex. (Wang Xinhua)

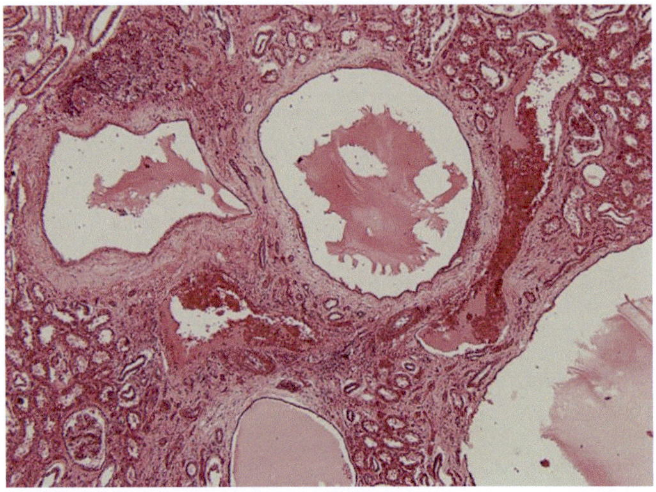

Fig. 10.18 Cystic kidney. Pig kidney. Cystic cavities are highly dilated renal tubules containing proteinaceous substance. The interstitial connective tissue is hyperplastic, with lymphocyte infiltration. HE ×100. (Chen Huaitao)

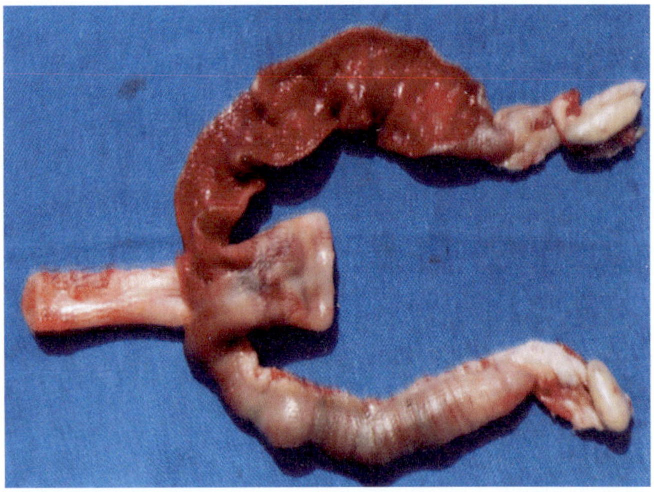

Fig. 10.19 Acute catarrhal endometritis. Rabbit uterus. The uterus is slightly enlarged in appearance, and the uterine mucosa is congested as well as flushing with some swelling. Some cloudy, maroon exudate is attached to the mucosal surface. (Chen Huaitao, Li Xiaoming)

4.1 Acute Catarrhal Endometritis (Figs. 10.19 and 10.20)

4.2 Chronic Endometritis

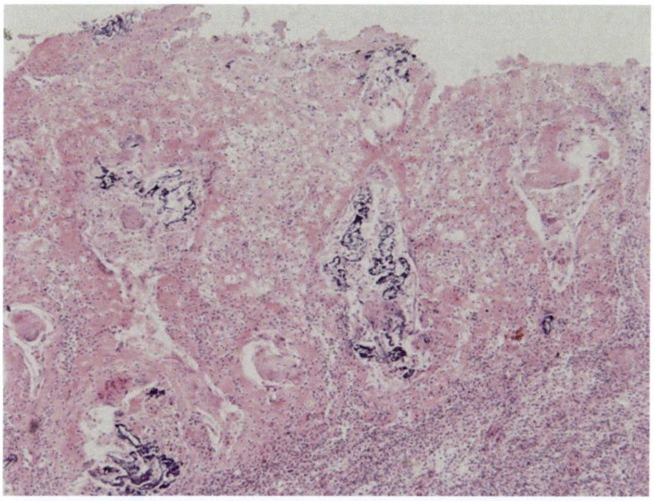

Fig. 10.20 Acute catarrhal endometritis. Bovine endometrial epithelium is degenerated, necrotized, and exfoliated. The mucosal tissue is congested, hemorrhagic, and edematous with neutrophil infiltration as well as uterine gland necrosis. HE ×100. (Chen Huaitao)

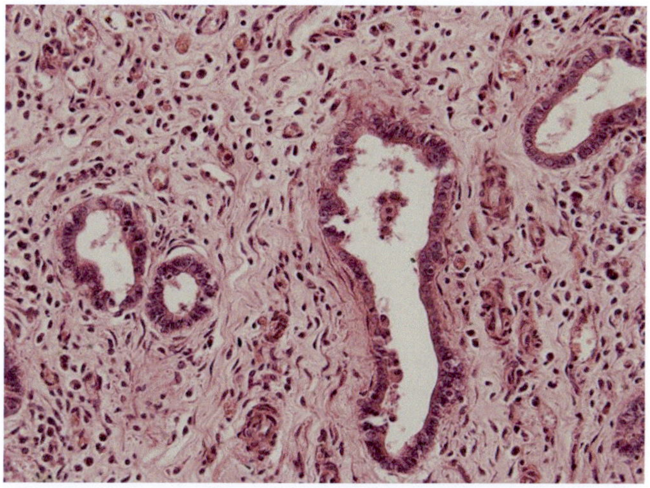

Fig. 10.22 Chronic catarrhal endometritis. Bovine endometrium shows a marked hyperplasia of connective tissue, infiltration of lymphocytes and plasma cells, and mostly atrophied uterine glands. HE ×400. (Chen Huaitao)

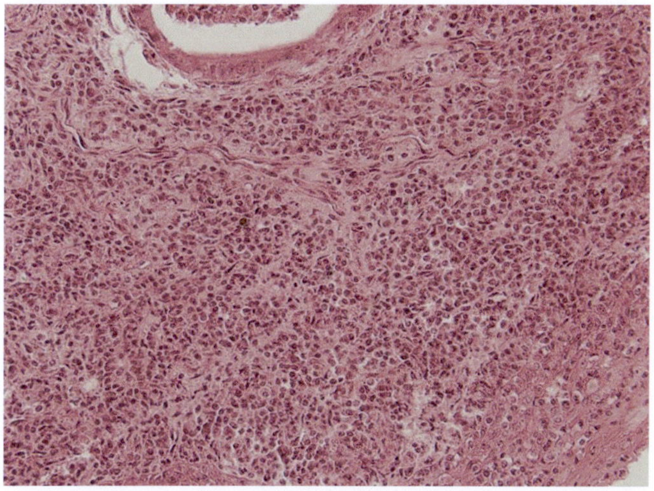

Fig. 10.21 Chronic catarrhal endometritis. Bovine endometrium is infiltrated by massive lymphocytes and plasma cells, with hyperplasia of a small amount of connective tissue and atrophy of the uterine glands. HE ×200. (Chen Huaitao)

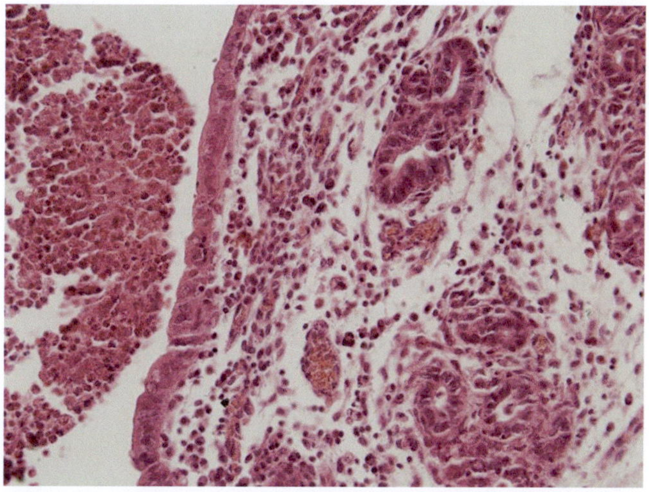

Fig. 10.23 Chronic suppurative endometritis. Rabbit uterus. A large number of pus cells accumulate in the uterine cavity (left side) and the endometrium is infiltrated with lymphocytes, plasma cells, and neutrophils. HE ×400. (Veterinary Pathology Unit, Gansu Agricultural University)

4.2.1 Chronic Catarrhal Endometritis (Figs. 10.21 and 10.22)

4.2.2 Chronic Suppurative Endometritis (Fig. 10.23)

5 Mastitis (Figs. 10.24, 10.25 and 10.26)

Mastitis occurs in a variety of animals, more often in cattle and sheep, and is characterized by various inflammatory processes in the mammary tissue. The causes of mastitis are complex, and it is mainly caused by multiple bacterial infections. The classification is not very well defined, and the common ones are serous mastitis, suppurative mastitis, chronic mastitis, and atopic (granulomatous) mastitis.

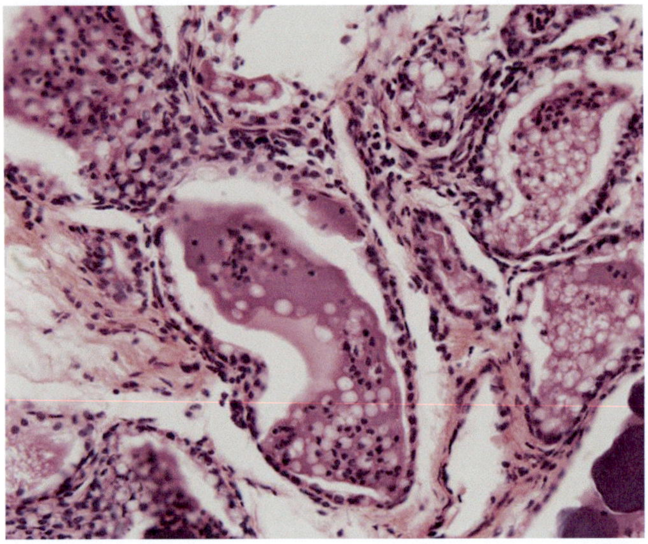

Fig. 10.24 Serous mastitis. Bovine mammary gland. Serum (containing fat droplets), neutrophils, and detached epithelial cells are present in the acini. The glandular epithelial cells are degenerated and detached, and the interstitium is edematous with inflammatory cell infiltration. HE × 400. (Chen Huaitao)

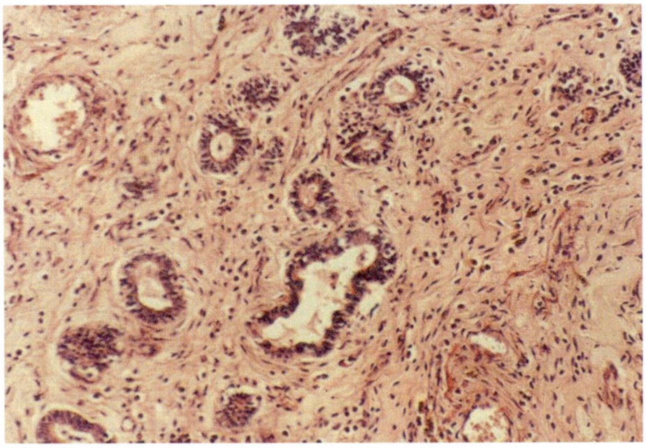

Fig. 10.25 Chronic mastitis. Bovine mammary gland. Inter-acinar connective tissue is significantly hyperplastic with infiltration of lymphocytes and plasma cells. The inter-acinar gaps are widened, and the acini are mostly atrophied, but some are dilated. HE ×400. (Chen Huaitao)

6 Orchitis and Epididymitis (Fig. 10.27, 10.28, 10.29, 10.30, and 10.31)

Orchitis is caused by an injury infection or accompanied or secondary to other diseases, such as various suppurative infections and some granulomatous diseases (brucellosis, tuberculosis, etc.), and the inflammation manifests itself as an acute or chronic process. Epididymitis is one of the more common diseases of the reproductive organs in male animals, occurring most frequently in rams and characterized by sperm degeneration and sperm granulomas.

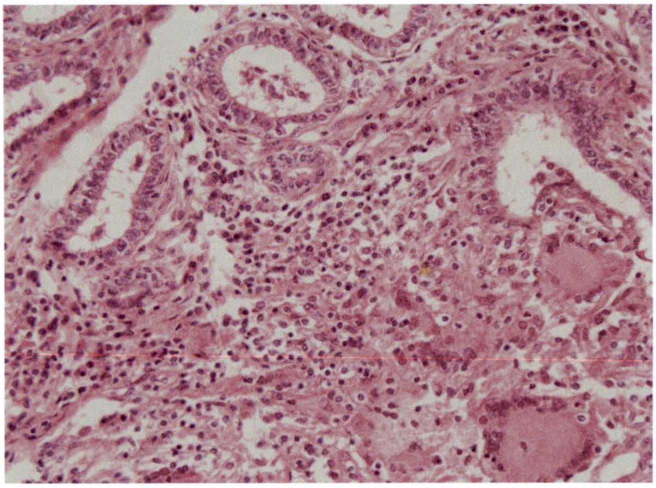

Fig. 10.26 Specific mastitis. Bovine tuberculosis. Epithelioid cells and Langhans giant cells are markedly hyperplastic in the mammary tissue. HE ×400. (Chen Huaitao)

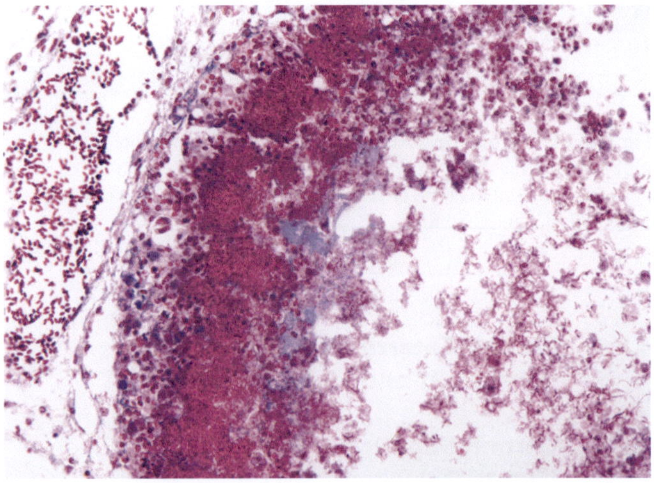

Fig. 10.27 Orchitis. Salmonellosis in a rooster. Suppurative orchitis: the epithelium of the testicular seminiferous tubules (shown only in the upper left) has mostly necrotized and coagulated into a purplish-red substance, with only some epithelium remaining near the basement membrane. Inflammatory cell infiltration is obvious in the necrotic substance, and a small amount of necrotic substance are present in the tubules. HE ×400. (Chen Huaitao)

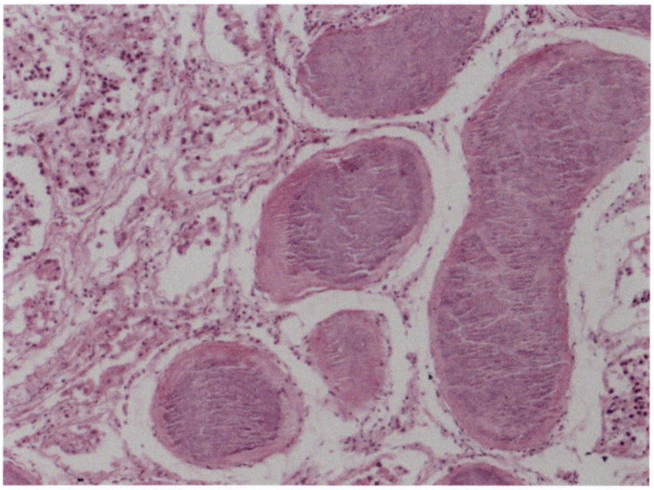

Fig. 10.28 Spermatozoal cysts. Spermatozoal cysts in the testis of goats: some fine sperm ducts dilated into a sac, which was filled with sperm; some fine sperm ducts on the left side had necrotic epithelium and the lumen was filled with necrotic substance. HE ×200. (Chen Huaitao)

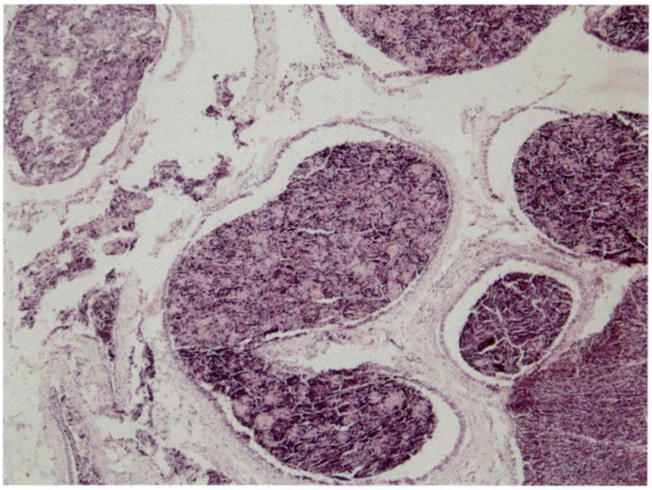

Fig. 10.29 Spermatozoal cysts. Epididymal spermatozoa cysts in goats: the epididymal ducts are cystically enlarged, the walls of the ducts are thinned, and they are filled with sperm; if the spermatozoa come into contact with the extra-tubular tissue, they can provoke the formation of sperm granulomas. HE ×100. (Chen Huaitao)

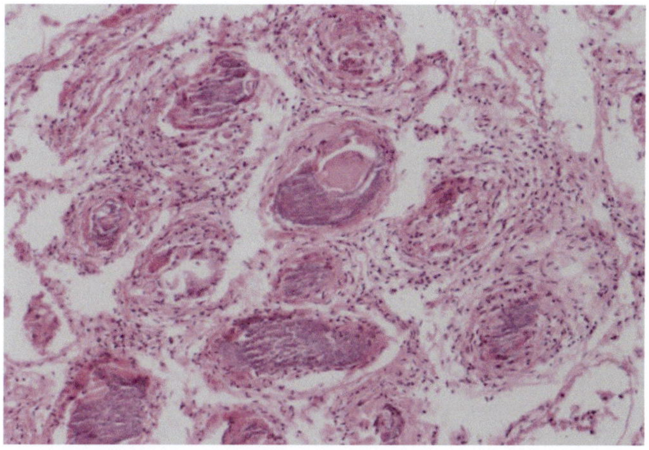

Fig. 10.30 Sperm granuloma. Sperm granuloma of the testis of goats: at the site of several fine sperm ducts where sperm cysts had originally occurred, granuloma formation had occurred, with very few sperms in the ducts, also with damaged walls and proliferating cells at the periphery. HE ×200. (Chen Huaitao)

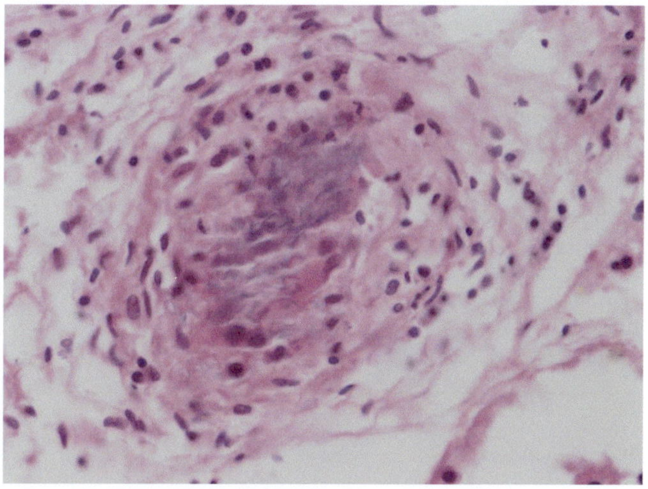

Fig. 10.31 Sperm granuloma. Sperm granuloma of goat testis: the center of the granuloma shows a sperm necrotic mass, a few spermatozoa are also visible, and its periphery shows some epithelioid cells and giant cells. HE ×400. (Chen Huaitao)

Bibliography

1. Henmin C, editor. Pathological anatomy of domestic animals. 4th ed. China Agricultural Press; 2018.
2. Lirang Q, editor. Pathological anatomy of domestic animal systems. Beijing: China Agricultural Press; 1992.

11 Pathology of the Nervous System

1 Pathological Changes of Brain

1.1 Pathological Changes of Neuron

1.1.1 Neuronal Vacuolar Degeneration (Fig. 11.1)

1.1.2 Central Chromatolysis (Figs. 11.2 and 11.3)

1.1.3 Acute Neuronal Swelling (Figs. 11.4 and 11.5)

1.1.4 Shrinkage or Coagulation of Neurons (Fig. 11.6)

1.1.5 Karyorrhexis and Karyolysis (Figs. 11.7 and 11.8)

1.1.6 Neuronolysis (Fig. 11.9)

1.2 Encephalitis

Encephalitis is complex and the classification is not quite defined; it can be classified into viral encephalitis, bacterial encephalitis, parasitic encephalitis, and salt toxic encephalitis, depending on the etiology.

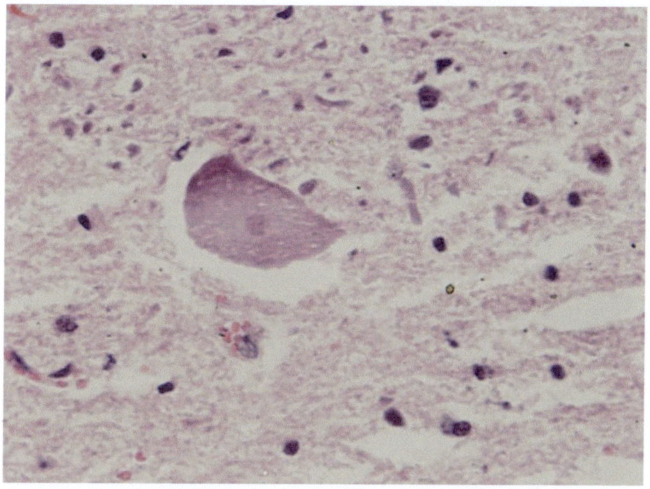

Fig. 11.1 Neuronal vacuolar degeneration. Locoweed poisoning in sheep. Many small vacuoles are present in the cytoplasm of neurons, and the nuclei are lysed and faintly stained, with only nuclear shadows visible. HE ×400. (Chen Huaitao)

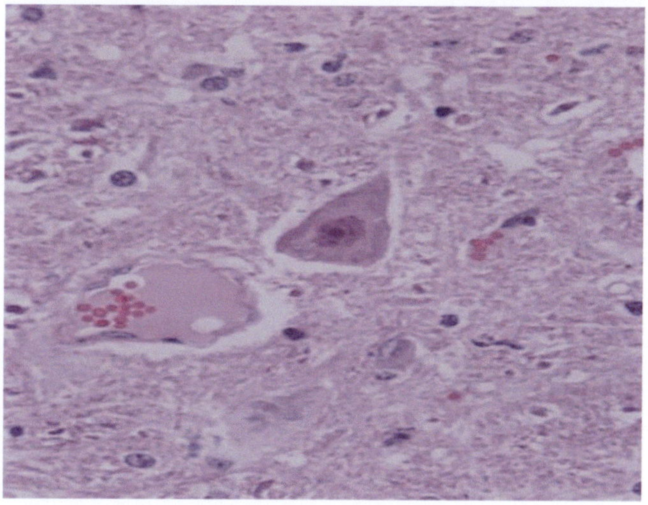

Fig. 11.2 Central chromatolysis. Chromatin lysis occurs around the nucleus of a neuron in the center of the figure. It is stained pale with the peripheral chromatin still recognizable and the nucleus relatively intact. HE ×400. (Chen Huaitao)

H. Chen, *Color Atlas of Veterinary Pathology*, https://doi.org/10.1007/978-981-96-7617-0_11

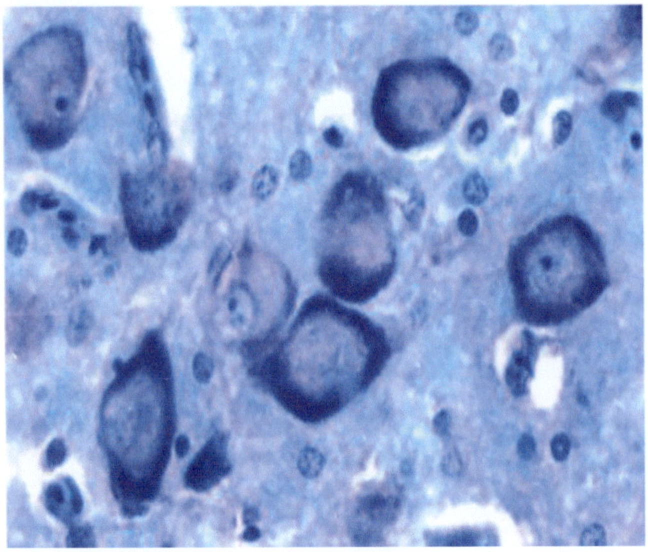

Fig. 11.3 Central chromatolysis. Encephalomyelitis in a chick. Within the round nucleus of the midbrain, chromatin lysis can be observed in the central region of several neurons. Some of the nuclei have lysed and disappeared. Toluidine blue staining ×400. (Zhao Zhenhua)

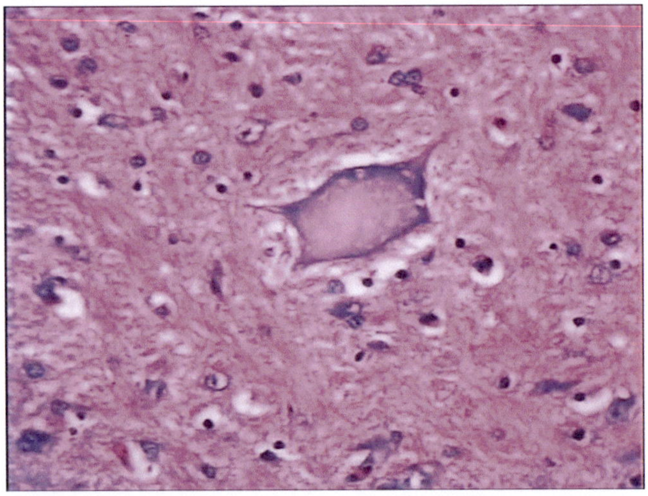

Fig. 11.4 Acute swelling. Neurons are enlarged, with shortened neuritis. Most of the chromatin is lysed and the cytoplasm is lightly stained. HE ×400. (Hu Xueying)

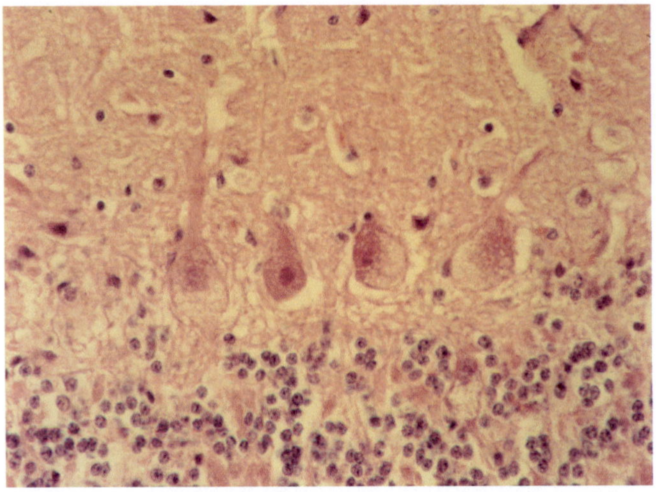

Fig. 11.5 Acute swelling. Cerebellar Purkinje cells are enlarged and rounded, with lightly stained cytoplasm and remaining nuclei. HE ×400. (Chen Huaitao)

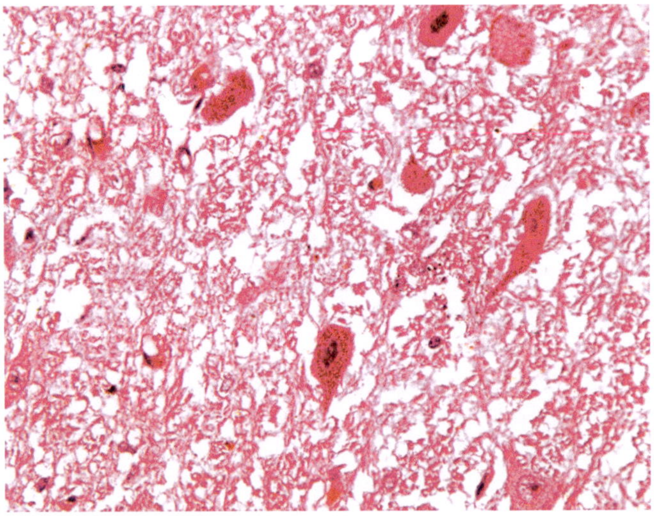

Fig. 11.6 Cell concentration. Neurons are thinned, lack of cytoplasm, darkly eosin stained, and homogeneous. The nuclei are small and darkly stained, poorly defined, or disappeared, and nucleoli are not recognizable. HE ×400. (Chen Huaitao)

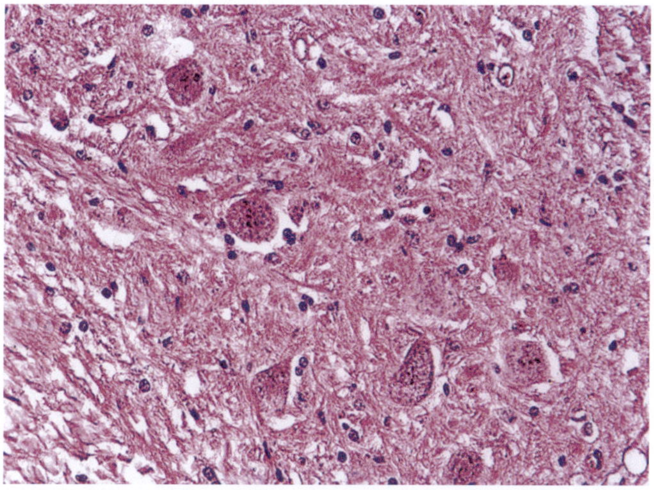

Fig. 11.7 Karyorrhexis. Several neurons have undergone karyorrhexis, and the nuclei have disintegrated into fragments of varying sizes scattered in the cytoplasm. HE ×400. (Chen Huaitao)

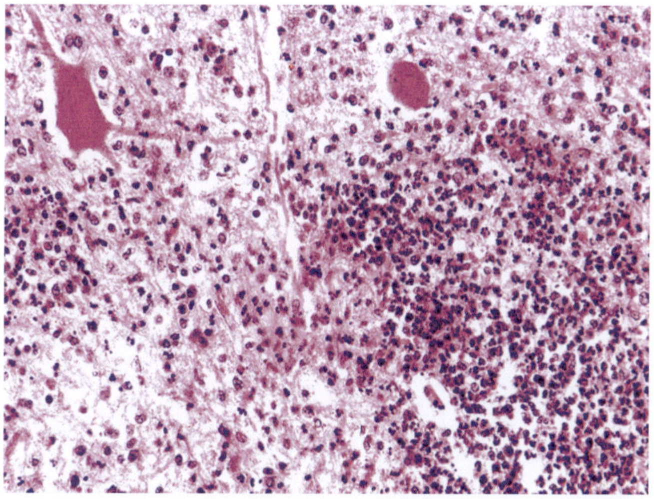

Fig. 11.8 Karyolysis. This image shows that two neurons have undergone karyolysis and disappeared. In addition, the purulent process is present in the brain tissue. HE ×400. (Chen Huaitao)

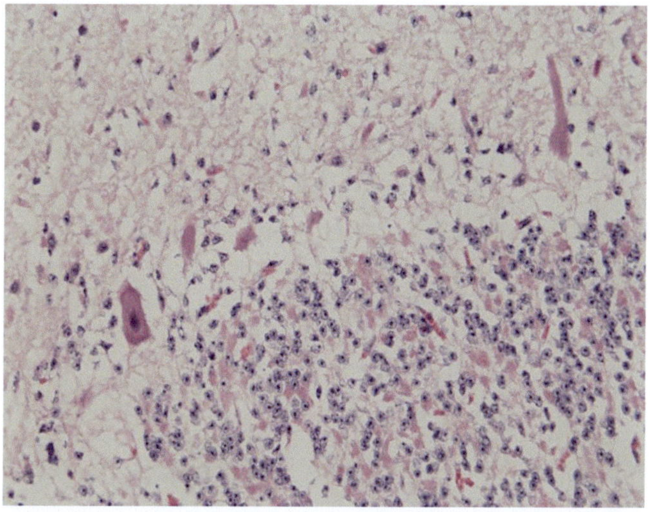

Fig. 11.9 Necrosis of Purkinje cells. In this figure, most of the cerebellar Purkinje's cells have been necrotic and lysed, and some of them remain only as remnants, and the brain tissue, especially the ganglion cell layer, is obviously edematous. HE ×400. (Chen Huaitao)

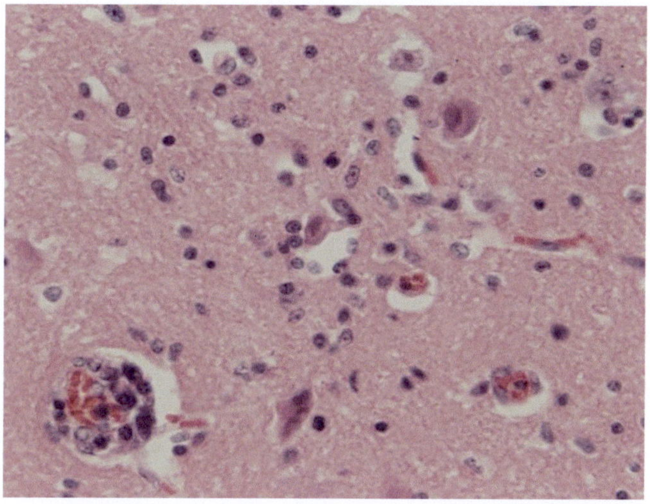

Fig. 11.10 Nonsuppurative encephalitis. Cerebral edema: cerebral vessels are congested, perivascular space is dilated and edematous; neuronal cells are degenerated with glial cells proliferation. HE ×400. (Chen Huaitao)

1.2.1 Viral Encephalitis (Figs. 11.10, 11.11, 11.12, 11.13, 11.14 and 11.15)

Viral encephalitis, or nonsuppurative encephalitis, is a subacute inflammatory process of brain tissue caused by a variety of viruses and is characterized by changes such as degenerative necrosis of neural tissue and vascular reactions with glial cell proliferation.

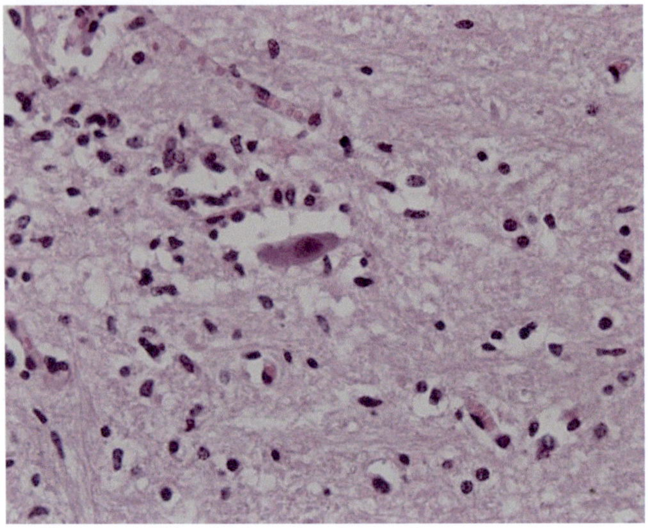

Fig. 11.11 Nonsuppurative encephalitis. Satellitosis: In the center of the figure, a degenerated necrotic nerve cell is surrounded by several microglia and oligodendrocytes . HE ×400. (Chen Huaitao)

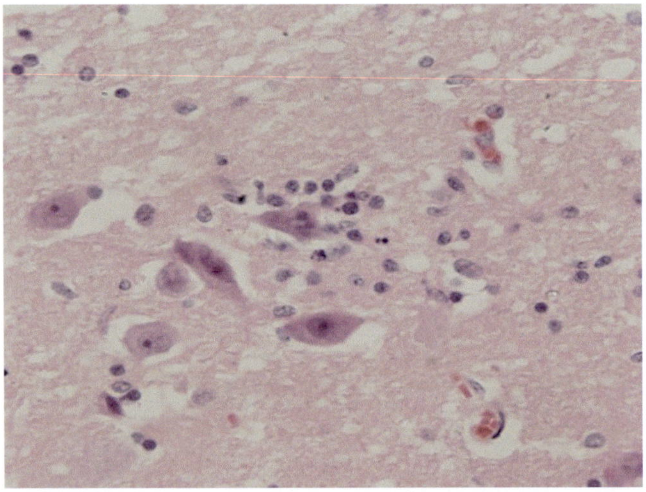

Fig. 11.12 Nonsuppurative encephalitis. The phenomenon of neuronophagia: a necrotic neuron in the center of the figure is engulfed and cleared by microglia. HE ×400. (Chen Huaitao)

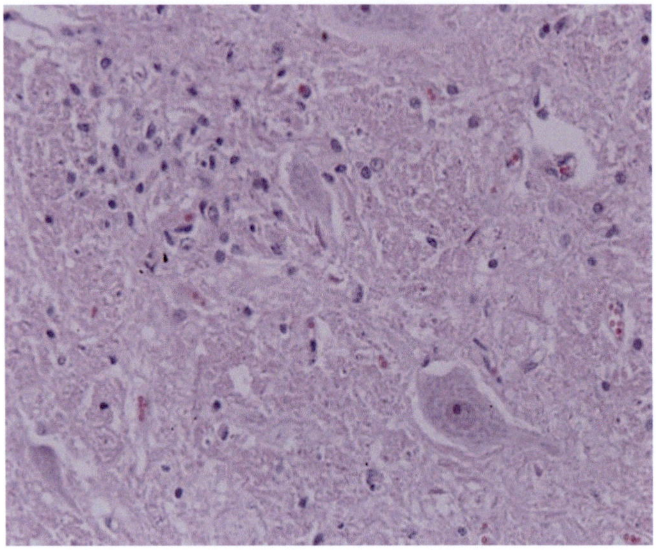

Fig. 11.13 Nonsuppurative encephalitis. Glial nodules: microglia proliferate to form a cellular mass (top left of the figure), with necrosis and lysis of a nearby nerve cell. HE ×400. (Chen Huaitao)

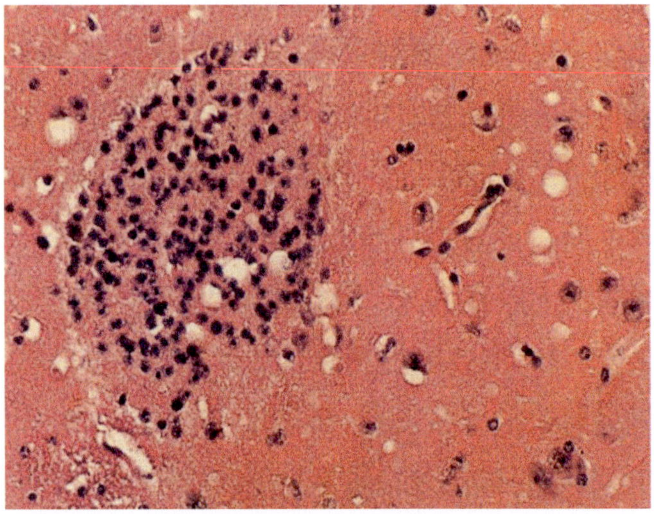

Fig. 11.14 Nonsuppurative encephalitis. Glial cell nodules: In the lenticular nucleus of the striatum of the ovine scrapie sheep's brain, astrocytes proliferate locally and form clumps. HE ×400. (Feng Zeguang)

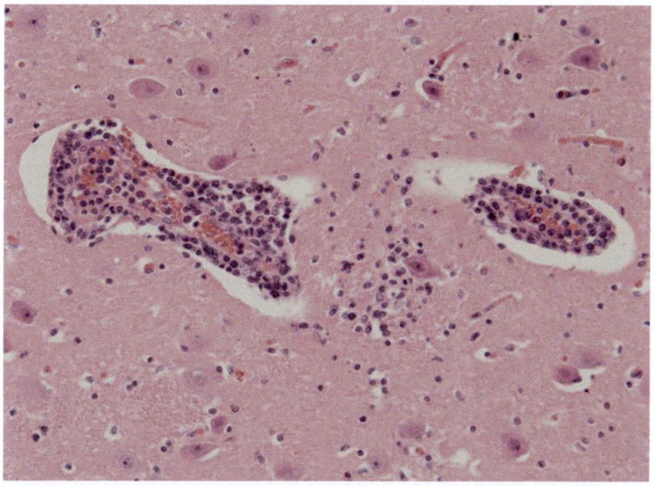

Fig. 11.15 Nonsuppurative encephalitis. Perivascular cuffing: on the cross-section of both vessels, many lymphocytes surrounding the canal can be observed, forming a vascular cuff; a small nodule of glial cells remains in the brain tissue between the vessels, and central chromatinolysis occurs in the nerve cells near the periphery. HE ×400. (Chen Huaitao)

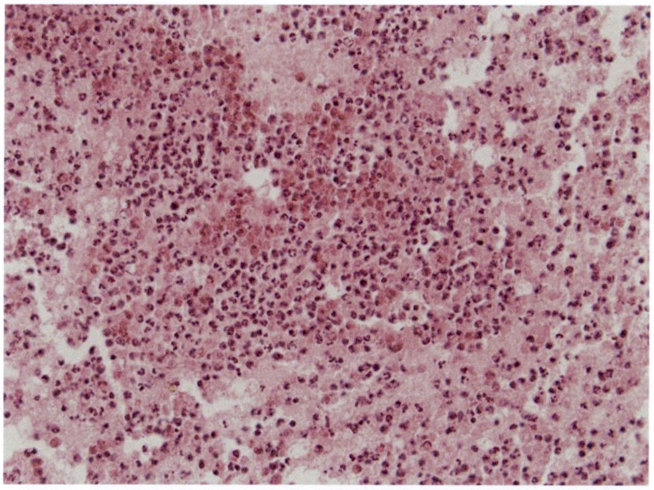

Fig. 11.16 Bacterial encephalitis. Suppurative focus: There is a septic focus in the brain tissue with many neutrophils and other white blood cells (white blood cells) accumulation. Local tissue starts to dissolve and liquefy, so the tissue structure is indistince. HE ×400. (Chen Huaitao)

1.2.2 Bacterial Encephalitis (Figs. 11.16, 11.17, 11.18, 11.19 and 11.20)

Bacterial encephalitis, or suppurative encephalitis, is caused by suppurative bacteria and characterized by the presence of massive neutrophil exudation and septic lysis, or even abscess formation, often accompanied by an inflammatory process in the meninges.

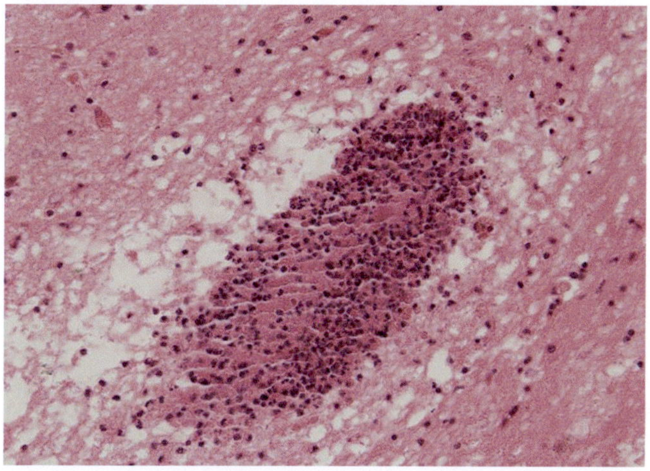

Fig. 11.17 Bacterial encephalitis. Small abscess: an oval abscess is formed in the brain tissue with a large number of pus cells (pus cells). The local tissue is necrotized and lysed, and the brain tissue around the abscess shows a reticular structure. HE ×400. (Chen Huaitao)

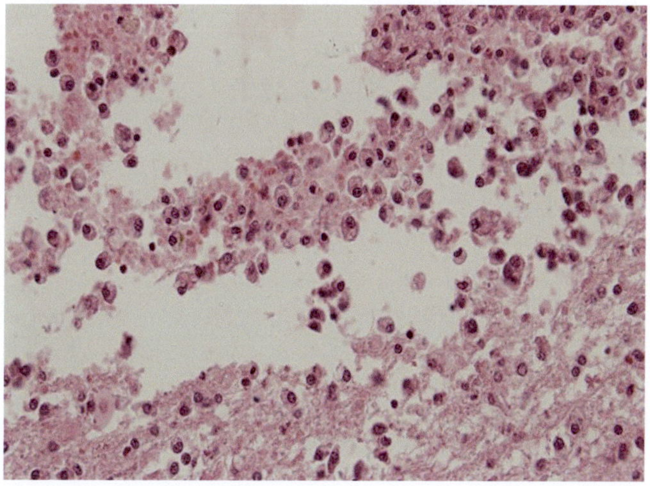

Fig. 11.18 Suppurative encephalitis. Cavity formation: After the pus-containing lipid is phagocytosed by macrophages locally, a cavity is left, in which many macrophages phagocytosing lipid, which are foam cells or gitter cells, can be observed. HE ×400. (Chen Huaitao)

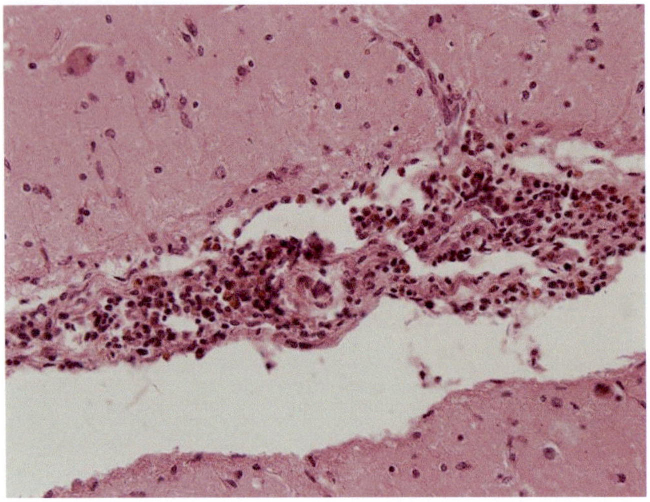

Fig. 11.19 Suppurative encephalitis. Suppurative meningitis: The meninges are thickened with massive neutrophils infiltration, vascular congestion, and edema around them. HE ×400. (Chen Huaitao)

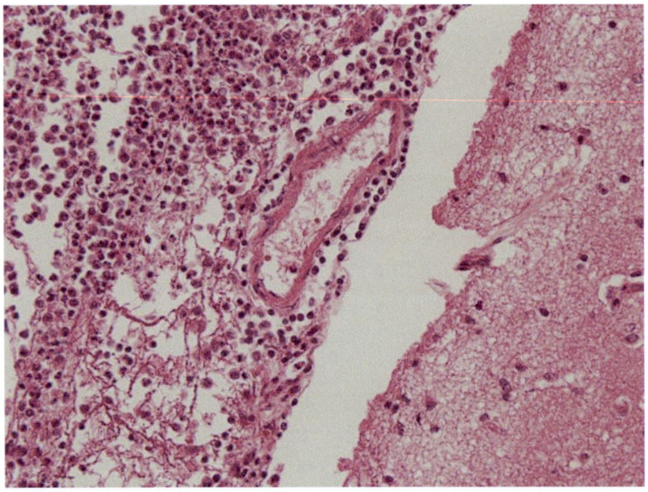

Fig. 11.20 Suppurative encephalitis. Suppurative meningitis: There are a large amount of neutrophils, pus cells, and fibrin exudate in the meninges with vasodilatation and congestion. HE ×400. (Chen Huaitao)

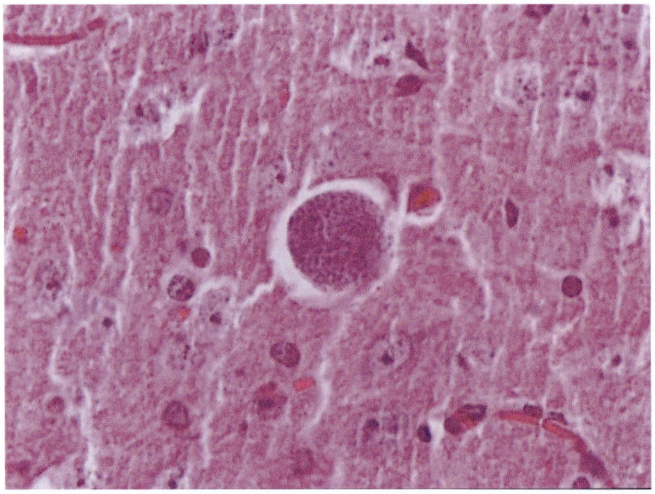

Fig. 11.21 Parasitic encephalitis. Toxoplasmosis in mice. Endothelial cells and epidermis of cerebral vessels proliferate, and glial cells also proliferate. There may be a pseudocyst of *Toxoplasma gondii* in brain tissue. HE ×400. (Chen Huaitao)

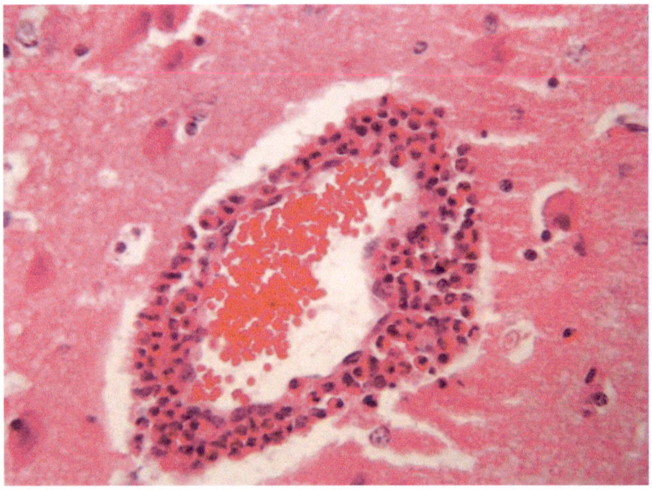

Fig. 11.22 Salt toxic encephalitis. Salt poisoning in pigs. The eosinophilic vascular cuffing is present around gray matter vessels in the brain. HE ×400. (Xu Yimin)

1.2.3 Parasitic Encephalitis (Fig. 11.21)

Parasitic encephalitis is an encephalitis caused by certain species of parasites (e.g., protozoa, cysticercus, nematodes, trematodes), which varies widely in pathology and is characterized by certain changes in non-suppurative encephalitis and, in the presence of infection, a suppurative process. In this type of encephalitis, the presence of the pathogenic parasites is common with eosinophilic infiltration.

1.2.4 Salt Toxic Encephalitis (Eosinophilic Encephalitis) (Fig. 11.22)

1.3 Encephalomalacia (Fig. 11.23)

Encephalomalacia is the process by which brain tissue breaks down and liquefies after necrosis.

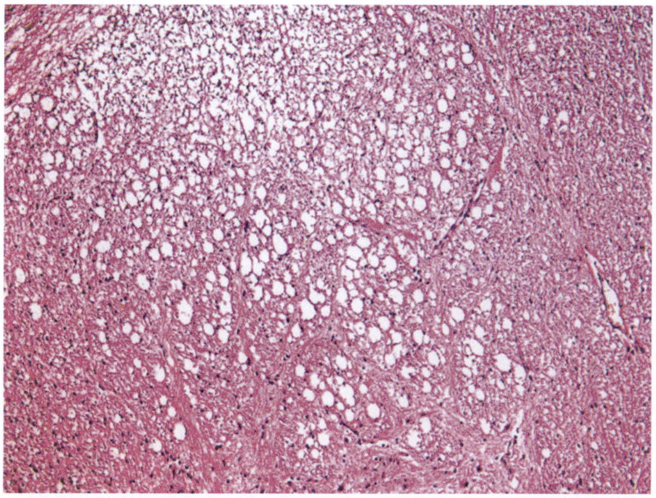

Fig. 11.23 Encephalomalacia. Ovine locoweed poisoning. Spongiform degeneration of the retinal nerve fiber network is observed with cerebral softening and a porous spongy appearance. HE ×100. (Chen Huaitao)

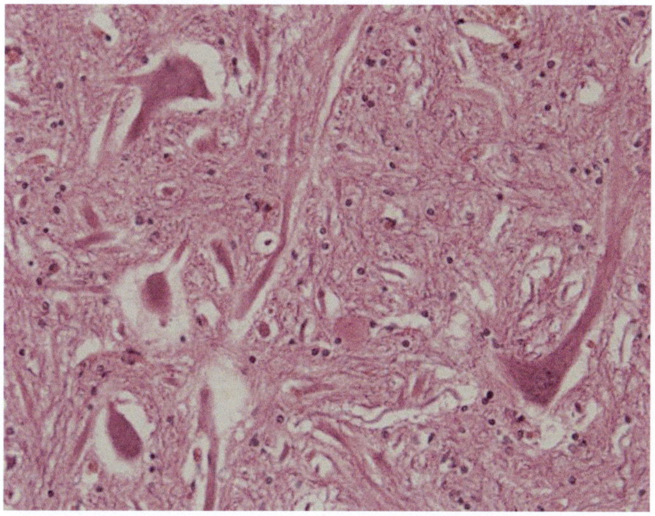

Fig. 11.24 Spinal cord nerve cell necrosis. Necrosis and lysis of nerve cells can be observed in the gray matter of the spinal cord with indistinct boundaries. HE ×400. (Chen Huaitao)

2 Pathological Changes of Spinal Cord (Figs. 11.24 and 11.25)

The lesions of the spinal cord are basically similar to those of the brain and are accompanied by lesions of the brain (e.g., encephalitis). The lesions of the spinal cord include mainly degenerative changes in neurons and nerve fibers, proliferation of glial cells, and vascular reactions.

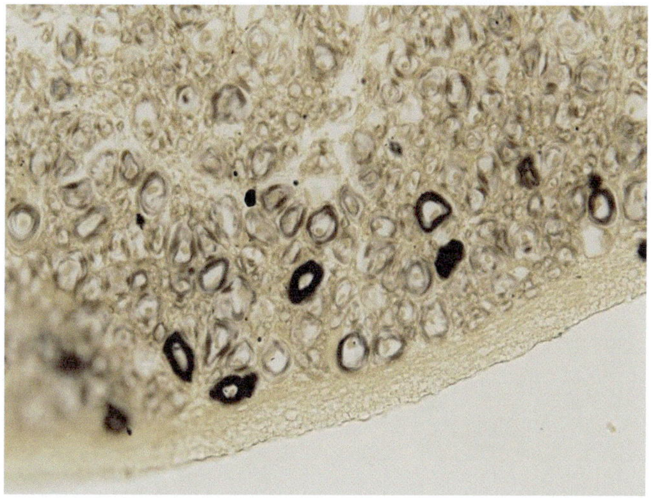

Fig. 11.25 Demyelination of nerve fibers in the white matter of the spinal cord. Normal nerve fibers are stained black at the myelin sheath, but the demyelinated nerve fibers cannot be stained. Myelin staining ×400. (Chen Huaitao)

3 Pathological Changes of Peripheral Nerves

3.1 Wallerian Degeneration (Figs. 11.26, 11.27 and 11.28)

Waller's degeneration or axonal degeneration is a degenerative process that occurs after injury to myelinated nerve fibers (trauma, inflammation, etc.) and detachment from the cytosol, manifested by a series of morphological changes in the axon (irregular swelling, fracture, disintegration), loss of myelin sheath, and subsequent cellular reactions. Macrophages containing fat droplets and myelin debris after engulfing, which is gitter cells or foam cells are present after Phagocytes engulf axons with myelin debris.

3.2 Demyelination (Figs. 11.29, 11.30, 11.31, 11.32, 11.33 and 11.34)

Demyelination or myelin loss is an important pathological change in nerve fibers of the spinal cord, which is classified into primary and secondary lesions. The former means the axons of nerve cells are not injured, but only myelin is degenerated and lost, which is rare in animals; the latter occurs after axonal degeneration and is often part of the pathological changes of axonal degeneration. Demyelination occurs in many inflammatory and noninflammatory pathological processes.

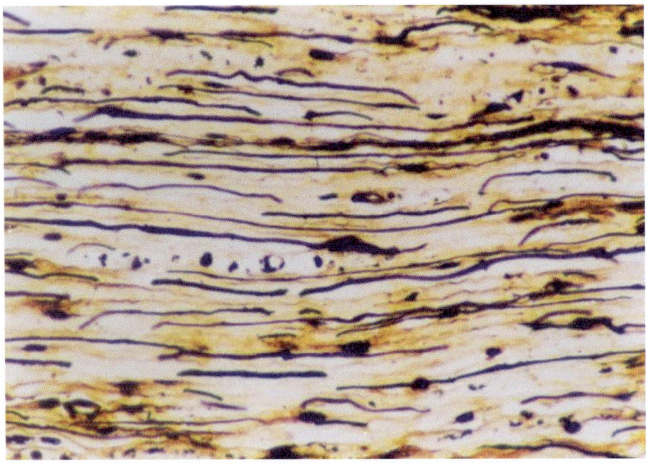

Fig. 11.26 Axonal degeneration. The axons are deformed and fractured. Marsland's silver plating staining ×400. (Wang Wenhui)

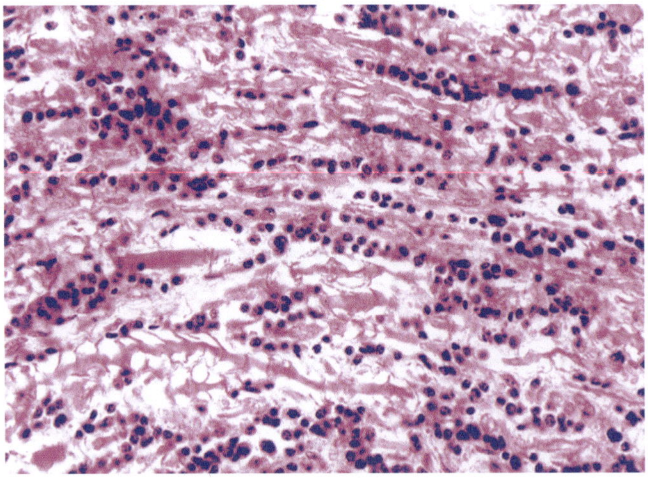

Fig. 11.27 Axonal degeneration. Chicken Marek's disease. There are a large number of polymorphic tumor cells infiltrating among the sciatic nerve fibers. Severe demyelination of the nerve fibers and degeneration of the axons can be observed which manifests by uneven thickness, variable sizes, twisting, fracture, disintegration, or even dissolution and disappearance of the axon. HE ×400. (Chen Huaitao)

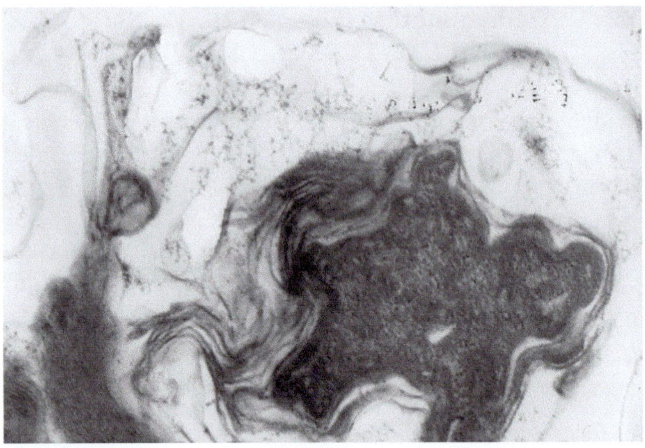

Fig. 11.28 Axonal degeneration. Transverse section of axon: The axon is deformed, bend at the periphery with the formation of protrusions. ×33,000. (Wang Wenhui)

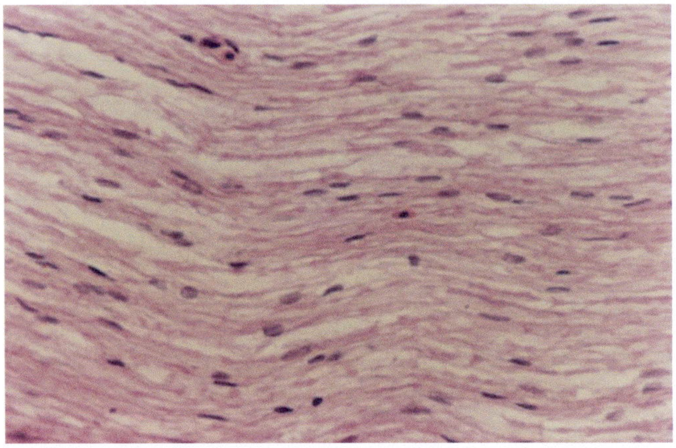

Fig. 11.29 Demyelination of the sciatic nerve. The nerve fibers are stained lightly due to demyelination, and they are thin stripes resembling fish spines because only nerve axons and Schwann's cells remained. HE ×400. (Wang Wenhui)

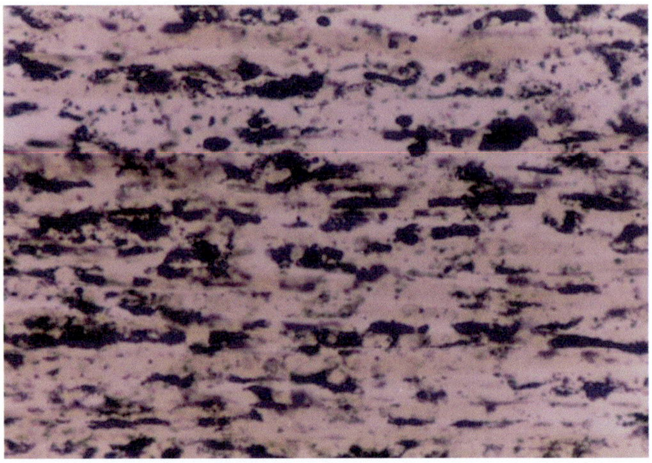

Fig. 11.30 Demyelination of the sciatic nerve. Myelin can be stained with osmium acid as irregular black masses after severe loss of myelin. Marchi staining ×400. (Wang Wenhui)

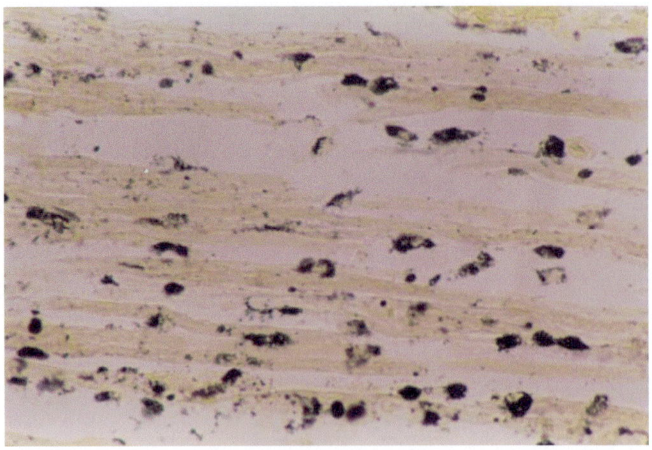

Fig. 11.31 Demyelination of the sciatic nerve. If myelin is phagocytosed by Schwann's cells after demyelination, dense black osmiophilic granules (for its phagocytosed degenerated myelin) can be observed in their cytoplasm. Marchi staining ×400. (Wang Wenhui)

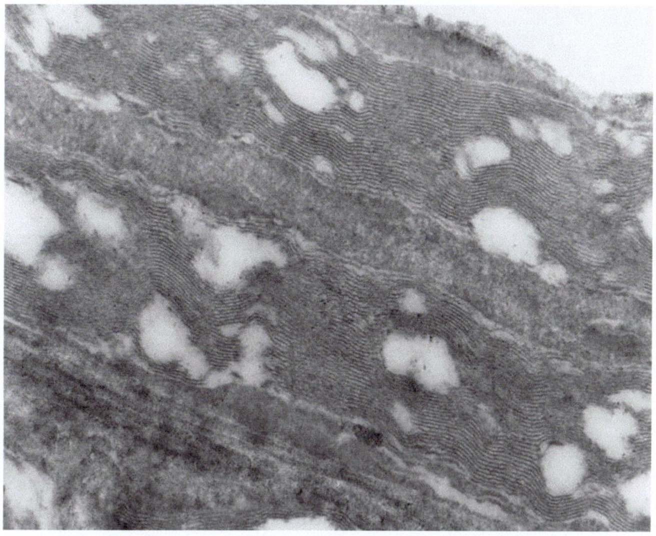

Fig. 11.32 Demyelination of the sciatic nerve. Longitudinal section of the sciatic nerve: in mild demyelination, only a few scattered gaps appear in the nerve. ×8000. (Wang Wenhui)

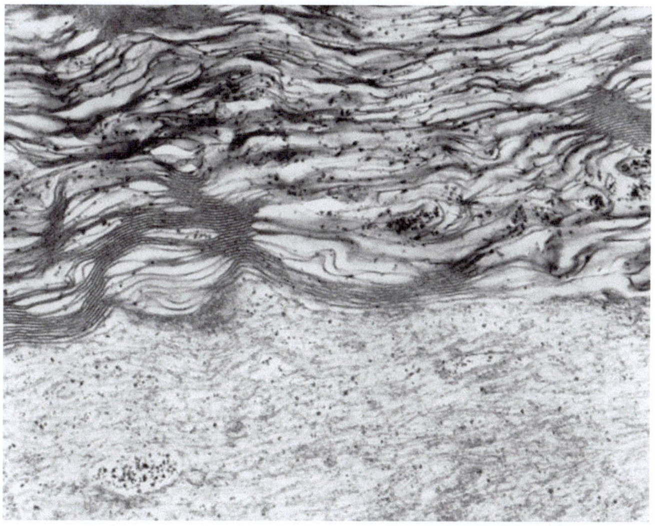

Fig. 11.33 Demyelination of the sciatic nerve. Longitudinal section of the sciatic nerve: if the demyelination is severe, the myelin laminae are separated from each other, forming distorted and deformed lacunae. Some fine particles with high electron density can also be observed. ×33,000. (Wang Wenhui)

3.3 Neuritis and Neural Edema (Figs. 11.35 and 11.36)

Neuritis is an inflammatory change in peripheral nerves characterized by varying degrees of inflammatory cell infiltration or proliferation in the interstitium along with nerve fiber degeneration. Neuroedema is present in inflammatory or non-inflammatory processes and is characterized by increased interstitial fluid and loosening of nerve fibers.

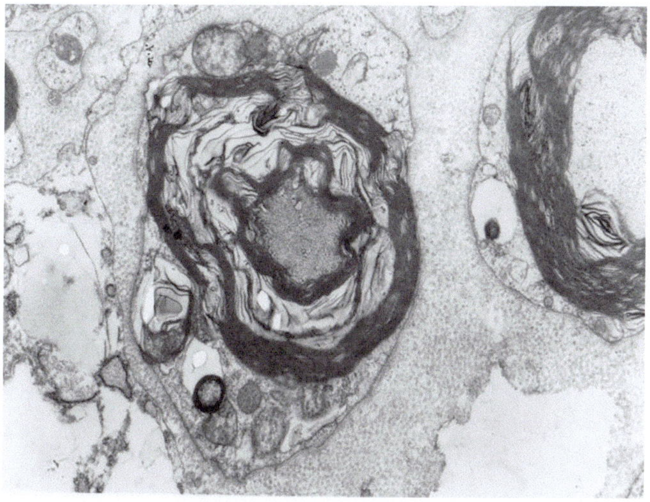

Fig. 11.34 Demyelination of the sciatic nerve. Transverse section of sciatic nerve: in addition to the above changes, myelin-like bodies can be observed in the cytoplasm of the Schwann's cells. ×20,000. (Wang Wenhui)

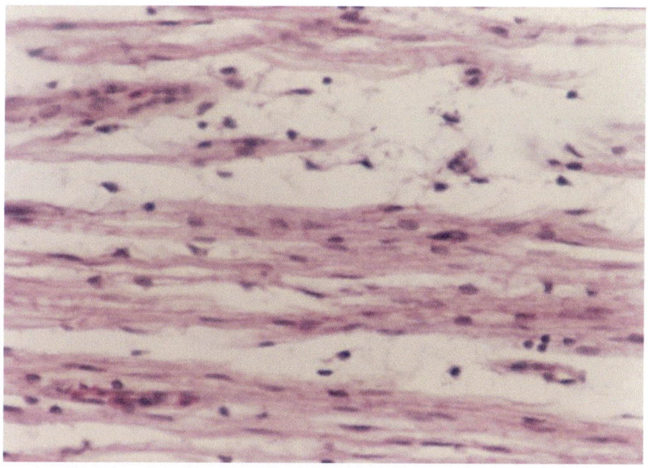

Fig. 11.35 Neuritis. Longitudinal section of sciatic nerve: The gaps among nerve fibers are widened with infiltration of serous and inflammatory cells. HE ×400. (Wang Wenhui)

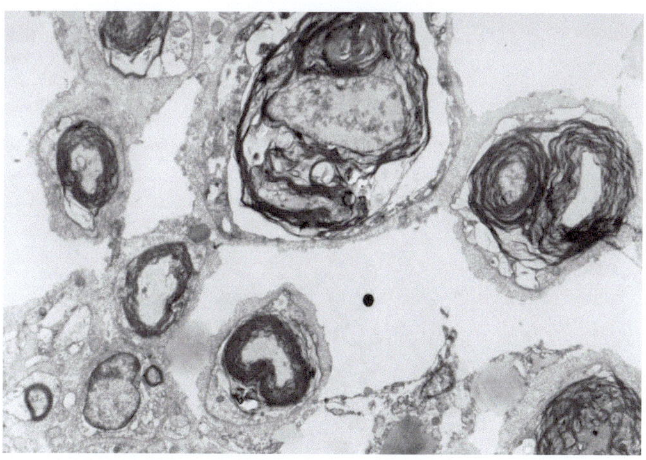

Fig. 11.36 Neural edema. Transverse section of sciatic nerve: nerve fibers are separated from each other due to edema and the gaps are widened. ×18,000. (Wang Wenhui)

Bibliography

1. Huaitao C, Deming Z, editors. Veterinary pathology. Beijing: China Agricultural Press; 2013.
2. Cheville NF. Cell pathology. 2nd ed. Ames: Iowa State University Press; 1983.

12 Pathology of the Skin and the Locomotor System

1 Dermatitis (Figs. 12.1, 12.2, and 12.3)

2 Myositis (Figs. 12.4 and 12.5)

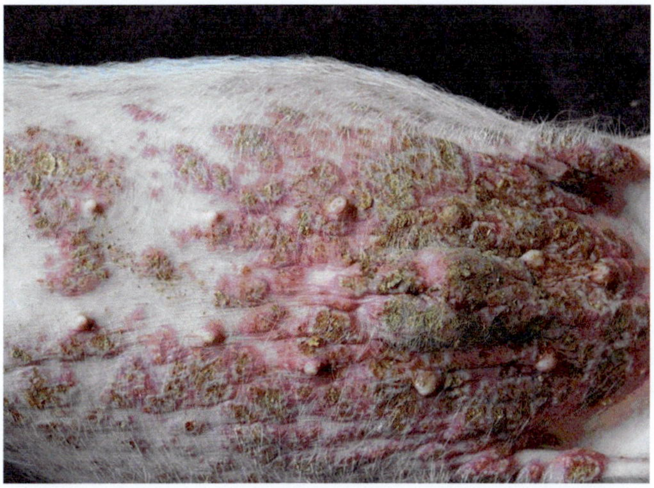

Fig. 12.1 Dermatitis. Multi-system failure syndrome in weaned piglets. Abdominal dermatitis is present with congested, hemorrhagic foci of inflammation, and a rough, uneven surface. (Wang Xinhua)

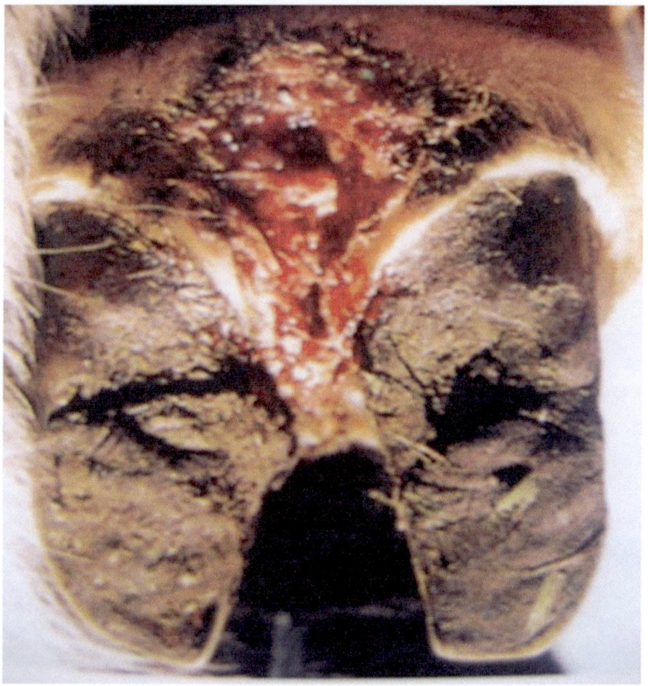

Fig. 12.2 Dermatitis. Interfinger (toe) cellulitis in a cow. The skin is necrotic and ruptured. (Zhou Qingguo)

H. Chen, *Color Atlas of Veterinary Pathology*, https://doi.org/10.1007/978-981-96-7617-0_12

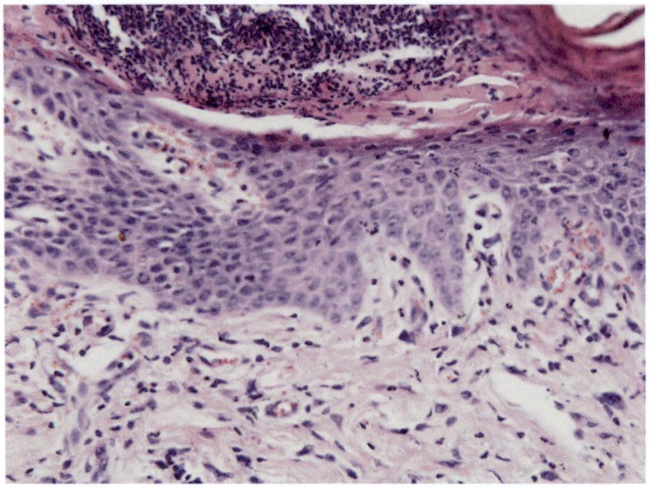

Fig. 12.3 Dermatitis. Suppurative epidermitis: The skin epidium is suppurative and necrotized with massive accumulation of pus cells. HE ×400. (Chen Huaitao)

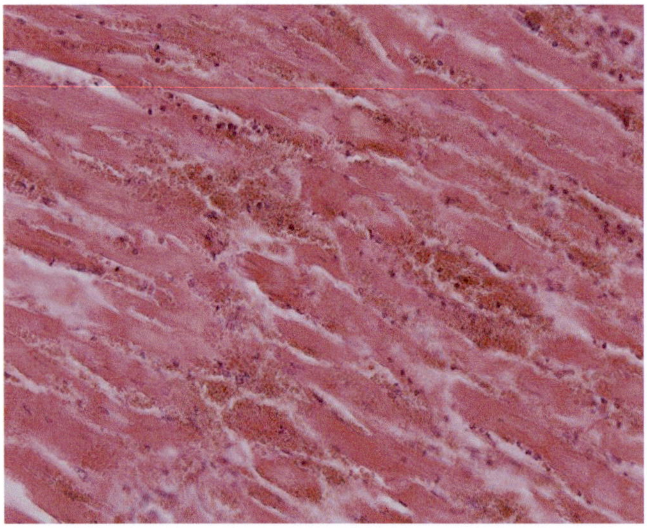

Fig. 12.4 Myositis. Hemorrhagic myositis: A large number of erythrocytes and neutrophils are present among myofibers with degeneration of myofibers. HE ×400. (Chen Huaitao)

3 Pathological Changes of Bone and Arthron (Figs. 12.6 and 12.7)

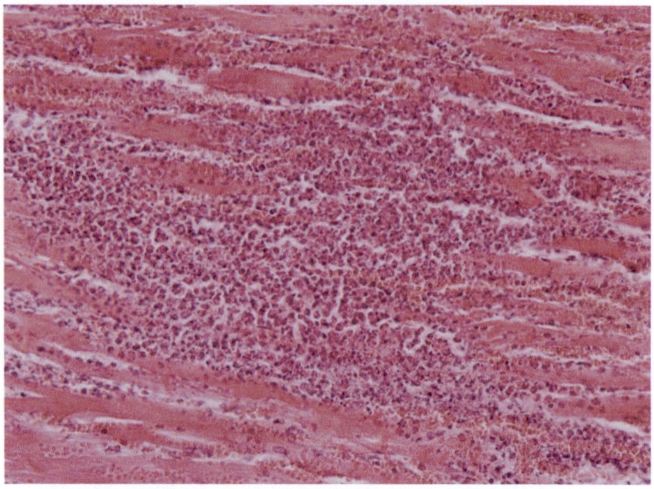

Fig. 12.5 Myositis. Suppurative myositis: A large number of neutrophils and pus cells are present among muscle fibers. Some muscle fibers have lysed and some have atrophied. HE ×400. (Chen Huaitao)

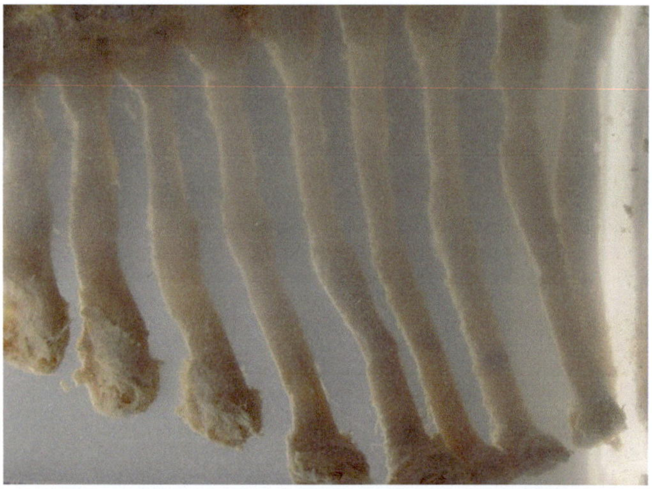

Fig. 12.6 Calcium deficiency. Pig. The rib cage is soft and easily reflexed, and the middle part of the backbone is expanded in spindle-shape in varying degrees. The deformation of the ribs is obvious. (Cui Hengmin)

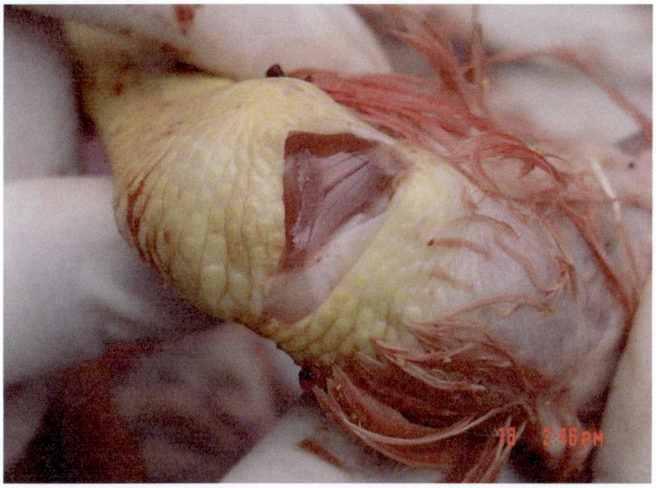

Fig. 12.7 Arthritis. Edema and effusion of tibiometatarsal joint of infected chicken

Selected References

1. Xuanren Z, editor. Pathological anatomy of domestic animals. Beijing: China Agricultural Press; 1988.
2. Huaitao C, Deming Z, editors. Veterinary pathology. Beijing: China Agricultural Press; 2013.
3. Jiye S, editor. Pathology. Beijing: Science Press; 2000.

Index

H. Chen, *Color Atlas of Veterinary Pathology*, https://doi.org/10.1007/978-981-96-7617-0_12

MIX
Papier aus verantwortungsvollen Quellen
Paper from responsible sources
FSC® C105338

If you have any concerns about our products,
you can contact us on
ProductSafety@springernature.com

In case Publisher is established outside the EU,
the EU authorized representative is:
Springer Nature Customer Service Center GmbH
Europaplatz 3, 69115 Heidelberg, Germany

Printed by Libri Plureos GmbH
in Hamburg, Germany